D1468054

Guided Brain Operations

Guided Brain Operations

Methodological and Clinical Developments in
Stereotactic Surgery
Contributions to the Physiology of Subcortical
Structures

Ernest A. Spiegel

with a contribution by *Philip L. Gildenberg*

67 figures and 3 tables, 1982

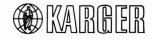

S. Karger · Basel · München · Paris · London · New York · Tokyo · Sydney

Ernest A. Spiegel

MD, Professor emeritus of Neurology and Chairman of the Department of Experimental Neurology, Temple University Medical School, Philadelphia, Pa. (USA)

Philip L. Gildenberg

MD, PhD, Professor and Chairman of the Division of Neurosurgery, University of Texas Medical School, Houston, Tex. (USA)

National Library of Medicine, Cataloging in Publication
   Spiegel, Ernest Adolf, 1895–
   Guided brain operations: methodological and clinical developments in stereotactic surgery: contributions
   to the physiology of subcortical structures
   Ernest A. Spiegel, with a contribution by Philip L. Gildenberg.– Basel; New York: Karger, 1982.
   1. Brain – physiology 2. Brain – surgery 3. Stereotactic Technics
   WL 368 S755g
   ISBN 3–8055–3451–5

Drug Dosage
   The authors and the publisher have exerted every effort to ensure that drug selection and dosage set forth in
   this text are in accord with current recommendations and practice at the time of publication. However, in
   view of ongoing research, changes in government regulations, and the constant flow of information relating
   to drug therapy and drug reactions, the reader is urged to check the package insert for each drug for any
   change in indications and dosage and for added warnings and precautions. This is particularly important
   when the recommended agent is a new and/or infrequently employed drug.

Contents

Contents

Acknowledgement

For permission to reproduce illustrations, the author is indebted to the following copyright owners: American Medical Association (fig. 9, 10, 15, 16, 23, 24, 31, 37, 38, 41, 44, 45, 49, 63, 64); Elsevier-North Holland Scientific Publishers (fig. 35, 36, 42, 43, 50–52, 56–58, 61, 62); Excerpta Medica (fig. 40); the office of the editor of Experimental Neurology, Dr. *C.B. Clemente* (fig. 28, 29, 53, 54); Grune and Stratton (fig. 17, 32); the editor of the Journal of Neuropathology and Experimental Neurology, Dr. *John Moossy* (fig. 47); the office of Dr. *H.G. Schwarz,* editor of the Journal Neurosurgery (fig. 2, 3, 18–22); Dr. *William S. Fields,* editor of Pathogenesis and Treatment of Parkinsonism (fig. 48); Dr. *Daniel E. Sheer,* editor of Electrical Stimulation of the Brain (fig. 11, 59, 60, 66); Williams and Wilkins Company (fig. 1).

Preface

Slightly over three decades have passed since the method of guided electrodes and other guided instruments was applied to the treatment of pathological disorders of the hitherto more or less inaccessible human subcortical regions and to the study of their physiology. During this period an astonishing number of neurosurgeons, clinical neurologists, electroencephalographers and neurophysiologists have become interested in this new discipline of stereoencephalotomy or stereotactic surgery. It seems, therefore, appropriate to survey their work in order to serve as an introduction to the methods and the possibilities of clinical and research applications, and also to aid in the perusal of the considerable literature. For the sake of completeness, some nonstereotactic procedures have also been included.

The reader interested in the rationale of the operative procedures may find it useful to review the details of the structure and connections of the thalamus and basal ganglia in the section dealing with physiological observations before studying the chapter describing the clinical applications.

These pages are dedicated to the memory of my late friend and surgical associate, *Henry T. Wycis,* MD, without whose faithful acceptance of my suggestions and enthusiastic cooperation, guided brain operations could not have been initiated and developed.

The author wishes to express his deep gratitude to Dr. *Philip L. Gildenberg* and to *Patricia O. Franklin* for their kind help in the preparation of the manuscript, and to Dr. *Helen Adolf* for proofreading.

E.A.S.

Introduction

Neurophysiology has not only greatly aided the understanding of clinical neurological signs and symptoms and their mechanisms, it has also fathered the development of important therapeutic and research techniques. This is particularly evident in the use of guided instruments, which has made it possible to apply surgery to pathologic conditions of subcortical regions with only minimal impairment of overlying structures, particularly the cortex, and to explore the functions of the subcortex not only in experimental animals, but also in humans.

The use of guided probes in neurophysiology goes back to the second half of the 19th century, when in *Ludwig's* laboratory a guiding device was applied to the medulla oblongata [*Dittmar,* 1873]. This technique reached a climax when *Horsley and Clarke* [1908] devised their so-called stereotaxic apparatus for the study of the deep cerebellar nuclei in experimental animals. It may seem astonishing that it took nearly four decades until this technique was applied to the human brain. The explanation may be found in the differences of variability between the skulls of cats and monkeys on the one hand, and those of humans on the other. In the former one may determine the coordinates of subcortical targets rather exactly in relation to reference points on the skull, since the dimensions of their skulls are relatively constant. In man the conditions are more complicated and variable; here we have brachy- and dolichocephalic skulls, and it is well known to roentgenologists that the position of an intracerebral structure, such as the pineal gland, in relation to the skull, may vary by as much as 10 mm or more. Therefore, in 1947 it became obvious to *Spiegel* that the use of cranial reference points was quite insufficient, when he proposed to *Wycis* to replace prefrontal lobotomy, with its extensive gross tissue damage and many undesirable side effects, by circumscribed lesions of the dorsomedial nucleus, the nodal point of thalamofrontal circuits. Cranial reference points were satisfactory when one wanted to reach a structure closely adjacent to the skull, such as the Gasserian ganglion [*Kirschner,* 1933], but not if one wanted to influence a subcortical cell group such as a thalamic nucleus.

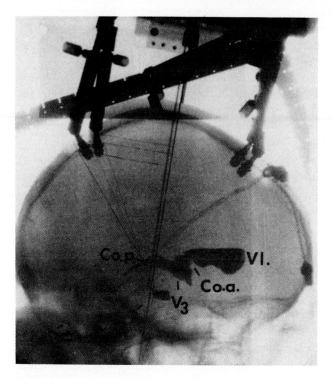

Fig. 1. Roentgenogram of Pantopaque filled anterior horn of lateral ventricle (Vl.), ventral part of 3rd ventricle (V₃), and aqueductus Sylvii. Anterior (Co.a.) and posterior (Co.p.) commissure. From *Spiegel and Wycis* [1967], reproduced with permission.

The cardinal difference between *Horsley and Clarke's* procedure in experimental animals and the use of guided instruments in the human sub-cortex is the *necessity,* in patients, *to use intracerebral reference points or lines.* These are chiefly structures around the third ventricle (pineal gland, anterior and posterior commissure, intercommissural line) [*Spiegel* et al., 1947; *Jasper and Hunter,* 1949; *Talairach* et al., 1949; *Leksell,* 1949, 1951; *Riechert and Wolff,* 1951] (fig. 1), and in some instances the inferior horn [*Talairach* et al., 1958; *Spiegel and Wycis,* 1962] for deep temporal lobe structures, or parts of the fourth ventricle for the deep cerebellar nuclei [*Heimburger and Whitlock,* 1965; *Nashold* et al., 1969].

Kim and Goettsching [1975] pointed out that the anatomical relationship of the amygdala to the temporal horn is extremely variable. Errors may occur when the temporal horn is not sufficiently filled. The authors advocated, therefore, different reference points and lines: the foramen of Monroe (FM), the temporal pole (TP), the crossing point of the clivus and the temporal base of the skull (TB), and the midpoint of the foramen ovale (FOV). In order to determine the coordinates of the midpoint of the amygdala, they ascertain the distance of FM from TB and the distance of the TP from a line connecting FM-TB on lateral roentgenograms, and the distance of the center of FOV from the midline. The coordinates of the amygdala are proportional to these reference lines [*Heimburger* et al., 1966].

The use of periventricular reference points was hardly possible in *Horsley and Clarke's* time[1]; it became feasible only with roentgenological contrast visualization of the ventricles using air, Pantopaque (Myodil) or Conray [*Campbell* et al., 1964; *Kandel and Chebotaryova, 1972*][2]. The term stereoencephalotomy was proposed for the human application of the technique in order to signify the methodological differences in experimental animals and in man [*Spiegel and Wycis, 1952*]. The expressions stereotaxy and stereotactic neurosurgery are frequently used also.

---

[1] The use of cranial reference points for determination of the coordinates of intracerebral targets [*Austin* et al., 1967; *Mundinger* et al., 1975] may be advantageous in patients in whom contrast filling of the ventricles is undesirable. *Mundinger* et al. [1975] chose the following cranial reference points: A = point of intersection of the squama frontalis and the partes orbitales ossis frontalis on the tabula interna; A[1] = point of intersection of the lambda with the sagittal suture on the tabula interna; B = point of intersection of the coronal with the sagittal suture on the tabula interna (= Bregma); B[1] = interclinoidal point, i.e., the interpolation between the anterior clinoidal processes of the sella at the transition to the tuberculum sellae. The calculations were carried out using a computer. *Birg* et al. [1977] point out that the coordinates of large areas, e.g., cingulum or pulvinar, can be determined with sufficient exactness, if the calculated coordinates fall within the range of a standard deviation of ± 1.5 mm from the true value. If this precision cannot be obtained, a ventriculogram is necessary.

[2] Of the 2 radiopaque contrast substances, Pantopaque (ethyl iodophenylundecylate) and Conray 60 (methylglucamine jothalamate), the latter is water-soluble and absorbable. *Campbell* et al. [1964] found it less toxic than other similar compounds when injected cisternally in rabbits. In order to avoid toxic reactions that are usually related to exposure of the cortical surface to the substance, no more than 5–6 ml of Conray should be employed. Usually 3 ml diluted with CSF or sterile water to 10 ml is sufficient for ventriculography. The patient should be positioned in such a way that hyperbaric flow of Conray over the cerebral cortex is minimized. It is usually visible radiographically in the ventricles for only half an hour.

Thus, a new subspecialty was born, promising a drastic reduction of mortality in subcortical procedures, e.g., a 10.0% mortality on open surgery of the basal ganglia by transventricular approach was experienced by *Meyers* [1958], while a 2.0% operative mortality of stereotactic pallidoansotomy was observed by *Spiegel and Wycis* [1962]. None of their 45 Parkinson patients subjected to lesion of Forel's field H died in the first postoperative weeks [*Spiegel and Wycis,* 1962; *Spiegel* et al., 1963a, b]. 2 of these patients with advanced tremor died several months postoperatively, but a certain relation with the operation could not be established. A mortality of 1.6% was reported by *Riechert* [1962b] for his first 1,500 stereotactic operations; after improvement of the thermocoagulation, this dropped to 0.82% for Parkinson's disease [*Hassler* et al., 1979]; for hyperkineses *Riechert* experienced a mortality of 1.4%. The figure of *Krayenbühl* et al. [1961], 1.8%, is not significantly different.

The first human stereotactic operation was performed by *Spiegel and Wycis* in the spring of 1947, and since that time investigators worldwide have applied the method: in France, *Talairach* et al. [1949], *Baudoin and Puech* [1949], *Rémond* [1952], *Guiot and Brion* [1953], *Wertheimer* et al. [1960], *Lapras* [1960], *Szikla* [with *Talairach,* 1962]; in Germany, *Riechert and Wolff* [1951], *Hassler and Riechert* [1954], *Riechert and Mundinger* [1955], *Umbach and Riechert* [1959], *Roeder and Orthner* [1961], *Schaltenbrand and Bailey* [1959], *Nittner* [1970]; in Sweden, *Leksell* [1949, 1951]; in England, *Lister and Sherwood* [1955], *Brierley and Beck* [1959], *McCaul* [1959], *Hughes* [1960], *Walsh and Till* [1960], *Watson and Naughton* [1960], *Woringer* et al. [1960], *Knight* [1964]; in Scotland, *Gillingham* [1962]; in Switzerland, *Monnier* [1952], *Krayenbühl* et al. [1961], *Siegfried and Fisch* [1967] and *Siegfried and Wiesendanger* [1967]; in the Netherlands, *Van Manen and Van Hoytema* [1962]; in Belgium, *Peluso and Gybels* [1969]; in Spain, *Obrador* et al. [1956], *Bravo* [*Cooper and Bravo,* 1958a, b]; in Russia, *Kandel* [1965], *Bechterewa* [1969]; in Denmark, *Broager* [1958]; in Norway, *Nordlie* et al. [1962]; in Finland, *Laitinen* [1963]; in Austria, *Ganglberger* [1961], *Diemath* et al. [1966]; in Czechoslovakia, *Nádvornik* et al. [1972]; in Hungary, *Tóth* [1961]; in Italy, *Maspes* et al. [1961], *Fasano* et al. [1961], *Pagni* et al. [1963], and *Fraioli* et al. [1973].

In the United States, *Adams* [1965], *Alberts* et al. [1961], *Andy* [1962], *Aronson* et al. [1959], *Bailey* [1951], *Burton* et al. [1966], *Campbell* et al. [1962], *Cooper* [1955], *Gildenberg* [1960], *Heimburger and Whitlock* [1965], *Housepian and Pool* [1960], *Mark* et al. [1960], *Meyers* et al. [1949], *Mullan* et al. [1967], *Nashold and Wilson* [1966], *Rand* [1961], *Sweet* et al.

[1960], *Voris and Whisler* [1975], *Walker* [1957] and *Zervas* [1965] became interested. This approach has also been used in Canada by *Jasper and Hunter* [1949], *Bertrand and Martinez* [1959], *Bertrand and Jasper* [1965], *Tasker and Emmers* [1969]; in Mexico by *Velasco-Suarez and Escobedo* [1967]; in Argentina by *Fairman* [1959]; in Brazil by *Niemeyer* [1955] and in Chile by *Asenjo* et al. [1964]. In Asia, stereotactic centers were developed by *Uchimura, Narabayashi* et al. [1950], *Sano* [1962], *Jinnai and Nishimoto* [1963] in Japan; by *Ramamurthi and Kalayanaraman* [1965] in India, and by *Chitanondh* [1966] in Thailand.

According to *Nashold* [1970], over 40,000 stereotactic operations had been performed during the previous 10 years. A survey prepared by *Gildenberg* [1975] revealed that 151 neurosurgeons in the United States and Canada performed stereotactic operations.

Methods

Localization and Elimination of the Target

Atlases

Previous atlases of the human brain did not permit one to determine exactly the relationship of subcortical structures to the intracerebral reference points and reference lines. The atlas of *Spiegel and Wycis* [1952] was the first to permit measurement of the distance between subcortical targets and some of the periventricular structures on frontal, sagittal and horizontal sections in millimeters; it also shows the variability in the position and size of the most important ganglia. Irregular shrinking of the tissue due to the embedding of the brain was taken into consideration by incising small notches into the brain stem preparations at distances of 10 mm preceding the embedding, and adjusting the millimeter scales framing the microphotographs according to the changes in these distances measured in the final stained sections. Subsequently excellent stereotactic atlases were prepared by *Talairach* et al. [1957] and by *Schaltenbrand and Bailey* [1959]. Particularly the one published by the latter authors has been most useful. Some more recent ones have been devoted to special regions, i.e., the basal ganglia [*Van Buren and Maccubin*, 1962], in parkinsonism [*Hassler* et al., 1979], the diencephalon [*Andrew and Watkins*, 1969; *Van Buren and Borke*, 1972; *Emmers and Tasker*, 1975], and the brain stem and cerebellar nuclei [*Afshar* et al., 1978].

Production of Lesions

Various methods have been employed to produce circumscribed *subcortical lesions*. Injection of *alcohol* was used by *Spiegel and Wycis* [1950b] only transitorily, because the size and shape of the lesions were unpredictable. Similar objections have to be made regarding injection of *Cooper's* [1955] *Etopalin* (mixture of ethylcellulose and ethanol).

Mechanical production of lesions, such as destruction by means of a *modified leukotome* or wire loop [*Obrador and Dierssen*, 1956], can hardly be recommended in view of the possible tearing of blood vessels that may result in hemorrhages. Less undesirable side effects accompany injection of a *procaine-oil-wax* mixture [*Narabayashi* et al., 1960]. *Cooper and Bravo* [1958a, b] attempted to produce a cavity by insertion of an *inflatable balloon* combined with alcohol injection. An examination by *Gildenberg* [1960] showed that irregular cavities surrounded by hemorrhages developed. As to the use of extreme temperatures, heat as well as cold have been advocated. So-called *inductive heating* was produced by a stereotactically implanted metallic pellet; the head was surrounded by the coil of a conductor carrying a high frequency current [*Riechert*, 1959; *Riechert* et al., 1967; *Burton* et al., 1966; *Walker and Burton* (radiofrequency telethermocoagulation), 1966]. *Riechert* [1980] considered the method indicated especially in patients in whom gradual lesioning of tissue is required because of age or physical condition. In trigeminal neuralgia, reversible and irreversible lesions of nerves were attempted.

Low temperatures were originally applied by *Trendelenburg* [1910] on the cerebral cortex of experimental animals and by *Bárány* [1913] on the cerebellar cortex of patients in order to induce transient paralysis or depression of function. For production of subcortical lesions, localized cooling was used by *Mark* et al. [1961] and particularly by *Cooper* [1961]. *Cooper* [1961] pointed out that a reversible depression of function can be obtained by temperatures between +18 and +5 °C. Such a transient depression of function may be useful in order to check the proper position of a subsequently produced permanent elimination of activity of an area. *Cooper* et al. [1965] emphasized that freezing below −50 °C produces a hemostatic congelation. The absence of hemorrhages, however, is controversial, since *Mark* et al. [1965] showed that freezing may be accompanied by hemorrhages. The variability of the lesions produced by cooling [*Miyazaki* et al., 1963] also should not be overlooked.

Electrical methods became particularly useful for the elimination of circumscribed areas. *Horsley and Clarke* [1908] destroyed deep cerebellar nuclei in cats by electrolysis induced *around the anode* of a direct current. In order to avoid undesirable side effects caused by the variability of such lesions, *Spiegel and Wycis* [1962] used *fractionated electrolysis.* Following each period of electrolysis (10 s), undesirable effects were ascertained and the motor power of the hand on the affected side was tested.

High frequency *(radiofrequency)* coagulation using pure sine waves was introduced by *Wyss* [1945] and *Hunsperger and Wyss* [1953]. *Mundinger* et al. [1960] built a thermocouple in their electrode; thus it became possible to regulate the output of the current according to the temperature and to avoid hemorrhage and scab formation. The radiofrequency (RF) lesion technique mostly using 100,000–500,000 Hz has become the most popular method. A survey prepared by *Gildenberg* [1975] including centers in the USA and Canada shows that RF has been used by 192 of 260 neurosurgeons (partly also for nonstereotactic procedures). *Organ* [1976/77] pointed out the difference between electrocautery and RF techniques. The former method applies a heated electrode tip to the tissue. With the RF technique a high frequency AC flows from the tip of the electrode into the tissue; 'ionic agitation' is produced in the tissue about the tip of the electrode resulting in frictional heating of the tissue rather than of the electrode itself. During the production of a lesion the current as well as the temperature should be monitored. The physical parameters of RF lesions were discussed by *Aronow* [1960]. For details of the technique and various applications a recent symposium edited by *Gildenberg* [1976/77] supplies excellent information. It is of practical importance that lesions produced by high frequency currents spread more easily in the white matter (fiber systems such as the internal capsule) than in the gray matter [*Dieckmann* et al., 1966].

Ultrasound has been developed to a high degree of perfection, particularly by *Meyers* et al. [1959]. It requires, however, a complicated and expensive apparatus and a lengthy operation, including a craniectomy, to avoid cerebral cortical injuries caused by differences in density between the skull and the brain. Echo lesions may be produced on the ventral surface of the brain if the beams strike concave parts of the base of the skull [*Bakay* et al., 1956].

Deep-seated lesions may be produced with the skull intact by various forms of *radiation,* e.g., roentgen rays [*Leksell* et al., 1955], deuterons [*Tobias* et al., 1955], or proton beams [*Leksell* et al., 1960; *Kjellberg* et al., 1962, 1979]. There occur, unfortunately, undesirable long-range effects. The risk of hemorrhage and malignant degeneration after roentgen irradiation should not be overlooked. Up to 3 months after proton beam irradiation, the well-demarcated lesions were restricted to the path of the beam. After 3 months, the lesions became broader than the beam; after 23 weeks telangiectasis developed in the irradiated zone. It seems that the lesion does not reach its final shape even after 1 year [*Leksell* et al., 1960; *Rexed* et al., 1960]. Delayed radionecrosis developed also after *betatron* irradiation so that *Arnold* et al. [1954] felt that this technique should primarily be applied to the treatment of tumors.

In choosing *radioactive isotopes* for therapeutic purposes (destruction

Table I. Therapeutically useful radioactive isotopes

Isotope	Rays emitted	Half-life	Energy, MeV
^{198}Au (gold)	beta, gamma	2.7 days	0.41
^{60}Co (cobalt)	chiefly gamma, some beta	5.3 years	1.13–1.17
^{192}Ir (iridium)	chiefly gamma	74 days	0.3–0.6
^{32}P (phosphorus)	beta	14.3 days	1.69
^{103}Pd (palladium)	beta	17 days	0.02
^{182}Ta (tantalum)	gamma, beta (filtered by platinum)	111 days	1.22
^{90}Y (yttrium)	beta	2.5 days	2.18–2.24

After *Evans* [1944], *Mundinger and Riechert* [1967], and *Riechert* [1980].

of normal tissue, e.g., in functional hypophysectomy, or of tumors), one has to consider their physical characteristics shown in the above table I, the type of rays emitted, their half-life and their energy. There are three types of radiations: alpha rays (helium nuclei), beta rays (electrons), and gamma rays (electromagnetic radiations similar to X-rays) [*Evans,* 1944]. It is important to consider the half-life of the various isotopes, i.e., the time required for half of the initial stock of the atoms to decay (table I).

The range of effect of the alpha emitters reaches only fractions of millimeters, that of beta emitters a few millimeters. The latter isotopes, e.g., ^{90}Y, produce a sharply limited necrosis, leaving the surrounding tissue intact. A gamma emitter like ^{60}Co, with its great energy, reaches deep into the tissue, which is useful for irradiation of large tumors. Isotopes with a short half-life are applied for relatively fast tissue destruction, e.g., hypophysectomy; they are left permanently in the tissue. ^{192}Ir, with a half-life of 74 days, is used for protracted tissue destruction. An isotope with a long half-life, such as ^{60}Co, must be removed as soon as the required dosage is reached.

It is of practical importance to note that the lesions usually develop gradually, reaching a maximum size after several days [e.g., experiments by *Boyesen and Campbell,* 1955]. Thus, observation during operation does not enable one to determine whether a lesion produced in the vicinity of a physiologically important structure will encroach upon it. The application of radioisotopes, therefore, has become restricted chiefly to the treatment of tumors and to hypophysectomy [*Talairach* et al., 1955, 1956; *Riechert,*

1957a, b, 1980; *Mundinger and Riechert,* 1967]. The same applies to radon, a gaseous decay product of radium, which is inserted in glass or gold seeds. In *Bagg's* [1921] experiments, for instance, after exposure of the central nervous system to radon for 30 min, it took several days until the destructive effect upon the tissue became manifest. Radioisotopes have rarely been used for production of lesions in the central nervous system. *Mullan* et al. [1963] employed radioactive strontium needles for destruction of the spinothalamic tract, *Knight* [1964] radioactive yttrium for production of subcaudate lesions.

Models of Stereoencephalotomes

Over three dozen models of stereoencephalotomes have been developed since 1947, and it would be beyond the scope of this survey to enumerate all the apparatuses described in the literature. They can be classified into three groups, and it may suffice to describe the characteristics of each group and to quote a few examples.

Type I. A cuboid or rectangular frame carries the electrode holder which can be moved in an anteroposterior and/or lateral direction and be rotated in sagittal and in frontal planes. The cuboid shape of the frame or a cuboid attachment to the rectangular frame permits one easily to place the film parallel or perpendicular to the median plane of the skull. The central beam of the X-rays can also easily be directed perpendicularly to the film and in constant relationship to the third ventricle. On the film the position of the target in relation to the ventriculogram is drawn according to the data found in a stereotactic atlas, and its coordinates in relation to the zero position of the electrode are determined. *Spiegel and Wycis'* models III (fig. 2) and V (fig. 3–5) correspond to this type.

Type II. The electrode holder rides in a lateral direction on a semicircular arc that surrounds the skull. This arc can be rotated around a transverse axis; it is attached to a sagittal arc in the desired position. The whole system is fixed to a basal ring [*Riechert and Mundinger,* 1955]. The user may avoid calculations of the position and direction of the electrode and of the depth of its tip by using a phantom apparatus (fig. 6, 7). The basal ring of the phantom carries a coordinate system on which the coordinates of the target obtained on the roentgenogram are duplicated. The target is represented by the tip of the vertical coordinate. On this phantom model the arc with the electrode holder is placed in the desired position, and the electrode is directed so that its tip reaches the target point. The data read on this phantom model are used in the actual operation. *Birg and Mundinger* [1973] adapted *Riechert-Mundinger's* model

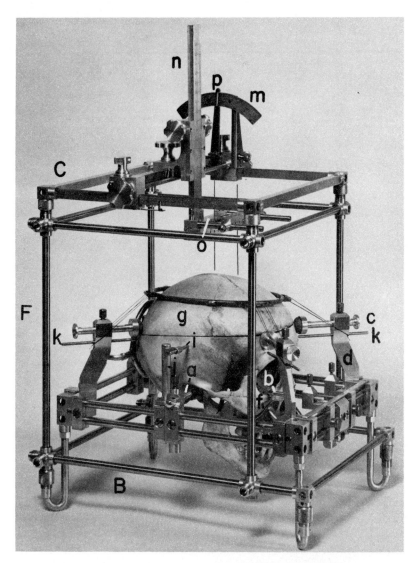

Fig. 2. Stereoencephalotome (SET), model III of *Spiegel and Wycis.* The base (B) has to be aligned parallel to Reid's baseline by application of the ear plugs (a) and orbital bars (b). SET is fixed to the head by stops (c) on supports (d), an occipital rest, a maxillary support (f) and a ring (g) suspending the apparatus. A cuboid frame (F) is attached to B. The square electrode carrier C can be placed on top of F, on its posterior or lateral aspects. i, j = removable upright support; k = graduated pins; m = protractor; n = upright bar; o = transverse bar of electrode holder; p = pointer. After *Spiegel* et al. [1951c]; reproduced with permission.

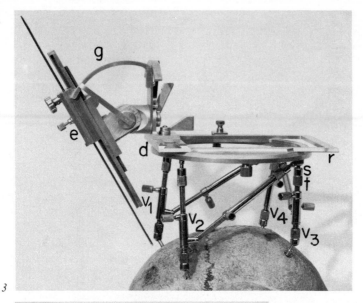

Fig. 3. Stereoencephalotome, model V of *Spiegel
and Wycis.* The electrode
holder (e) is shown placed on
the outside of the frame (r).
r can be moved forward or
backward and rotated in a
ring. The latter rests on
vertical (V_1–V_4) and oblique
posts and ball and socket
mechanisms.
g = Graduated arc;
s = spring socket;
t = threaded collar.
From *Spiegel* et al. [1956d];
reproduced with permission.

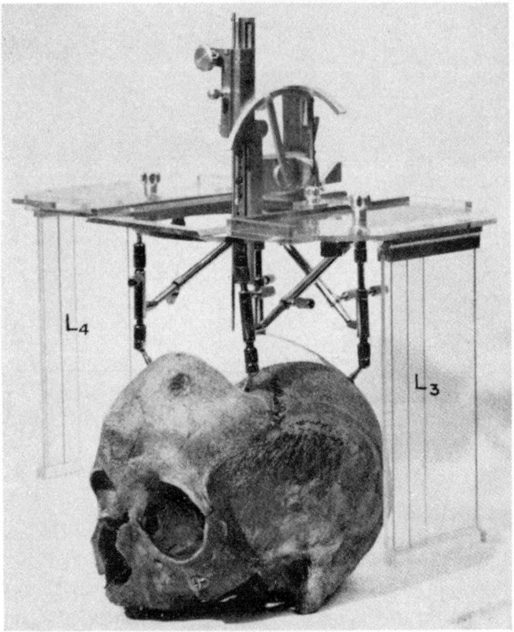

Fig. 4. Stereoencephalotome V, oblique side view with lateral plates carrying mov-
able lead marks (L_3, L_4) for proper positioning of the central X-ray beam. (In figures 4 and
5 the electrode holder is seen inside the frame r.) From *Spiegel* et al. [1957b].

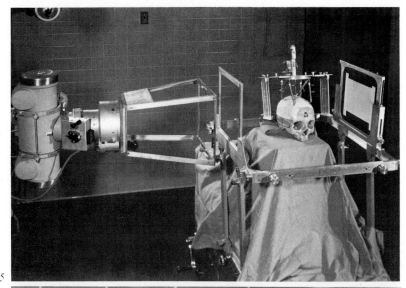

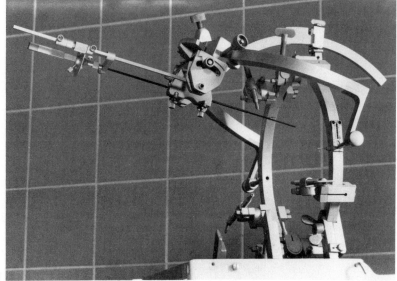

Fig. 5. Alignment of the head with the stereoencephalotome (SET), so that the median sagittal plane of the head and the plastic plates on each side of the SET are parallel to the film cassette (on the right) and to the front of the pyramidal frame (on the left) that is attached to the roentgen apparatus. After *Henny* et al. [1961].

Fig. 6. Riechert and Mundinger's stereotactic apparatus modified by *Birg and Mundinger* [1973].

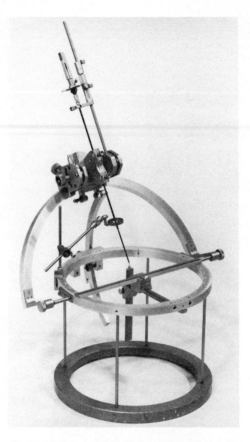

Fig. 7. Riechert and Mundinger's phantom apparatus.

for computer calculation, so that the phantom model became dispensable. The principle of an arc carrying the electrode holder is also used in the apparatus devised by *Leksell* [1949, 1951], whose method combines the features of a rectangular frame and of a semicircular electrode carrier, and in those constructed by *Schaltenbrand and Bailey* [1959] and by *Todd-Wells* [*Todd,* 1967] (fig. 8). According to *Gildenberg's* [1975] statistics, in recent years the latter model is the most frequently used (by 92 neurosurgeons) in the USA and Canada.

Type III. A simplified device is fixed in or above a trephine opening in the skull. It permits rotation of the electrode only in frontal and sagittal planes (e.g., *Rand's* [1961] model) or in any direction around a fulcrum

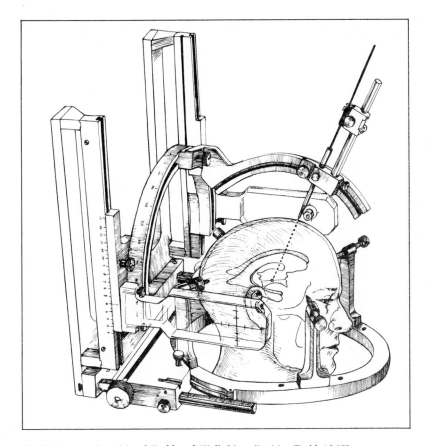

Fig. 8. Stereotaxic guide of *Todd and Wells* [described by *Todd,* 1967].

located, for instance, on the dural surface [*Spiegel* et al., 1953a]; Austin's ball and socket apparatus [*Austin and Lee,* 1958]). The proper position of the trephine hole is chosen after determination of the target and of the direction of the path of the electrode on the film with the ventriculogram. Usually, however, it is necessary to make several corrections in order to direct the electrode exactly to the target point [*Austin and Lee,* 1958]. Auxiliary equipment is needed so that the X-ray film is positioned in proper relation to the median plane of the patient's skull and at the desired, constant distance from the skull and from the X-ray tube and to direct the central beam of the roentgen rays perpendicularly to the film and in constant relation to the third ventricle.

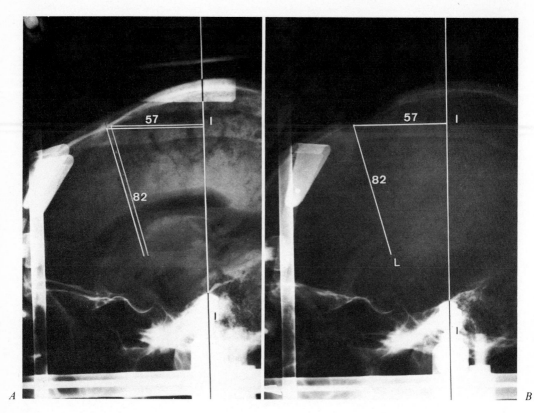

Fig. 9. Comparison of the direction and length of the planned puncture and of the position of the lesion (pallidoansotomy) in pre- *(A)* and postoperative *(B)* roentgenograms of a Parkinson patient. *A* Lateral roentgenograms with air filling of the ventricles and visualization of the foramen of Monro; coordinates and direction of the punctures reaching the anterior commissure and a point 3 mm behind it. *B* Postoperative X-ray study, showing location of a droplet of ethyl iodophenyl undecylate (Pantopaque), injected corresponding to the posterior puncture (at L); I to I = interaural line. From *Spiegel and Wycis* [1954]; reproduced with permission.

The *exactness of the localization* can be tested, fortunately only rarely, at autopsy. The position of the lesion can be identified, however, in vivo by injection of a droplet of Pantopaque at the site where the lesion had been produced, and by comparing the location of the Pantopaque droplet, seen on postoperative roentgenograms, with the position of the end of the planned puncture canal drawn on preoperative roentgenograms (fig. 9). From such studies *Spiegel and Wycis* [1952] concluded that the lesion usually could be placed with an error of 1–2 mm, frequently even less than 1 mm. Analyzing their autopsy material, *Hassler* et al. [1979] calculated that the median total error of accuracy in reaching the predetermined target was 1.23 ± 1.48 mm in the vertical, 1.68 ± 1.20 mm in the frontal, and 1.10 ± 0.92 mm in the sagittal coordinates.

Apparatuses for stereotactic spinal surgery have been devised by *Hitchcock* [1969b] and by *Lipton* et al. [1974]. Instead of the generally used rectangular coordinate system, *Turner and Shaw* [1974] developed a cylindrical coordinate system. It can be likened to a cylindrical hatbox lying on its side. The point of reference of the system is located on the long axis of the cylinder. The target is situated at a point at the rim of the hatbox. Similar to *Riechert and Mundinger,* he uses a mechanical analogue on which the radiologic measurements (relations to structures seen on the roentgenogram of the third ventricle) are plotted and from which the data for placement of the electrode can be obtained, so that calculations are not necessary.

Aids to Localization

Depth Electroencephalography

It was early recognized that the coordinates of a target found in a stereotactic atlas alone do not indicate with sufficient accuracy the site and extent of a planned subcortical lesion in view of the variability of the location and of the dimensions of subcortical structures. Consequently, it became necessary, preceding the production of a lesion, to check its intended placement by depth electroencephalography using multilead electrodes and by electric stimulation. For recording, macro- or microelectrodes were applied. Often multiple electrodes were inserted, a method termed *'stereoelectroencephalography'* by *Bancaud, Talairach* et al. [1965].

The insertion of *chronic electrodes* permits observation beyond the period when irritative phenomena may appear that are caused by the trauma of electrode insertion and are particularly seen in areas with a low convulsive threshold, such as the hippocampus. Chronic electrodes enable one to study an area under various functional conditions and to produce subcortical lesions gradually, thus reducing the incidence of complications. Several authors have used such electrodes [*Meyers,* 1949; *Heath,* 1954;

Spiegel et al., 1958a; *Sem-Jacobsen and Torkildsen,* 1960; *Walter and Crow,* 1964; *Bechterewa,* 1969] in order to determine the constancy of epileptogenic foci. Particularly after insertion of multiple electrodes, *Bechterewa* [1969] noticed in the first postoperative days transient increased intracranial pressure, slight headache and nausea due to cerebral edema lasting up to 10 days. She left the electrodes in place as long as 8 months.

Electrograms described in the older literature, which were obtained by introducing the recording electrode by hand and without roentgenographic control showing the relation of the electrodes to the ventricles, did not permit one, of course, to determine the nuclear area, the discharges of which were recorded. Such precautions as X-ray control were observed by *Wycis* et al. [1949], *Hayne* et al. [1949], *Rémond* et al. [1958], and *Umbach* [1966]. Originally macroelectrodes were used. The findings in cats that (1) the macroelectrograms of the various thalamic nuclei are not specific, so that the pattern of the record usually could not be used for localization, and (2) that there is a relative independence of the EEG and the electrothalamogram (EThG) [*Spiegel,* 1937], applied also to electrograms of human subcortical areas, not only to records taken during operation, but also to chronic records [*Heath,* 1954]. A certain difference between the EThG and the electrostriatogram seems to exist, in that the rhythm of the latter is slower [*Meyers* et al., 1949] than that of the former. In a correlation analysis of depth recordings, *Brazier and Barlow* [1956] found that the rhythms of the intrinsic activities of the basal ganglia appeared to be independent of each other and of the cortical rhythm.

Unit Discharges

Extracellular recording of unit discharges with microelectrodes in the human subcortex was practiced by *Albe-Fessard* et al. [1962], *Guiot* et al. [1962], *Jasper and Bertrand* [1964], *Gaze* et al. [1964], and *Umbach* [1966]. *Albe-Fessard* et al. [1962] and *Guiot* et al. [1962] reported that unit discharges recorded with microelectrodes permitted one to discern localizing differences between various thalamic nuclei. The discharges of the white matter were lower than those of the gray matter, and discharges were absent on passage through the ventricles.

Gillingham et al. [1977] pointed out that the amplitude of the discharges is lower from the pulvinar than from the anteriorly adjacent sensory nucleus, so that the extent of the pulvinar can be clearly defined. Similarly, *Fukamachi* et al. [1977] estimated the neural noise pattern (the background fast activity) using unit recording and amplitude averaging. Different

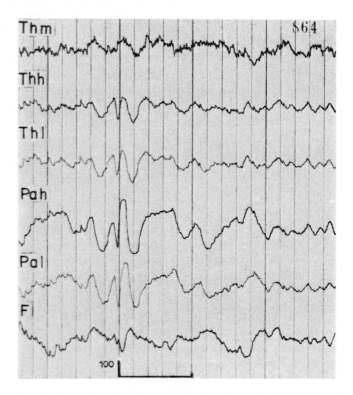

Fig. 10. Convulsions in tuberous sclerosis. Monopolar depth electroencephalogram from the right thalamus (Th; m = middle; h = upper; l = lower electrode), and from the right pallidum (Pa; h = upper; l = lower electrode); F = frontal scalp lead. Time: 1 s; calibration in microvolts. Roentgenograms revealed a nodule in the vicinity of the maximal seizure discharges in the caudate nucleus. Its elimination stopped the seizure. From *Spiegel* et al. [1956b]; reproduced with permission.

regions have a different amplitude of neural noise, e.g., when the electrode enters the VL, and still more marked in the Vim, one notices a steep increase of the noise level. *Buño* et al. [1977] processed the unit discharges by a digital computer; they found pulvinar units firing in rhythmic bursts at 3–7 Hz and units firing at random. About 20% of the units showed a phase relationship with voluntary movements, suggesting a possible role of the pulvinar in motor activity.

Depth electrography also became a valuable tool for localization of *subcortical seizure foci* (fig. 10). For an evaluation of such recordings the experience became important that multiple subcortical discharging foci are found in epileptics [*Walker and Marshall,* 1961]. 'Will-o'-the-wisp' patterns are often seen. Before using such recordings as a guide for placing lesions in the hope of eliminating or at least reducing seizures it is, therefore, necessary to ascertain by repeated testing [*Spiegel* et al., 1958a, b] whether a certain subcortical area is the site of constant seizure discharges. It was noted, for instance, that psychomotor attacks usually are initiated by spikes in the amygdala and hippocampus, from where the excitation may spread to the temporal or inferior frontal cortex [*Walker and Marshall,* 1961].

Stimulation

In addition to depth electrography, *stimulation* proved helpful in an attempt to find a subcortical focus. On stimulation of the amygdala, behavior automatisms, complex movements, disturbances of consciousness, followed by amnesia were observed, associated with low voltage, rapid cortical discharges [see review by *Feindel,* 1961]. On application of threshold stimuli and using concentric needle electrodes, a correlation of stimulated areas not only with motor effects (movements, change of tremor, automatic behavior) but also with subjective sensations (paresthesias, pain, anxiety, dizziness, clouding of consciousness, memory defects) proved important. For the somesthetic thalamus, *Emmers and Tasker* [1975] published maps showing the coupling of particular thalamic sites with specific peripheral fields to which the patients project paresthesias on stimulation of these areas.

Evoked Potentials

A further help in localization became the determination of sites that react by *evoked responses* to stimulation of the skin, e.g., with a pin, or to electrical stimulation of peripheral nerves (fig. 11, 12). For such recordings macroelectrodes proved sufficient, as was also pointed out by *Albe-Fessard* et al. [1962]. It could be ascertained whether responses were evoked in certain cortical or overlying scalp regions on stimulation of thalamic nuclei. Smelling evokes spikes in the medial amygdala [*Narabayashi* et al., 1963].

Regarding the practically important determination of the *border between* the nuclei in the ventrolateral area of the *thalamus and the internal capsule,* weak bipolar stimulation seems sufficient, as we found in agreement with *Hassler* [1960], and microelectrode recording seems to be unnec-

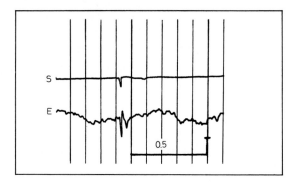

Fig. 11. Evoked potential in the right spinothalamic tract induced by stimulation of the left ulnar nerve. S = Stimulus signal; E = evoked potential. Recording electrode is in the right spinothalamic tract at the level of the posterior commissure. Stimulus: pulse duration 2 ms, 5 V; calibration: 100 µV; time: 0.5 s. From *Spiegel and Wycis* [1961]; reproduced with permission.

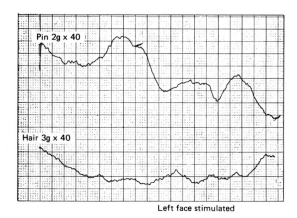

Fig. 12. Averaged responses from the base of the right thalamus to 40 stimuli by a pin (2 g) and by a v. Fry hair (3 g) applied to the face on the left side. Duration of sweep 250 ms. From *Spiegel and Wycis* [1966].

essary. Using single pulse depth stimulation at a rate of 1 Hz, *Bickford* et al. [1961] could continue recording on a 16-channel oscillograph during stimulation. An interesting technique using an implanted receiver coil and electrode unit for intracerebral *stimulation and recording in completely free-*

moving patients was developed by *Delgado* et al. [1968] and *Mark* et al. [1969a, b]. Two-way communication with the brain of free-moving subjects was refined by using radio links to send electrical stimulation or to record cerebral electrical activity [for technical details see *Delgado* et al., 1973].

Electromyography

The importance of *electromyography* and *microelectroneurography* for analyzing the effect of central stimulation as well as of stereotactic lesions is emphasized by *Struppler* [1982]. He recorded the muscle spindle activity in relaxed muscles during intracerebral subthreshold stimulation and studied the modification of alpha-gamma relations by stereotactic lesions.

Impedance

Differences of the impedance measured when the electrode tip is advanced from the white matter into a nuclear area or, conversely, from the gray into the white matter, or from the brain tissue into the ventricle filled with cerebrospinal fluid or with air, proved occasionally useful to monitor the progress of an inserted electrode [*Robinson and Tompkins*, 1964]. For the determination of the border between a tumor and the brain substance, depth electrographic recordings were more reliable than measurement of the impedance [*Laitinen and Toivakka*, 1972].

Transient Depression of Function

Production of a transient depression of function, e.g., by mild cooling (to +5 °C) preceding the definite elimination of a target, was useful to *Cooper and Lee* [1961] as a test of the proper selection of an area for destruction and of proper instrument position. Local injection of 0.25–0.50 cm^3 of a 0.5–1% solution of procaine served a similar purpose in our work [*Spiegel and Wycis*, 1962].

Computer Techniques

The application of computer techniques initiated a new stage of stereo-encephalotomy. It has been useful in three ways: in the plotting of the electrode track in relation to subcortical structures on a stereotactic atlas, in recording and processing physiological observations, and in the visualization of the location and size of a therapeutic lesion. Methods to provide visualization of the electrode against a stereotactic atlas have been developed by *Bertrand* et al. [1974], *Birg* et al. [1977] and *Barcia-Salorio* et al. [1977]. *Bechterewa* [1969] used a computer devised by *V.V. Usov* to calculate the stereotactic coordinates and the direction of electrodes inserted into the brain. Computer calculation of two-target trajectories was reported by *Peluso and Gybels* [1969].

An analysis of electrophysiological data from the human thalamus by computer technique was developed by *Bates* [1974]. He showed that a three-dimensional map of the functional properties of the thalamus and neighboring structures can be constructed. A superimposition of functional probability maps with the probabilities based on anatomical data can be achieved. Automatic exploration of unit discharges along the electrode track through the thalamus and on-line processing of pulse and analog signals obtained from the same electrode were developed by *Saito and Ohye* [1974].

An on-line computer system, developed by *Tasker* et al. [1977], combines the possibility of following the progress of a stereotactic probe through successive brain structures with a graphic display of physiological data resulting from subcortical stimulation. The possibility of data storage and of selective display of pooled material permits a refinement of stereotactic techniques and an advanced study of the functional organization of the brain. *Obrador's* group [*Buño* et al., 1977] processed spontaneous thalamic unit discharges by using a digital computer to obtain histograms showing the unit firing patterns. The knowledge of specific patterns of unit activity within the thalamic nuclei supplies additional information useful for localization of the target. The thalamic distribution of neurons responding to tactile stimuli, pressure, and limb movements was studied by *Bertrand and Hardy* [1977], continuing experiments with *Jasper* [*Jasper and Bertrand*, 1964, 1966]. Depth recordings, visual-evoked potentials and 'readiness' motor potentials were analyzed by *Ohmoto* et al. [1978].

By use of *computerized tomography* (CT) not only the localization but also the size of stereotactic RF lesions could be studied by *Kullberg* et al. [1980]. Lesions in the ventrolateral nucleus of the thalamus appeared as a discrete central core of increased attenuation surrounded by an area of decreased attenuation. Following lesions of the amygdala, the cingulum or the internal capsule, the changes were less consistent. In the initial stage after production of RF lesions, these lesions were unexpectedly large, perhaps due to edema.

Stereoscopic-stereotactic *teleangiography* is advocated by *Szikla* et al. [1979a, b]. It permits one a three-dimensional view of the cerebral vascular system and helps in localizing underlying normal or pathologically distorted cortical structures.

In view of the increasing importance of computerized tomography for stereotactic neurosurgery, I invited Dr. *P.L. Gildenberg* to write a special chapter on this subject.

Computerized Tomography and Stereotactic Surgery
by *Philip L. Gildenberg*, MD, PhD

The field of stereotactic surgery has been influenced periodically by developments outside its immediate realm. For example, the development of tranquilizers made unnecessary many stereotactic psychosurgical procedures. The development of more efficient medical management for Parkinson's disease provided alternative therapy for a large group of patients who ordinarily would have been candidates for stereotactic surgery. The development of implantable electronic stimulation devices added stimulation of both the brain and spinal cord to the classical ablation procedures.

We are on the threshold of another significant change in the course of stereotactic surgery which has come about through the development of a technique in a related field. Computerized tomography (CT scanning) enhances radiologic visualization by computer reconstruction of tomographic images representing a series of cross sections through the brain. The head or other body part is placed in the center of a rotating X-ray beam. Multiple detectors around the periphery allow accumulation of data indicating the radiodensity as the beam passes through the body at a multitude of angles. These data are manipulated by computer to allow the reconstruction of the image, as though one were looking at the slice of tissues through which the X-ray beam has passed. The patient is moved further into the gantry at a measured distance and the procedure is repeated, resulting in a series of slices which together constitute a three-dimensional picture of the head or body part [*Greitz and Bergstrom,* 1981]. Because the identification of differences in radiodensity is far more sensitive than with conventional radiographic films, one can identify the anatomy of the soft tissue structures within the head, such as ventricles, cisterns, or major blood vessels. The more sophisticated scanners can define neurologic structures such as the thalamus, caudate nucleus, internal capsule, or cortical gyri and sulci. Processes within the brain, such as tumors or hematomas, can be directly visualized on CT scanning with a reliability and definition not previously possible.

Because images are produced in anatomically accurate configurations which can be precisely measured, the utilization of the multitude of data derived from CT scans to calculate the stereotactic introduction of various probes facilitates a host of stereotactic procedures and permits many new procedures. CT stereotaxis makes it possible to introduce a probe accurately into any lesion or anatomical structure visualized on CT scanning for biopsy, aspiration, electrode implantation, etc. [*Gildenberg* et al., 1982].

Since it is possible to visualize the ventricular system without the use of contrast material, it becomes possible to relate target points to the ventricular system without a ventriculostomy. However, because CT scans are taken in transverse planes, the structures about the third ventricle which ordinarily serve as landmarks for stereotactic surgery are not directly visualized, so it is difficult to utilize the usual techniques to refer CT images to a stereotactic atlas or calculate stereotactic coordinates. Since images are generally scanned at slices greater than 1 cm apart, usual midsagittal reconstruction does not give the resolution to accurately identify landmarks about the third ventricle, such as the anterior and posterior commissure. Consequently, CT stereotaxis is presently used more for introducing probes into visualized cerebral lesions than for functional neurosurgery, but it is certain that techniques will evolve to allow accurate calculation of coordinates from CT data [*Burchiel* et al., 1980].

Most techniques for CT stereotaxis have depended on the development of a stereotactic apparatus attached to a CT scanner or the incorporation of an existing apparatus. These have the advantages of establishing a precise and definite relationship between the scan and the electrode carrier to optimize the accuracy of the system, making it possible to verify probe placement by performing the electrode insertion while the patient's head is within the scanner, and allowing progress to be followed by repeated scans, which is especially helpful with such procedures as aspiration of cysts or hematomas. The greatest disadvantage is that such systems are costly. Either a CT scanner must be dedicated to stereotactic surgery – and present utilization makes questionable the cost-effectiveness of such an arrangement – or a nondedicated scanner must be tied up for long periods while the stereotactic procedure is being performed – frequently an impractical consideration in an institution where the scanner must be kept operational many hours a day to meet diagnostic demands. In addition, most scanners are housed in the radiology department, often in rooms of marginal size and facilities, where it is inadvisable to perform major surgery because of the lack of immediately available emergency equipment or increased risk of infection.

Other systems involve the calculation of stereotactic coordinates from the CT scan and the subsequent use of those coordinates to insert a probe in the operating room at the time of stereotactic surgery. Thus, the scan and the surgery are performed as two separate procedures at different times. Advantages include cost-effectiveness and efficient use of facilities. It is not necessary to obtain a stereotactic apparatus designed specifically for CT procedures. Usually, the equipment required for the determination of stereotactic coordinates is not expensive, or there may not be a need for specialized equipment at all. The CT scanner is required for little more time than the CT scan itself. Surgery is performed in the operating room where facilities are more appropriate for an invasive procedure. Disadvantages include inaccuracies that result from errors in relating the CT image to the patient's head, or errors may result from even minor movement of the patient's head between successive scans [*Kaufman and Gildenberg,* 1980].

Perhaps the most widely employed CT stereotactic techniques involve modifications of the Leksell stereotactic apparatus [*Leksell and Jernberg,* 1980]. A baseplate may be used which can be accurately secured to the CT scanner and then, in the operating room, to the Leksell frame. Since the relationship between the baseplate and the target can be calculated accurately, and the relationship between the baseplate and the frame is known, the relationship of the target point to the frame can be ascertained. Alternatively, the stereotactic frame can be secured to the patient's head and, in turn, to the CT scanner, so that the scans are taken with the frame in place. When coordinates have been determined, the patient's head is removed from the CT scanner, the arc secured to the frame, and the probe introduced to the target point.

The baseplate or frame can be secured to the patient's head either through the direct method of inserting pins through the scalp, or a helmet can be constructed of light orthopedic casting material, and the head frame secured to the helmet [*Greitz* et al., 1980]. The vertical coordinate is determined by the height of the selected CT section from the baseplate, and the other coordinates are measured in the transverse section bearing the target. The Leksell apparatus is attached to the baseplate to perform insertion of the probe [*Boëthius* et al., 1980a-c]. Leksell has also designed an apparatus which focuses gamma irradiation from multiple sources on a small target. The level of radiation is sufficient to make a lesion of approximately 1 cm^3 with minimal irradiation to the surrounding brain tissue. By using the technique described above to marry the Leksell stereotactic apparatus to CT scanning, the Leksell gamma unit can be used to direct focused radiation to lesions visualized on the CT scan [*Boëthius* et al., 1980a-c; *Bergstrom and Greitz,* 1976]. Another system to adapt the Leksell stereotactic apparatus for CT scanning employs a three-sided, polyethylene cube ('helmet') with slotted corners that permits precise and reproducible placement of the conventional Leksell stereotactic frame over the cube [*Law and Cacak,* 1980; *Kingsley* et al., 1980]. The patient wears the plastic cube fixed to the skull with nylon screws during the scan, and the stereotactic frame is fixed to the cube for the surgery.

The base ring of the Riechert-Mundinger stereotactic apparatus can be adapted to the CT table. The computer of the CT scanner can calculate the position at which the arc and electrode carrier are attached to the base ring to assure accurate insertion of the probe [*Birg and Mundinger,* 1982]. Another technique [*Colombo* et al., 1980, 1981] employs three acrylic screws with lead markers placed in the patient's skull prior to scanning, which are used to establish a reference plane. The basal ring of a stereotactic apparatus is attached to the screws, and calculations are performed by computer. A motorized apparatus driven by the stereotactic-assisting computer has been described which will completely automate the procedure. It is based on the principle of adjusting the target to the center of a spherical system, but the motorized arm bearing the electrode carrier is placed outside of the scanning plane, so it does not intrude on the confines of the CT scanner.

Another system uses a modified Leksell stereotactic apparatus which is fixed to the table of a GE 8800 CT scanner [*Lunsford,* 1982; *Rosenbaum* et al., 1980; *Perry* et al., 1980; *Maroon* et al., 1977]. The Koslow system [*Koslow* et al., 1981, 1982; *Koslow and Abele,* 1980] is based on a newly designed frame incorporated into a CT scanner which has been modified to use solely for stereotactic surgery. Appropriate landmarks are identified on the scan and a series of mathematical steps resident in the CT computer are used to transfer the landmark coordinate frame of reference to the anatomical frame of reference. An ingenious stereotactic frame consisting of two interlocking arcs has been devised by *Brown, Roberts and Osborne* for use with CT scanner. The frame is attached during the scanning and a small programmable calculator is used to interrelate the frame and the CT geometry to indicate the position at which each arc must be set, in order to aim the apparatus precisely at any visualized target [*Brown,* 1981, 1979a, b; *Brown* et al., 1980, 1981; *Roberts and Brown,* 1980]. A particularly sophisticated system employs computer processing of CT scanner data from the regions of interest by filtering, magnifying, color-coding, and three-dimensional reconstruction. The stereotactic coordinates are calculated by the computer and fed into a modified head fixation system. A binocular endoscope directed by the stereotactic frame can be used to remove or treat small CNS lesions [*Jacques* et al., 1980a, b; *Shelden* et al., 1980].

By using a ball-pivot type of stereotactic apparatus which is secured to a burr hole and remains outside the scanning plane, a probe can be inserted while verifying its progress on repeated scans [*Rushworth, 1980*].

Gildenberg employs a procedure to calculate coordinates from the CT scan, which are later employed in stereotactic surgery in the operating room, using the GE 8800 scanner [*Gildenberg* et al., 1982; *Gildenberg and Kaufman*, 1982]. The key to this system is the ScoutView, a reconstruction that appears like a lateral skull X-ray with each scanning plane marked, which can be used to establish the vertical (Z) coordinate. A CT scan is performed in the usual fashion with the gantry at 90°. A target point within each lesion is marked on the appropriate CT scans. The slice closest to the majority of targets is taken as the 'zero' slice, and, on that slice, the distance between the frontal and occipital bones is bisected, to provide a zero point from which anterior-posterior measurements are made. The image of the zero slice with the cursor at the zero point in the midline is photographed for future reference. The zero point is established on each slice bearing a target by displaying the zero slice with the cursor at the zero point on the console, and then changing the image to the slice bearing the target without moving the cursor, so that the zero point appears at the appropriate place on each slice.

The anteroposterior (Y) coordinates are measured by moving the cursor from the zero point in the midline to a point directly medial to the target, and the resident program for measuring the distance is used. The cursor is then moved lateral to the target and the lateral (X) coordinate is measured. Since the distance between slices is known from the scanning program, the distance from the zero slice to each target slice (Z) is known.

Later, in the operating room, the initial lateral X-ray is taken, and one of the planes intersecting identifiable landmarks near the base of the skull, as seen on the ScoutView, is drawn on the lateral X-ray. The distance from that plane to the zero slice is reconstructed on the lateral X-ray, so that the zero slice can also be marked. The zero point is marked on that line, half-way between the intersection with the frontal and occipital bones, so that the anteroposterior measurements can be made on the zero slice. Lines representing the other target-bearing slices are likewise made, and a line intersecting the zero slice at the zero point is drawn at right angles to intersect each target-bearing plane at its zero point. Thus, the vertical (Z) and anteroposterior (Y) coordinates are made on the lateral film to be used as the stereotactic targets. The distance from the midline is measured directly. The stereotactic surgery is then performed in the usual fashion in the operating room depending on the type of apparatus employed.

Other systems employ visualization during CT examinations of air grooves or wires within an acrylic plate [*Barcia-Salorio* et al., 1982], with a duplicate plate with wires used during ScoutView radiography, in order to calculate the vertical (Z) coordinates [*Lee* et al., 1978; *Piskun,* 1979; *Wester* et al., 1981]. A similar system involves the use of wooden scales containing wires placed at angles to obtain the Z coordinate [*Bergstrom* et al., 1978], or a reference ring on the patient's head that is used to establish the Z coordinate in relation to the tip of the biopsy needle [*Huk and Baer,* 1980]. Several systems require estimating the plane of the CT slices on lateral X-rays taken at the time of stereotactic surgery [*Cail and Morris,* 1979; *Penn* et al., 1978].

Indications for CT stereotaxis are numerous. *Biopsy* can be done in those patients whose lesion is not accessible to open surgery, particularly in those patients whose tumor may not be resectable and who do not have the mass effect which would require even partial resection, but in whom a tissue diagnosis is desirable prior to institution of radiotherapy or chemotherapy. Stereotactic biopsy of those lesions makes possible definitive diagnoses of many lesions where only a presumptive diagnosis could be made previously. This is particularly helpful in lesions of the brain stem, in which CT scanning may be the most sensitive means of identifying a lesion.

Certain lesions may be managed completely by *stereotactic aspiration.* Primary among these are abscesses, where aspiration of well walled-off lesions may constitute the only required treatment, although the abscess cavity may be irrigated with saline or antibiotic solutions, if desired. Colloid cysts may likewise be aspirated, often with complete resolution, obviating the need for transventricular surgery [*Bosch* et al., 1978]. Hematomas may be evacuated by the use of a mandrel, which may allow alleviation of the mass effect with minimal disruption of overlying tissue [*Higgins and Nashold,* 1980a, b; *Higgins* et al., 1982]. A catheter may be left in place for the installation of streptokinase for gradual dissolution of the clot and repeated later aspiration.

The CT scan may be used to define the lesion in three dimensions [*Jacques* et al., 1980a; *Shelden* et al., 1982], so that calculations might be made for the optimal positioning of stereotactically inserted radioisotopes [*Mundinger* et al., 1980]. In patients who require ventriculostomy but who may have small ventricles due to cerebral edema or shifted ventricles due to a mass lesion, the ventricle may be tapped accurately by the use of CT stereotaxis, possibly combined with impedance monitoring [*Boëthius* et al., 1979; *Broggi and Franzini,* 1981]. A microelectrode may be inserted into the plane of a CT scan, and as the trajectory of the electrode insertion is noted on the scan image, it is possible to correlate the neural activity of deep structures with their anatomical location as seen on the CT scan [*Ohye* et al., 1980].

When stereotaxis is used to approach lesions seen on CT scanning, the edge of the lesion may be verified by monitoring electrical impedance [*Benabid* et al., 1979] or recording *electrical activity* as the probe crosses the interface into the lesion [*Nakajima and Ohye,* 1980; *Ohye* et al., 1980]. Tissue surrounding a tumor may produce abnormal electrical activity, e.g., slow wave activity, but electrical silence is encountered within the lesion itself. With a side-arm electrode it is possible to explore the area surrounding the trajectory to define the edge of a lesion which may have an irregular border or to determine the dimensions of a small lesion. Such electrical recordings might also be used if CT directed stereotaxis is employed for functional neurosurgery, for instance to introduce an electrode into visualized structures with characteristic electrical activity, such as the amygdaloid nucleus [*Burchiel* et al., 1980].

The safety and efficacy for diagnoses of brain *biopsies* has been well demonstrated [*Edner,* 1981]. In one series of nonstereotactic biopsies, there was a total morbidity and mortality rate of 13%, with abnormal tissue noted in 85% of the specimens [*Kaufman and Catalano,* 1979]. In one series of stereotactic biopsies for glioma, abnormality was noted in 12 out of 13 cases with a correct morphologic diagnosis in 11 and no adverse effects reported. In another series [*Gildenberg* et al., 1982], all biopsies taken in 7 patients were diagnostic; 2 patients had brain abscesses that were treated with aspiration at the time of establishing the diagnosis, 1 patient with six brain abscesses and another with two. CT directed stereotaxis has been used to obtain smear preparations, which, in the proper hands, can provide an accurate diagnosis [*Mundinger* et al., 1980; *Ostertag* et al., 1980, 1981]. Other series depend on tissue specimens obtained by biopsy forceps and diagnosed by the usual pathology techniques [*Gildenberg* et al., 1982; *Norén and Collins,* 1980; *Gildenberg and Kaufman,* 1982; *Rougier* et al., 1982; *Edner,* 1979; *Boëthius* et al., 1978] or involve the development of new neuropathological criteria [*Dumas-Duport* et al., 1982]. The opportunity to obtain multiple biopsies from various points within a single tumor or to obtain biopsies over time has made possible new studies of the histological characteristics of brain tumors and their biochemical make-up [*Boëthius* et al., 1980a-c].

Because CT scanning allows diagnosis of cerebral lesions with definition and accuracy not previously attainable, new indications for biopsy of cerebral lesions are being developed. (1) Lesions that could not previously be identified are seen clearly with CT scanning. (2) Since lesions can be identified earlier, new indications must be developed for the management of small lesions. (3) Even those lesions which cannot be resected with open surgery can be localized with precision and biopsied. (4) Lesions which are localized in areas that were previously considered to be too risky for surgery can be localized with CT scanning, which is particularly sensitive in many of those areas, to invite tissue diagnosis. (5) As new nonsurgical means of treatment become available, stereotactic biopsy may obviate the need for more extensive surgery, particularly if the cerebral lesion is a manifestation of systemic or generalized malignant disease which might best be treated with chemotherapy or radiation. (6) Some lesions, such as abscesses or hematomas, can be treated solely with stereotactic aspiration and medical management. (7) Even those patients who have a primarily intracerebral tumor may be candidates for stereotactic biopsy prior to craniotomy in order to plan surgery with as much definite information as possible [*Bergstrom* et al., 1978, 1981; *Boëthius* et al., 1980; *Bosch*, 1980a, b; *Lewander* et al., 1978; *Mundinger* et al., 1980; *Norén and Collins*, 1980].

With more lenient indications for biopsy of deep cerebral lesions, various techniques to obtain biopsy specimens must be reconsidered. Lesions of different vascularity or different firmness may require different biopsy techniques.

Biopsy forceps are still the most efficient means of obtaining tissue. However, if the cup is less than 1.0–1.5 mm in length, the specimen may be inadequate, unless the lesion is firm and cellular, or unless a smear preparation is used [*Mundinger* et al., 1980; *Ostertag* et al., 1980]. A biopsy forceps of 1.5–1.8 mm has been found to be more satisfactory, and it has been consistently possible to obtain a tissue diagnosis. Because biopsy forceps vary considerably in their cross-section configuration, some forceps require a rather large cannula through which the forceps can be inserted. Ideally, a cannula and forceps are matched for optimal utilization of cross-sectional diameter, which allows one to obtain the largest possible tissue specimen through the smallest diameter cannula. It is an additional advantage for the cannula to be matched to the various types of electrodes which may be employed to perform electrical or impedance monitoring prior to obtaining the specimen.[3]

If the tumor is quite firm, satisfactory biopsy can frequently be made with a corkscrew type of instrument which burrows into the tumor and pulls it back against the edge of a cannula to obtain the specimen. A theoretical advantage of this system is improved safety because of less threat to vascular structures. In addition, there is less crushing of tissue, so that the specimen may be more satisfactory for histologic preparation.

Satisfactory biopsy can sometimes be obtained by the use of a cannula with a sharpened edge [*Hahn* et al., 1979] or specialized biopsy needle [*Colombo* et al., 1980]. The cannula is inserted with the obturator in place until it lies 5–10 mm short of the target point, at which time the obturator is removed. Suction with a specimen trap is applied to the cannula while it is advanced sharply to the target or a point just beyond. With continuous suction the cannula bearing the tissue specimen may be withdrawn. This technique is especially advantageous for very soft friable tumors or tumors in the vicinity of vascular structures.

Additional information to assist the evaluation and management of tumors can be obtained from the combination of CT scanning and stereotactic surgery [*Lobato* et al., 1982; *Scarabin* et al., 1978]. The tumor volume may be calculated from CT programs involving boundary detection, which can be verified by impedance or deep brain electroencephalographic recording [*Broggi and Franzini,* 1981; *Cerroni* et al., 1979; *Mundinger* et al., 1980]. Progression of the tumor or response to treatment can be estimated. Three-dimensional reconstruction of a lesion by computer can define the shape and volume accurately, as well as the relationship to nearby vital structures, which may assist in planning surgery or evaluating progression of the tumor [*Cerroni* et al., 1979; *Mundinger* et al., 1980; *Shelden* et al., 1982; *Schlegel* et al., 1981]. The information about configuration of the tumor can be used to plan radiation treatment, either by stereotactic implantation of multiple sources at precisely determined points to optimize the distribution of radiation [*Mun-*

---

[3] An integrated stereotactic biopsy kit designed by the author is available from Radionics Inc., Burlington, Mass.

dinger et al., 1980], or by the use of an external source of focused irradiation [*Backlund and Leksell,* 1971].

An integrated system can be employed for biopsy or aspiration and insertion of radioisotopes for interstitial radiotherapy of deep-seated tumors, but radiation treatment should not be considered without histologic confirmation, which can be performed through the same cannula [*Mundinger* et al., 1978, 1980; *Birg and Mundinger,* 1982]. The sites of administration and dosage of the interstitial source of radiation can be calculated by using the information obtained from the CT image [*Mundinger* et al., 1980; *Kelly* et al., 1978]. Alternatively, multiple stereotactic radiofrequency lesions may be used to treat the tumor [*Gleason* et al., 1978].

Patients with *epilepsy* should have CT scans as part of their general evaluation. A number of these patients demonstrate abnormalities on CT scanning which might invite stereotactic biopsy, particularly since lesions associated with epilepsy are frequently not indications for craniotomy [*Nakajima and Ohye,* 1980].

Intracerebral *hematomas* have been successfully evacuated with a cannula into which a helical mandrel is inserted. The mandrel is rotated to break up the blood clot and to help drive it into the cannula, through which a combination of irrigation and suction propel it [*Backlund and Von Holst,* 1978; *Higgins and Nashold,* 1980a, b; *Broseta* et al., 1982]. *Abscesses* can be treated successfully by aspiration of pus, which is then also available for diagnosis and culture. Aspiration alone may allow resolution of the mass effect, or the abscess may be irrigated with saline or antibiotic solution, which is often curative when combined with systemic antibiotic administration [*Moran* et al., 1979; *Mundinger* et al., 1980; *Wise and Gleason,* 1979; *Gildenberg* et al., 1982; *Walsh* et al., 1980].

CT stereotaxis can be a valuable *adjunct to open surgical procedures.* Small tumors, malformations, cysts, or vessels feeding tumors or arteriovenous malformations are often identified most readily by CT scanning. In order to identify and clip feeding vessels of malformations prior to resection of the entire malformation, they may be used as target points and appropriate coordinates calculated. At stereotactic surgery a section of radiopaque tubing may be inserted to the target along the desired approach for open surgery. The stereotactic frame may be used as the surgical headholder, if it is the appropriate type, or the patient's head may be secured in a more appropriate headholder. A small craniotomy or craniectomy may be performed so that the deep-seated lesion is approached through a narrow opening guided by the tubing, to minimize damage to overlying brain or to avoid functional areas. If it is desired to return the patient for surgery on another day, the tubing can be sutured to the pericranium at the edge of the burr hole and folded under the skin prior to closure so that no tubing extrudes. A reasonable resection can be made through a core of brain tissue retracted by a small speculum. Resection of the tumor may be accomplished by a stereotactically directed laser beam, so that the entire visualized mass of the tumor may be resected [*Kelly and Alker,* 1980]. The use of coordinates to establish the boundaries of resection plus repeated CT scanning may maximize the amount of tumor resected.

Clinical Applications

Disturbances of Emotions and Behavior

Dorsomedial Thalamotomy

It has been mentioned that stereotactic lesions of the *dorsomedial nuclei* (fig. 13) of the thalamus were originally performed as an alternative to prefrontal leukotomy, since these nuclei send fibers to and receive impulses chiefly from the orbital surface of the frontal lobes [*Spiegel* et al., 1947] (see fig. 55). Thus, the indications for operations on these nuclei were the same as for prefrontal leukotomy, especially anxiety, tension, agitated depression, involutional melancholia, or obsessive-compulsive disturbances. Results of dorsomedial thalamotomy were followed in 77 patients for 1–8 years after operation [*Spiegel* et al., 1956c]. They were classified as follows: Group A: institutionalized patients who had gained more or less full working capacity outside the hospital or noninstitutionalized patients who were completely relieved of their emotional disturbances without side effects. Group B: patients who returned home but with definitely reduced working capacity, or nonhospitalized patients in whom relief of most emotional disturbances was obtained, and slight side effects such as memory defects, decreased initiative were noticeable. Group C: remained hospitalized, but became less agitated and assaultive and more manageable; or nonhospitalized patients in whom the emotional disorder was only slightly relieved. Group D were unimproved and group E became worse.

In the nonschizophrenic patients the results were more satisfactory (47.5% in groups A and B) than in schizophrenics (21.4% in groups A and B). Within the schizophrenic groups, better results were obtained in the catatonic type (5 of 10 patients in groups A, B and C) than in the paranoid type (14 of 36 patients in groups A, B and C). Within the nonschizophrenic groups, the best results were observed in severe anxiety neurosis (5 out of 7 in group A) and in depressive states (3 out of 4 in groups A and B). In the manic types (1 out of 3 in group B) and the obsessive-compulsive neurotics (1 out of 4 in group A) the results were less satisfactory. Thus, the best

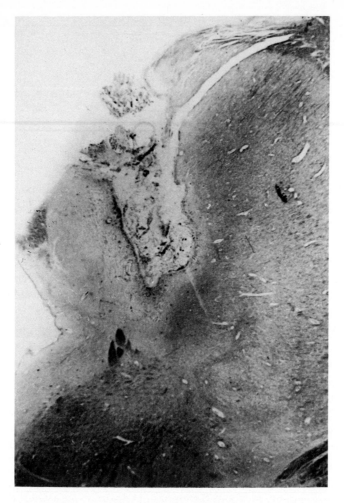

Fig. 13. Electrolytic lesion in the dorsomedial nucleus of a schizophrenic patient.
Death caused by pyelonephritis and vascular hypertension 5½ years postoperatively.

long-range effects in cases refractory to nonoperative procedures in use at
that time were obtained in severe anxiety neurosis and in depression.
Relapses appeared in 23% of the schizophrenics after time intervals lasting
up to 2 years. *Baudoin and Puech* [1949], *Monnier* [1952], *Riechert* [1953a]
and *Wada and Endo* [1951] obtained favorable results after dorsomedial
thalamotomy. The relapses may be compared with those after frontal lobo-

tomies; *Freeman and Watts* [1950] reported that 12 of 20 patients relapsed during an observation period of 10 years.

Remarkable effects were reported by *Talairach* [1952] in 22 psychotics, chiefly schizophrenics, after lesions of the *nucleus ventralis anterior*. In 20 schizophrenics he attained in 15% complete social readaptation, 20% corresponded to the above described group B and 40% more or less to the group C or relapsed. The observation period lasted from 1 to 4 years postoperatively. These very favorable results probably are because the lesion was placed in an area where all the fibers coming from the dorsomedial nucleus to the frontal lobe could be cut; the relatively short duration of observation also should be considered.

Further experiences showed that, besides frontothalamic connections, other systems play an important role in the mechanism of emotions, and the therapeutic effects of their interruption were tested.

Anterior Thalamotomy

In addition or as an alternative to elimination of the dorsomedial nuclei, lesions of the *anterior nuclei* were devised because these nuclei are part of the Papez circuit [see p. 169]. In 21 patients subjected to anterior thalamotomy, the results could be classified as follows: 1 belonged to group A, 3 to group B, 5 to group C and 3 relapsed after an improvement corresponding to group C [*Spiegel and Wycis*, 1951, 1952, 1962]. Favorable results were also reported by *Mark* [1970] and by *Arjona* [1974].

Hypothalamotomy

In cases of relapse of aggressive schizophrenics following dorsomedial and/or anterior nuclear lesions, later also independently, hypothalamic lesions were produced [*Spiegel and Wycis*, 1951, 1953b, 1962][4]. Since it is known from animal experiments that bilateral hypothalamic lesions cause a decrease of emotional reactions, 1–3 small electrolytic lesions of the lateral hypothalamus and overlying subthalamus were produced in 25 patients; 10 had relapsed after dorsomedial or anterior thalamotomy; in 13 it was combined with dorsomedial thalamotomy; in 2 instances only hypothalamic lesions were placed. Of the 23 cases, 4 showed results belonging to group B, but 2 of these relapsed; 13 belonged to group C. In the 2 patients in whom hypothalamotomy alone was performed, the results were as follows: The

---

[4] In the literature, the erroneous statement is frequently found that *Sano* [1962] initiated hypothalamotomy in psychiatric surgery.

paranoid schizophrenic became more manageable. The manic-depressive, manic type, with grandiose ideas and paranoid trends had still become occasionally assaultive after bilateral transorbital lobotomy and needed repeated electroshock treatment. Following bilateral hypothalamotomy, he was still euphoric, but no longer a problem in supervision, was without EST, and could be permitted restricted home visits. Success of posteromedial hypothalamotomy was reported by *Sano* [1962] and *Black* et al. [1975]. Preoperative stimulation produced horror and marked sympathetic response.

While *Nádvornik* et al. [1973] stated that posterior hypothalamotomy seemed to give the best results in the treatment of the aggressive syndrome, *Kim and Umbach* [1973] found it insufficient in periodic terror and sudden outbreaks of violence and combined it with medial amygdalotomy.

Based upon the finding of *Doerner* et al. [1969] that a lesion of the nucleus ventromedialis hypothalami could abolish neuroendocrine male homosexuality in the rat, *Roeder* [1966] and *Roeder* et al. [with *Orthner and Müller,* 1971, 1972a, b] performed unilateral lesions of the *nucleus ventromedialis (Cajal)* on the nondominant side in 10 *sexual offenders.* This nucleus is regarded as a 'sexual behavior center'. Since its depth below the intercommissural line varies from 7 to 11 mm, they stimulated the optic tract and used the appearance of light flashes as an aid to localization. Following the unilateral lesions, the sexual drive of the patients was weakened, but, in contrast to the effect of castration, the gonads continued to function normally, and the patients did not exhibit depression and feelings of inferiority that appear after castration. Metabolic side effects (eunuchoid obesity, diabetes insipidus) did not occur. Initiative and intellectual capacity were not impaired. Potency was weakened, but preserved after unilateral lesions. Bilateral lesions performed in 1 patient, who was cured of previously intractable exhibitionism, abolished potency. Of 3 patients with *pedophilic homosexuality,* reported by *Roeder and Mueller* [1969], 2 were cured by the procedure and 1 has shown a diminution of the sexual drive.

Dieckmann and Hassler's [1975] target in 3 cases of *pedophilic homosexuality* was also the *ventromedial hypothalamic nucleus* on the nondominant side, especially its basal part.[5] They point out that, according to animal experiments [*Doerner* et al., 1968], the ventromedial nucleus represents the

_____

[5] I am happy to note that these two groups developed this special application of hypothalamotomy belonging to a type of procedures first performed by *Spiegel and Wycis* in psychic anomalies, and that they used the side string electrode introduced in stereotactic operations by these authors.

female sexual behavior center. This nucleus and the tuberomammillar complex are gonadotropically active. Accordingly, *Dieckmann and Hassler* [1975] included the *tuberomammillar complex* in their lesion. In 3 other sexual delinquents they enlarged the lesion rostrally so that it included the *preoptic area,* where *Doerner* et al. [1968] located the gonadotropically inactive male sexual behavior center. This additional lesion reduced the patient's pathologically enhanced sexual drive. In the 3 homosexuals, complete loss of all homosexual activity was obtained; the pedophilic interests of the patients were not completely abolished. In the 3 other cases with violent hypersexuality, the results were classified good in 2 (marked reduction of their sexual drive) and fair in 1. Immediately after the operation, 3 patients showed strong feelings of hunger and verbal aggressiveness for a few hours. Diabetes insipidus or visual disturbances did not occur. The authors consider the effect of the stereotactic surgery much stronger and longer lasting than that of medication with antiandrogen. The indications of this operation are, of course, limited to patients in whom prolonged conservative treatment has been ineffective; it seems justified particularly when criminal offences were committed.

Roeder [1974] found unilateral lesions of the ventromedial nucleus insufficient in *alcohol and drug addictions.* He reported bilateral hypothalamotomy in this region in 11 addicted patients. There were side effects (signs of deficiency as well as of stimulation) of variable duration: confusion, impaired memory for recent events, somnolence, voracity and aggressiveness analogous to experiences in animal experiments, diabetes insipidus, and increase in body weight. The addiction and the sexual drive were reduced or abolished following the procedure. Although the results were encouraging, *Roeder* emphasized that the possibility of relapses has to be considered; he recommended postoperative psychiatric treatment and placement of the patient in a safe environment where he no longer could secure intoxication. In the discussion of *Roeder's* lecture, *D. Müller* even advocated postoperative commitment to a closed psychiatric institution for at least 8 weeks.

In one of *Dieckmann and Hassler's* [1975] sexual deviants, unilateral coagulation in the hypothalamic ventromedial and tuberomammillar regions stopped excessive smoking. *Dieckmann and Schneider* [1978] also coagulated the ventromedial nucleus bilaterally in alcoholism and drug addiction in 6 of 15 patients. The lasting side effects of the bilateral procedure, however, were considerable. These operations should be considered, of course, as treatment of last resort, particularly the application of the bilateral procedure. *Arjona* [1974] reported that in *erethitic* children (agitated idiocy) stereotactic hypothalamotomy was the only procedure which brought persistent relief.

Lesions of the Intralaminar Nuclei and of the Centrum medianum

Extending the coagulation of the dorsomedial nucleus to the *intralaminar nuclei* and the *lamella medialis thalami, Hassler and Dieckmann* [1967] improved the relief of the aggressiveness, destructiveness and agitation of erethitic imbecile children and of compulsive and obsessive symptoms of adults, compared with lesions restricted to the dorsomedial nuclei. The lesions of the dorsomedial nuclei were enlarged in the rostral and ventral direction. Unilateral intervention had a transient effect. Prolonged observations beyond the authors' observation period of 2 years will have to ascertain how long the favorable therapeutic effect of bilateral lesions may last. Their illustration shows that the lesions interrupted also the mammillothalamic tract to the anterior nucleus, and they explain the transitory amnesia of the patients by lesions of this bundle. Apparently their lesions also interrupted the Papez circuit [see p. 169]. Further studies seem to be required to decide whether their lesions had an effect different from that of combined lesions of the dorsomedial and anterior nuclei, and whether lesions of the dorsomedial plus intralaminar nuclei (leaving the Vicq d'Azyr bundle intact) have a favorable therapeutic effect similar to that reported by the authors.

Hassler and Dieckmann [1967] believed that the *Gilles de la Tourette syndrome* (multiple tics, obsessive motor compulsions and coprolalia [obscene language]) belongs to the group of obsessions and recommended thalamotomy. Accordingly, *de Divitiis* et al. [1977] placed lesions in the dorsomedial and intralaminar nuclei, but obtained only transient remission and considered the procedure not successful in this syndrome. *Hassler* improved the operative results by adding coagulation of the Voi.

Haloperidol (starting with 1 mg daily, gradually increased to an optimum clinical effect, maximum 10 mg daily) or clonidine hydrochloride (0.05–0.3 mg/day) should be tried [*Cohen* et al., 1980]. The possibility of development of Parkinson-like symptoms, of tardive dyskinesia (involuntary movements performed chiefly by the oral, lingual, facial, and cervical muscles), of dystonia or akathisia on use of haloperidol should not be overlooked [*Klawans* et al., 1980]. For treatment of extrapyramidal side effects of haloperidol, *Borison and Davis* [1980] recommended amantadine (100–300 mg daily), which proved superior to benztropine mesylate (Cogentin, 1–2 mg once or twice daily) in treating extrapyramidal side effects without producing discomforting anticholinergic effects.

The *centrum medianum,* a cell group adjacent to the lamina medullaris interna (see fig. 55), was chosen by *Andy* [1970] as the target in patients suffering from aggressive behavior or hyperactivity. The behavior of all 5 cases subjected to lesions of the centrum medianum was improved; 2 of them became rehabilitated, a third socially well adjusted.

Anterior Capsulotomy

The fact that the frontothalamic pathways form a discrete tract in the anterior limb of the internal capsule suggested interruption of this system by stereotactic anterior capsulotomy as an alternative to prefrontal leukotomy. Obsessional states were particularly benefited by this procedure [*Herner* (an associate of *Leksell*), 1961], so that *Bingley* et al. [1973] recommend this safe procedure as a routine method for treatment of severe obsessive-compulsive neurosis with anxiety. It was successful in 70% of 17 cases. There was a transient postoperative loss of initiative and in 2 cases a mild tendency to inactivity [similarly *Kullberg,* 1977]. The operation was successful in 90% of *Riechert's* [1980] patients with obsessional neurosis.

Cingulectomy and Cingulotomy

Originally, the Papez circuit was severed by nonstereotactic ablation of the anterior part of the gyrus cinguli (anterior cingulectomy) [*Ward,* 1948; *Cairns* et al., 1952; *Whitty* et al., 1952; *Le Beau,* 1952; *Livingston,* 1953]. This was the forerunner of stereotactic interruption of the cingulum (cingulotomy) [*Foltz and White,* 1962; *Ballantine* et al., 1967; *Brown and Lighthill,* 1968]. One has to bear in mind that anterior cingulectomy and cingulotomy differ in the extent of the lesions. While the anterior cingulectomy is more or less restricted to the cortical area 24, the stereotactic cingulotomy severs not only cingulum fibers connecting areas within the limbic system, but also connections with area 32, with the posterior orbital cortex and with other frontal lobe regions, as pointed out by *Lewin* [1973] and *Scoville* [1973].

Initially, anterior cingulectomy was performed in emotional-behavioral disturbances including aggressiveness and obsessional symptoms; in these latter conditions, however, relapses were rather frequent [*Lewin,* 1973]. Stereotactic cingulotomy proved to be more efficient, particularly in anxiety, depression and emotionally charged pain. *Balasubramaniam* et al. [1973] found cingulotomy useful in drug addiction and obsession.

Orbital Undercutting; Subcaudate Tractotomy

Orbital undercutting [*Scoville,* 1949] interrupts orbitothalamic and orbitotemporal connections. It was replaced by *Knight* [1964, 1973] with stereotactic implantation of radioactive ^{90}Y seeds in the subcaudate zone above cortical area 13 (subcaudate tractotomy). The lesion is located in and/or in front of the substantia innominata [*Newcombe,* 1975].

While *Scoville* [1949, 1973] applied the orbital undercutting to all forms of mental disease, *Knight* [1964] found the subcaudate tractotomy successful mainly in chronic depression and in anxiety states with a depressive element. Comparing 600 cases of orbital undercutting with 450 cases of stereotactic implantation of radioactive ^{90}Y, *Knight* noted identical clinical changes. The postoperative side effects, however, were missing after the stereotactic procedure.[6] In cases of unsuccessful subcaudate tractotomy, additional cingulotomy could relieve extremely tense and depressed patients. *King* [1961] pointed out that these operations rarely improve obsessional neuroses. He found such neuroses of early onset and without depression difficult to eradicate. Combined bilateral subcaudate tractotomy and cingulectomy improved 76% of obsessional neurotics [*Heggs* et al., 1977].

Anterior Mesoloviotomy

Laitinen [1972] and *Laitinen and Vilkki* [1973] combined bilateral stereotactic rostral cingulotomy in front and below the knee of the corpus callosum with bilateral coagulation of the superficial layers of the knee of the corpus callosum, 5–7 mm from the midline. These superficial layers of the corpus callosum consist of transcallosal cingulostriate fibers. The procedure, called anterior mesoloviotomy (mesolovion = corpus callosum), was efficient against anxiety, tension and fear of neurotic, schizophrenic and epileptic origin and schizophrenic catatonia, but ineffective against depression and obsessive-compulsive symptoms. Intelligence was not affected. It is presumed that in anxiety, tension and schizophrenic catatonia, the interhemispheric cingulostriate fibers are hyperactive; they may constitute a link between the emotional integrative system and its motor output. Electric stimulation of the rostral-most part of the cingulum with 6 Hz produced evoked potentials in the contralateral frontopolar scalp EEG. It has been

---

[6] In view of the risks inherent in the use of radioactive isotopes, stereotactic electrocoagulation of the subcaudate region may be preferable.

suggested by *Lewin* [1973] that the cingulotomy of *Laitinen and Vilkki* [1973] interrupted fibers from the posterior orbital cortex to the anterior part of the cingulum.

Amygdalotomy

The favorable effect of lesions of the amygdala [*Narabayashi* et al., 1963, 1970; *Narabayashi,* 1972, 1976; *Mark* et al., 1972] in uncontrollable unsocial behavior, outbursts of violence and aggressiveness of adults, in hyperactivity of erethitic, feebleminded children may be due to an influence upon the Papez circuit by way of the hippocampus or to an influence upon the hypothalamus by way of the stria terminalis or of ventral amygdalohypothalamic fibers.

Narabayashi selected patients with severely disturbed behavior and emotional problems associated with epileptic seizures of grand mal or temporal lobe type, patients without clear fits but with definite epileptic EEG anomalies, and children with nonprogressive feeblemindedness which suggested organic brain damage. He excluded patients with only behavior problems and emotional problems of different origin. Postoperatively the children could be more easily educated; nonspeaking epileptic children began to talk, some epileptic traits improved; spikes disappeared in the EEG. There was a slight increase of appetite for several weeks. The absence of a Klüver-Bucy syndrome (except 1 case), of changes of sexual behavior, memory loss, or olfactory or taste defects is emphasized. *Kim and Umbach* [1973] selected the medial part of the amygdala as the primary and the posteromedial hypothalamus as an additional target, if the first operation was not sufficient, in cases of pronounced violence and aggression. After coagulation of the amygdala, the patients' mood was elevated, their appetite and libido increased, and they gained weight. Very few cognitive changes, subtle transitory memory defects were detected by *Hitchcock* et al. [1973] after bilateral amygdalotomy. Stereotactic amygdalectomy and subcaudate tractotomy were useful in psychotics with aggressive behavior [*Vaernet and Madsen,* 1970]. Speech improved in disturbed children [*Ito* et al., 1972].

1 year after bilateral amygdalotomy, *Siegfried and Ben-Shmuel* [1973] found complete absence of aggressive behavior only in 1 of 8 patients and reasonable improvement in 4 cases. They consider the limited effect encouraging, since these cases were resistant to all conservative therapy. *Chitanondh* [1966] performed amygdalotomy in psychiatric disorders with olfactory hallucinations. Amygdalotomy on one side was combined with a

lesion of the opposite dorsomedial nucleus in erethitic children by *Diemath and Nievoll* [1966].

When faced by a patient with aggressive behavior, it is desirable, of course, that pharmacotherapy should be attempted, as in other psychiatric disorders, before surgery is considered. Regarding pathology due to hyperactivity of the amygdala, experiments reported by *Grossman* [1963] seem to be important. Microinjection of acetylcholine in doses as small as 1 µg into the basolateral part of the amygdala of cats induced rapidly spreading spike discharges, psychomotor seizures and behavioral changes. After a single microinjection of carbamyl choline chloride (carbachol) into the cat's amygdala, vicious behavior developed that persisted for observation periods of 5 months. It may be worthwhile, therefore, to study the effects of centrally acting anticholinergic drugs in aggressive patients. Furthermore, relatively high concentrations of endorphins and/or enkephalins have been found in the hypothalamus [*Bloom* et al., 1978; *Akil* et al., 1978] and of enkephalins in the amygdala [*Yang* et al., 1978] and in one of its efferent systems, the stria terminalis [*Uhl* et al., 1978]. It may be interesting to ascertain, preceding amygdalotomy, whether an opiate antagonist, naloxone HCl, could influence the assaultive behavior. If operation becomes necessary, one could ascertain, before performing a lesion, which amygdaloid or hypothalamic stimulation effects may be reduced or abolished by blocking the effects of endogenous opiate peptides. In performing such studies, one should bear in mind that for antagonizing endorphins much higher doses of naloxone are required than for blocking opiate alkaloids; e.g., 10 mg naloxone HCl was injected by *Akil* et al. in schizophrenics [*Watson* et al., 1979].

Lesions of the Stria terminalis

Inspired by animal experiments in which aggressive reactions produced by stimulation of the dorsomedial part of the amydgala were abolished by interruption of the stria terminalis [*Fernandez-Molina and Hunsperger,* 1962], *Burzaco* [1973] chose the precommissural and commissural components of the stria terminalis as an optional target in sedative stereotactic surgery. He suggested the procedure when bilateral lesions are considered necessary and amygdalotomy or posteromedial hypothalamotomy is to be done on the contralateral side after unsuccessful amygdalotomy or hypothalamotomy, or in cases of temporal lobe epilepsy where the focus is bilateral. One has to remember, however, that the blocking effect of interruption of the stria terminalis upon defensive reactions induced by amygdaloid stimulation proved transitory in animal experiments [*Hilton and Zbrozyna,* 1963], while defense reactions could no longer be obtained on amygdaloid stimulation after complete section of the ventral amygdalofugal fibers. After severance of the stria terminalis in mid-course, defense reactions could be evoked only on stimulation of the amygdaloid portion of the stria terminalis (i.e., of its afferent fibers to the amygdala), but not on stimulation of the hypothalamic portion (i.e., of efferent amygdalohypothalamic fibers). Apparently the ventral amygdalofugal fibers are more important than the efferent fibers of the stria for transmission of amygdalofugal impulses inducing defense responses to the hypothalamus.

Combined Lesions

Brown [1973] advocated multiple bilateral lesions involving the cingulum, the substantia innominata and the amygdala for treatment of schizophrenics with aggression. Such combined lesions offered more favorable results than lesions of either target alone [*Cox and Brown,* 1977].

While the success of pharmacotherapy has eliminated the need or justification of operative procedures in the majority of emotional and behavioral disturbances, it cannot be overlooked that pharmaca are by no means efficient in all instances. According to an editorial by *Callan* [1979], tricyclic medications alleviate symptoms of depression only in from one-half to two-thirds, monoamine oxidase inhibitors benefit only one-third and electroconvulsive therapy usually cures only three-fourths of depressed patients. The patients of *Roeder* et al. [1972b], relieved of their sexual abnormalities by hypothalamic interventions, had suffered for years from their deviations without help by any conservative therapy.

It may be astonishing and disturbing that emotional and behavioral disorders could be influenced by interventions at many different parts of the central nervous system. The explanation is given by the fact that emotions do not depend on one single area but on several circuits, so that they have a multiple representation [*Spiegel and Wycis,* 1968].

In his survey of psychosurgery, *Rylander* [1973] pointed out that the standard lobotomy became unpopular due to the undesirable personality changes, but that renewed interest developed with the introduction of restricted operations such as cortical undercutting and stereotactic operations in the thalamus. 'Thus a seed was planted that slowly would grow and initiate a new type of operation, to a great extent contributing to the renaissance of psychosurgery.'

Procedures no longer or only rarely practiced have been included briefly in this and in subsequent chapters because the experiences gathered are of unique value for an understanding of the normal physiology and the pathophysiology of subcortical areas in the human brain.

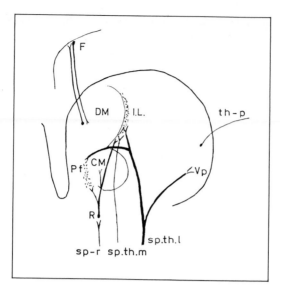

Fig. 14. Systems participating in the central mechanism of pain. CM = Centrum medianum; DM = dorsomedial nucleus; F = frontal lobe; I.L. = intralaminar nuclei; Pf = nucleus parafascicularis; R = cells of the reticular formation; sp-r = spinoreticular pathways; sp.th.l. = lateral spinothalamic tract; sp.th.m. = medial spinothalamic tract; th-p = thalamoparietal fibers; Vp = nuclei ventrales posteriores. The thickness of the lines in this diagram is not related to the diameter of the fibers in the respective systems. From *Spiegel and Wycis* [1966].

Chronic, So-Called Intractable Pain

Pain Conduction

It may be recalled briefly that pain is conducted centripetally in the central nervous system by two fiber tracts: by the phylogenetically old medial spinothalamic and spinoreticulothalamic systems (paleospinothalamic system) [*Bishop*, 1959] and by the phylogenetically young lateral spinothalamic (neospinothalamic) system partly shown in figure 14.

The former consists of the small diameter (1–2 µm) unmyelinated, slowly conducting (0.6–2 m/s) C fibers, the latter of thinly myelinated A delta and epsilon fibers (diameter 2–4 µm, conducting velocity 10–20 m/s) and of C fibers. The threshold of these systems varies inversely with the diameter: the larger diameter fibers are more easily stimulated (by weak stimuli) than the small diameter fibers that react only to strong stimuli.

Brief noxious peripheral stimuli induce a sensation of pricking conducted by myelinated fibers, prolonged noxious stimuli a burning, unpleasant, 'protopathic' sensation conveyed by unmyelinated C fibers [*Sweet,* 1959].

There is some antagonism between the faster and the slowly conducting systems, the former inhibiting the latter, so that elimination of the fast system induces a hyperpathia, as seen in causalgia or in thalamic pain [*Hassler,* 1975]. The fast conducting fibers end chiefly in the posterior ventral thalamic nuclei, the slowly conducting, forming multisynaptic chains, end in the centrum medianum, the parafascicular complex, the intralaminar nuclei, the posterior nuclear thalamic group, the nucleus limitans (cell groups forming a band between the habenula and the nucleus suprageniculatus), the periaqueductal and periventricular gray, the pulvinar, the posterior hypothalamus.

Therapeutic Lesions

The pain conducting systems have been interrupted, for pain relief, at various levels: in the spinal cord, the medulla oblongata, the midbrain, the diencephalon, or in the cerebral hemispheres. Circuits participating in the mechanism of emotions were also interfered with in an attempt to diminish the emotional reaction to pain.

At the level between the first and second cervical vertebra, the lateral spinothalamic tract was severed by *percutaneous chordotomy* with a strontium needle [*Mullan* et al., 1963] or with a RF current [*Rosomoff* et al., 1965]. In view of the danger of interfering with tracts descending from the respiratory center on high cervical chordotomy, *Lin* et al. [1966] made the incision at low cervical segments (between C5 and C6).

Midsagittal section of the spinal cord has been practiced at the level of the first cervical segment [*Hitchcock,* 1969a; *Schvarcz,* 1976] or at the thoracolumbar junction [*Gildenberg and Hirshberg,* 1979]. Alleviation of pain was obtained bilaterally in lower parts of the body in spite of the fact that the midline section was performed above the crossing of the spinothalamic fibers. It has been suggested that the beneficial effect may be due to the interruption of an ascending spinoreticular pathway [*Hitchcock, Schvarcz, Gildenberg*] located close to the midline. In cases of brachial pain due to avulsion of cervical roots, *Nashold and Ostdahl* [1980] obtained good relief in 67% of the patients by *coagulation of the dorsal root entry zone.*

For relief of *trigeminal neuralgia* in cases not benefited by Tegretol, alcohol injection into individual branches, or peripheral neurectomy, *percutaneous electrocoagulation of the Gasserian ganglion and trigeminal root* has been developed as a relatively simple, safe and effective method [*Kirschner*, 1933; *Sweet*, in *White and Sweet*, 1969; *Sweet and Wepsic*, 1974; *Onofrio*, 1975; *Tew*, 1978; *Rhoton* et al., 1977]. Although this is not strictly a stereotactic method, if the coagulating needle is inserted by hand through the foramen ovale under X-ray control, the practical importance of this procedure may justify a brief account.

Preceding the coagulation, the proper position of the electrode tip is checked by electrical stimulation in the conscious patient; it should produce paresthesia in the neuralgic zone. For coagulation, at present RF current is applied at 80–85 °C and lasts 0.5–1 min. Unconsciousness of the patient produced by intravenous injection of methohexital (Brevital) is necessary for a few minutes only.

Of 149 patients treated by *Rhoton* et al. [1977], 146 had immediate relief. There was no mortality. Although the recurrence rate, particularly after incomplete coagulation (18–25% reported by *Onofrio* [1975]; 53% experienced by *Stowsand* et al. [1973]) is higher than after craniotomy and intracranial root section, the ease of repeating the procedure, the shortness of the intraoperative unconsciousness and of the hospitalization seem to be definite advantages of the percutaneous coagulation, so that this procedure has become preferable to the classical retrogasserian rhizotomy. Complications appearing after either type of operation are numbness, paresthesia, pain (anesthesia dolorosa) in the anesthetic area, keratitis and corneal ulceration due to corneal anesthesia, transient paralysis of the motor branch of the trigeminus (paralysis of the muscles of mastication) and of the abducens. Complications noticed only after intracranial root section are transient facial paralysis and deafness, while puncture of the carotid artery, possibly inducing hemiplegia, occurred occasionally after percutaneous insertion of the coagulating needle.

In the hope of eliminating facial pain while preserving the sense of touch, and of avoiding neuroparalytic keratitis and corneal ulcers as well as facial paresthesia, the *descending trigeminal nucleus and tract* were stereotactically coagulated in the medulla oblongata [*Crue* et al., 1967; *Hitchcock*, 1970; *Schvarcz*, 1978], a replacement of *Sjöqvist's* intramedullary tractotomy.

In the *midbrain*, originally chiefly the long phylogenetically young lateral spinothalamic tract (neospinothalamic system, *Bishop*) was interrupted [*mesencephalotomy; Spiegel and Wycis*, 1948, 1953]. The lesions also included the quintothalamic tract and encroached upon the reticular formation dorsal to the nucleus ruber. Reviewing a 14-year period, *Wycis and*

Spiegel [1962] reported long-term relief in 31% of 54 patients. Later more extensive lesions were placed in the paleospinoreticulothalamic system located in the *medial mesencephalic reticular formation* by *Roeder and Orthner* [1961], *Nashold and Wilson* [1966] and *Amano* et al. [1980a]. In cases of pain in the head, neck and chest, *Voris and Whisler* [1975] consider mesencephalotomy preferable to extensive rhizotomies. Unilateral mesencephalotomy may relieve bilateral pain in these areas at least temporarily. These procedures have a high rate of complications which usually were not disabling.

Amano et al. [1980a] noted that they could produce pain on electrical stimulation of the medial reticular formation, but not on stimulation of the *periaqueductal gray. Schvarcz* [1977b] however, obtained relief in 4 of 5 cases of facial pain due to vascular insults of the brain stem by producing lesions in the contralateral *central gray* at the intercollicular level. Stimulation of this area produced a variety of sensory responses deep within the nasal and oral cavities, as well as emotional and autonomic reactions (blushing, sweating, piloerection). This is reminiscent of the crying, snarling, defense reactions elicited in cats by electrical and mechanical stimulation of the periaqueductal gray [*Spiegel* et al., 1954a]. The main problem with lesions in the medial tegmentum of the midbrain is the difficulty of avoiding roots of the oculomotor nerve. *Schvarcz* [1977b] also reported loss of upward gaze.

In the *thalamus,* the endings of the neospinothalamic pain conducting system in the *nuclei ventrales posteriores* as well as those of the paleospinoreticulothalamic system in the *centrum medianum* [*Hécaen, Talairach* et al., 1949], were chosen as targets.

By comparing the changes in the pain syndrome of their cancer patients induced by thalamic lesions with the histopathologic findings, *Mark* et al. [1963] could establish the differences between the effects of lesions of the endings of the neospinothalamic system and those of the paleospinoreticulothalamic system. Lesions of the ventral posterior thalamic nuclei produced sensory deficits but had little or no effect upon the cancer pain, while lesions of the intralaminar nuclei-centrum medianum-nucleus parafascicularis complex relieved the pain with little or no sensory deficit. Centrum medianum lesions are effective only when bilateral [*Voris and Whisler,* 1975].

Thalamic pain is considered by *Riechert* [1980] as due to a lesion of the rapidly conducting pain pathways, particularly of the nucleus ventralis caudalis parvicellularis, inducing a release of the nucleus limitans and of the intralaminar nuclei from inhibition. Therefore, the elimination of these released nuclei is recommended, in agreement with *Hassler* [1960].

Assuming that reverberating circuits between the lateral specific and the medial nonspecific sensory thalamic nuclei are responsible for thalamic pain, *Sano* et al. [1966a, b, 1967a, b] produced lesions in the region of the posterior part of the internal medullary lamina *(thalamolaminotomy)* in patients chiefly with central pain. This procedure caused incomplete lesions of the centrum medianum and the intralaminar nuclei. Apparently these lesions were quite similar to those reported by *Riechert* [1980], although the theoretical assumptions were somewhat different. *Riechert* intended to eliminate the hyperactive intralaminar nuclei and the nucleus limitans, while *Sano* planned to reduce the hyperirritability of the lateral specific nuclei. *Sano's* operation succeeded in relieving thalamic, tabetic and causalgic pain for prolonged periods, while pain due to malignancy recurred within several weeks or months.

Lesions of the medial part of the pulvinar *(pulvinotomy)* were initiated by *Kudo* et al. [1966], *Kudo and Yoshii* [1970], and *Yoshii* et al. [1975]. The procedure was successful in relieving pain, particularly cancer pain (in 15 of 16 cases), less in central pain following cerebrovascular accidents (in 2 of 11 cases). The pulvinar is reached by impulses induced by noxious stimuli on a multisynaptic pathway, since evoked responses were obtained in single cells of the pulvinar after latent periods of several hundred milliseconds [*Kudo* et al., 1968]. Stimulation of the pulvinar produces contralateral paresthesias in man without pain at low voltages, and severe discomfort at high voltages [*Richardson and Zorub,* 1970]. There seems to be agreement that pain relief can be obtained by pulvinotomy without sensory loss. Favorable results of the procedure were confirmed by *Richardson* [1967], *Siegfried* [1972], *Cooper* et al. [1973a, b], *Martin-Rodriguez and Obrador* [1975], *Laitinen* [1977]. Such results were obtained not only by lesions of the medial part of the pulvinar, but also by lesions of anterior areas *[Laitinen],* of anterior and basal parts *[Siegfried],* or of lateral parts of the pulvinar [*Cooper* et al., 1973a, b]. After unilateral lesions contralateral to the pain, *Laitinen* obtained complete relief in 19 of 39 patients, but *Fraioli and Guidetti* [1975] reported return of the pain following unilateral operation after 3 weeks. After bilateral pulvinotomy, the pain relief usually also lasted only several months up to somewhat over 1 year.

Since responses to noxious stimuli (pin pricks) could be recorded from single cells of the posteromedial hypothalamus in man, *Sano* et al. [1970a, 1973] initiated *posteromedial hypothalamotomy* in the treatment of intractable pain, obtaining relief in 11 of 13 cases of pain caused by tumor. Lesions of the *periventricular hypothalamic nuclei* were performed by *Fairman* [1971, 1976] for alleviation of intractable chronic pain due to malignant tumors with satisfactory results in 70%. This procedure is based on the notion that the hypothalamus coordinates the reticular activating system and regulates the level of cortical activity.

In addition to interruption of the pain conducting systems, *Spiegel and Wycis* [1948, 1953, 1966] added lesions of the *dorsomedial nuclei* of the thalamus in order to reduce the emotional component of the pain. *Riechert* [1966] added coagulation of the dorsomedial nucleus to lesions of the sensory thalamic nuclei when psychogenic factors predominated. *Martins and Umbach* [1975] combined lesions of medial parts of the dorsomedial nuclei with that of the basal parts of the centrum medianum, nucleus limitans and parafascicularis. In visceral pain caused by malignant tumors, *Kim and Umbach* [1973] extended lesions of the posterior ventral region of the thalamus into the mesencephalic tegmentum above the nucleus ruber; in severe cases they added lesions of the dorsomedial nucleus. In 70% of the patients they considered the results as satisfactory; this applied, however, to a survival time of 4–6 months.

Mundinger and Becker [1977] eliminated basal parts of the ventrocaudal thalamic nuclei (nucleus ventralis caudalis parvicellularis), the nucleus limitans and, in some cases, the dorsomedial nucleus. In a later series these authors ablated the ventrocaudal nuclei, the intralaminar nuclei with the lamina medialis and the centrum medianum, and, in some cases, the dorsomedial nucleus and the pulvinar as well. All patients with phantom pain and causalgia were improved; three-fifths were free of pain 4–6 years postoperatively. Seven-eighths of the patients with intractable trigeminal neuralgia, e.g., after herpes zoster, improved; half of them were pain free; three-fifths of them remained so after 1–2 years; four-fifths of patients with thalamic syndrome experienced satisfactory to good improvement [*Mundinger* et al., 1978]. A projection of the centrum medianum and the nucleus limitans into the *pallidum* has been described [*Hassler,* 1960]. In agreement with this finding, *Riechert* [1980] observed in a case of thalamic pain that pallidotomy reduced the intensity of the pain and altered it (preoperatively cramp-like, postoperatively stabbing pain).

There exist only few experiences suggesting a relation of the lateral part of the *amygdala* to pain mechanisms. *Jelasic* [1966] elicited retrobulbar pain by various stimulations of this area. In 2 of 4 patients, facial pain was relieved by bilateral lesions of this region. In the treatment of pain associated with anxiety and/or depression, many of the side effects of frontal leukotomy [*Freeman and Watts,* 1950] could be avoided by ablation of the *anterior part of the cingulate gyrus* [*Le Beau,* 1948, 1954] or by RF lesions of the *rostral cingulum* [*Foltz and White,* 1962; *Brown,* 1977, in pain with drug addiction]. Cingulotomy seldom gives long-term pain relief, but it may be beneficial in patients with emotional disturbances such as fear or depression associated with malignancy [*Voris and Whisler,* 1975]. The ability of patients subjected to cingulotomy by *Ballantine* to perform a wide range of tasks and to perceive sensory stimuli was demonstrated by *Teuber* et al. [1977]; the safety and efficacy of the procedure was also documented by *Corkin* et al. [1979]. One has to bear in mind, however, that pain relief in these cancer patients was limited to 37% if they survived less than 3 months, and to 11% if they survived longer [*Hurt and Ballantine,* 1974]. The experiences of *Wilson and Chang* [1974] after bilateral anterior cingulectomy for pain relief were less satisfactory. Favorable results in cancer patients regarding relief of pain and associated emotional disturbances were obtained by small RF lesions in the *subcaudate region* or in the *inferior posteromedial parts of the frontal lobes* [*Sweet,* 1980]. *Frontothalamic fibers* were interrupted by *Bertrand* et al. [1966] and *Martinez* et al. [1975] in the anterior limb of the *internal capsule,* and the *thalamoparietal* fibers in the corona radiata by *Talairach* et al. [1960] and by *Obrador and Dierssen* [1966]. Cutting of thalamofugal fibers to the supraclaustral region was abandoned by *Riechert* [1966] in view of its unconvincing effect. In summary, among the numerous attempts at pain relief by blocking central pain conduction or perception developed in recent years, those dealing with the pain conducting systems in the spinal cord seem to be the most simple and practical and deserve an initial trial where applicable.

As a consequence of the double neospinothalamic and paleospinoreticulothalamic pain conduction, there is no regular parallelism between the cutaneous analgesia and the relief of pain following section of the lateral spinothalamic tract. The pain may persist despite the development of cutaneous analgesia, and at least transitory pain relief may be obtained without cutaneous analgesia after interruption of the paleospinoreticulothalamic system.

Just as for the emotions, it became obvious regarding the biologically important pain mechanisms that a *multiple representation* in the central nervous systems exists [*Spiegel and Wycis,* 1968], so that even following extensive lesions of the pain conducting systems, e.g., at the base of the medial part of the thalamus [*Spiegel* et al., 1964a] a compensation and consequently a recurrence of the pain occurs. Thus, expectations of a really permanent success of these operations are hardly justified, and a satisfactory result is limited to patients with a relatively short life expectancy, for instance, sufferers from pain due to malignancy.

Therapeutic Stimulation

In recent years it has been recognized that pain can be controlled not only by elimination of pathways conducting nociceptive impulses and of cell groups participating in the perception of pain, but also by stimulation of certain regions, including systems that participate in the processes leading to pain perception. In this development the finding played an important role that impulses conveyed by large-diameter, fast-conducting, myelinated fibers (A fibers) are able to suppress or to diminish the primitive, undifferentiated, poorly localized, burning, emotionally charged pain sensation that is transmitted chiefly by the small-diameter unmyelinated, slowly conducting C fibers. Related to this antagonism between A and C fibers, recently reemphasized by *Hassler* [1975], is *Melzack and Wall's* [1965] gate theory which assumes that pain impulses entering the spinal cord are inhibited or modified in the substantia gelatinosa (partly by reticulospinal impulses) and *Sweet and Wepsic's* [1968] clinical experiments. The latter authors demonstrated that causalgia, atypical facial neuralgia, could be controlled by application of weak (0.1–0.5 mA), square wave, biphasic pulses of 0.1 ms duration to peripheral nerves; these weak stimuli set up impulses only in peripheral sensory fibers of the largest diameter which are the most excitable.

In these therapeutic stimulations reported by *Sweet and Wepsic* [1968], the importance of the frequency of the applied electric pulses could be demonstrated; the best subjective responses appeared in 1 case at 30–50 Hz, while at less than 20 Hz the affected area throbbed uncomfortably. Furthermore, the still poorly explained observation was made that the suppression of pain outlasted by about half an hour a stimulation of several minutes duration. In atypical facial neuralgia associated with disturbances of sensibility indicating trigeminal injury, *Meyerson and Hakansson* [1980] stimulated the *Gasserian ganglion* and the trigeminal rootlets via an implanted electrode. All 5 patients observed for 6 months to 2 years reported satisfactory pain relief. It became practically important that such results could also be obtained by easily applied *transcutaneous nerve stimulation* [*Wall and Sweet,* 1967; *Sheldon* et al., 1967; *Sweet and Wepsic,* 1968; *Shealy,* 1972, 1974; *Long,* 1974]. The long-term efficacy reported in the literature varies between 25 and 55% [*Ray,* 1975]. These experiences in the periphery were extended by *Shealy* et al. [1967, 1970] to the central nervous system. They found that stimulation of the large-diameter fibers of the *posterior columns,* so-called *dorsal column stimulation,* was able to relieve chronic pain without the functional impairment appearing after elimination of central structures [confirmed by *Nashold and Friedman,* 1972 and *Riechert* et al., 1973a, b].

Based upon experiments on rats, *Emmers* [1981] explains the analgetic effect of electric posterior column stimulation by an excitatory action of Goll's fasciculus upon the periaqueductal gray matter. This has a double effect, namely: (1) disorganization of the CM and of the cortical sensory area S_2, and (2) activation of the nucleus raphe magnus where a descending system originates that inhibits the spinothalamic tract. Furthermore, antidromic impulses descending in Goll's fasciculus inhibit, by way of collaterals, the cells where the spinothalamic tract originates.

It would be interesting to test this concept by studying the effect of posterior column stimulation upon thalamopetal and corticopetal conduction of pain impulses (elicited by sciatic stimulation) before and after destruction of the periaqueductal gray matter. In these experiments, the blocking of the spinothalamic system by impulses descending antidromically in Goll's fasciculus should be eliminated by section of this tract below the placement of the stimulating electrode. Section of the posterior column above the stimulating electrode is hardly an equivalent of elimination of the periaqueductal gray, since such a section interrupts not only the input into the periaqueductal gray, but also impulses reaching the thalamus via the medial lemniscus and cerebellopetal impulses.

It seems that probably multiple factors are involved in the mechanism of pain relief by posterior column stimulation. In patients suffering from chronic pain, the electrode is usually applied in upper thoracic or cervical levels, so that stimulation not only of Goll's but also of Burdach's fasciculus should be considered. This system carries impulses to the cerebellum, besides those continued by the medial lemniscus, so that participation of the cerebellar circuit discussed on page 137 should not be neglected. The possible role of cerebellar inhibition could be ascertained by studying the effect of stimulating the anterior lobe upon the potentials of CM elicited by sciatic stimulation.

In animal experiments, analgesia results from *periaqueductal stimulation,* so-called stimulation-produced analgesia [*Reynolds,* 1969; *Akil and Mayer,* 1972; *Besson and Oliveras,* 1979]. The clinical results of periaqueductal stimulation in man are controversial. In cancer pain with midline or bilateral distribution, *Boëthius and Meyerson* [1977] applied stimulation of the periaqueductal or periventricular gray as an adjunct to existing methods of pain treatment. *Schvarcz* [1979] obtained by similar stimulation significant pain relief in 2 and moderate relief in a further 2 of 6 cases of chronic pain followed for 6–38 months. Of 8 patients with chronic pain studied by *Gybels* et al. [1980], however, only 1 experienced a 60% reduction of pain. This report is particularly valuable because in 4 cases the electrode position was checked by autopsy. In *Hosobuchi's* [1980] experience, stimulation of the periaqueductal gray matter did not afford relief from deafferentation pain (thalamic syndrome, facial anesthesia dolorosa, postherpetic neuralgia, phantom limb pain), but was efficient in chronic pain of peripheral origin (cancer, low back pain, atypical facial pain).

Intermittent stimulation of the *area of the mesencephalic lemniscus medialis* introduced by *Mundinger* for chronic pain resulted in reduction of the pain in 53% of the patients observed by *Mundinger and Salomao* [1980] for 47 months. *Mundinger* [1977, 1978] was originally guided by the hypothesis that impulses in the fast-conducting, relatively large-diameter, myelinated A delta fibers are able to inhibit the slowly conducting, unmyelinated C fiber system that is responsible for the unbearable, usually not relievable, chronic pain that is experienced in causalgia, stump pain, phantom pain, postherpetic and thalamic pain. Using high frequency (50–200 Hz) electric pulses at 2–8 V, he stimulated for 20–30 min and obtained amelioration of the above-mentioned types of chronic pain, even in patients unresponsive to posterior column stimulation. The stimulation, however, affected not only the lemniscus medialis and the nucleus ventralis caudalis parvicellularis (ending of the neospinothalamic system), but also the nucleus limitans and centrum medianum [*Mundinger*, 1978] where the paleospinothalamic system ends; its C fibers are supposed to carry the primitive, burning pain that one wishes to suppress. It would seem, therefore, that his therapeutic successes should be attributed to a mechanism other than stimulation of the fast conducting A fiber system. Particularly considering that the pain relief or reduction outlasted the stimulation for 5–7 h, he recently seems to favor release of endorphins as an explanation [*Mundinger and Salomao, 1980*].

Mazars et al. [1975, 1980] reported that intermittent stimulation of the *nucleus ventralis posterolateralis* (2 ms pulses, 0.6–2.2 V, 16–20 Hz, applied for 1–3 min) proved a valuable method of treatment in pain after herpes zoster, plexus avulsion, amputations, and in anesthesia dolorosa. The relief lasted for one to several days. On stimulation of the nucleus ventralis posteromedialis, facial neuralgia could be benefitted [*Ray, 1975*]. *Adams* et al.

[1975] observed that stimulation of the sensory relay nuclei of the thalamus produced a tingling sensation which replaced pain; they applied this experience to the treatment of anesthesia dolorosa. Similarly, chronic pain could be relieved by stimulation of the *internal capsule* [*Adams* et al., 1974]. *Hosobuchi* [1980] reported stimulation of the lemniscus medialis, besides that of the sensory nuclei of the thalamus and of the internal capsule for pain treatment.

The principal targets of *Ray and Burton's* [1979] stimulations in cases of severe chronic pain were the *paraventricular* and *parafascicular nuclei* and the *centrum medianum* (CM). The stimulation reduced deep-seated agonizing pain and produced a sensation of warmth and in a few patients euphoria. The results were considered good to excellent in over 75% of 25 patients. Chronic *pulvinar* stimulation resulted, according to *Bechterewa* et al. [1972], in permanent relief of phantom pain.

In an attempt to analyze these various observations on diminution or elimination of pain induced by stimulation of a number of regions (some of which are even related to the conduction or perception of pain impulses), it seems that three mechanisms have to be considered. In one group of cases one deals with definite *inhibitory systems*. On stimulation of the striopallidum and of the internal capsule in cats, *Krauthamer and Albe-Fessard* [1965] could reduce the somatosensory potentials evoked in the CM. *Ervin* et al. [1966] found in cats a greater tendency for facilitation of CM-evoked responses when the dorsomedial part of the caudate nucleus was stimulated and a greater tendency for inhibition with stimulation of the dorsolateral caudate.

In a patient suffering from carcinoma of the pharynx and base of the skull, *Ervin* et al. [1966] induced, by stimulation of the caudate nucleus, with 1-ms pulses at frequencies of 10–40 Hz (optimum 30 Hz), mood elevation and absence of pain appearing after 15–20 min; after intermittent stimulation for 1–2 h the alleviation of pain lasted for 6–8 h. Electrical stimulation of the *septal area* was also able to relieve pain [*Gol,* 1967]. In a patient with phantom limb, transdermal stimulation of the septum and the head of the caudate nucleus diminished the otherwise intractable pain and decreased the hostility of the patient [*Delgado* et al., 1973]. Chronic stimulation of the posterior *perifornical septal region* [*Broseta* et al., 1980] was studied in an experimental model of 'painful and symbolic stress'. Decreases in gastric ulceration and plasma cortisol levels were observed. The finding that stimulation of the posterior limb of the *internal capsule* [*Adams* et al., 1974] may induce pain relief in thalamic syndrome and painful paraplegia is tentatively explained by activation of inhibitory fibers from the parietal cortex. Analgesia produced in rats by stimulating the periaqueductal gray [*Reynolds,* 1969] probably is mediated by fibers of the serotonin rich nucleus raphe magnus descending to the dorsal horn [see *Samanin and Valzelli,* 1971].

Regarding a second group, one has to remember that stimulation of a certain area may induce *opposite effects depending on the frequency* of stimuli without change of other stimulus parameters. For static innervation it was found that stimulation of the anterior lobe of the cerebellar cortex at a repetitive rate of 2–10 Hz increases, and at a rate of 30–300 Hz reduces ipsilateral decerebrate rigidity [*Moruzzi,* 1950]. For afferent peripheral nerves, *Sweet and Wepsic's* [1968] above-mentioned experiments may be quoted. Stimulation of the periaqueductal gray in cats at a rate of 30 Hz elicited pain-suggestive reactions [*Spiegel* et al., 1954a]. Stimulation of this region in rats at 60 Hz induced analgesia [*Akil and Mayer,* 1972]. In analogy with these animal experiments, RF stimulation of the periaqueductal gray inhibited pain in 14 of *Hosobuchi's* [1980] 20 patients. The effect of variations of the stimulus frequency, however, differs in different areas. 10–20 Hz pulses applied to the ventrolateral-subventrolateral thalamic area induced tremor and a sensation of electricity, higher frequencies caused discomfort and a sensation of warmth [*Johansson,* 1969].

A third mechanism to be considered is the production of analgesic substances. *Akil and Mayer* [1972] found that the *analgesia* produced by *periaqueductal stimulation* in rats is diminished by administration of the serotonin (5-HT) synthesis inhibitor *p*-chlorophenylalanine (*p*-CPA), similarly as morphine analgesia is affected by this substance. This stimulation-produced analgesia initially dropped from 100 to 12 %; it gradually recovered, so that it reached 80 % on the 18th day after drug administration. Disruption of the analgesia by *p*-CPA occurred only for electrode sites near the 5-HT-rich dorsal raphe nucleus. The experiments were interpreted as showing that stimulation-produced analgesia, like morphine analgesia, may depend on the integrity of serotoninergic transmission. It is pointed out that responses to noxious stimuli at different levels of the nervous system might be controlled by different systems of pain inhibition.

In man, morphine-like substances, found in the pituitary gland and the brain *(endorphins),* containing amino acid sequences, have been considered responsible for the pain reduction produced by stimulation of the periaqueductal gray, the medial pulvinar, and the region of the mesencephalic lemniscus medialis [*Mundinger and Salomoa,* 1980; *Schvarcz,* 1979]. These endorphins produce analgesia when injected into the brain, some also on intravenous injection; they are blocked by morphine antagonists such as naloxone.

The production of such substances would explain the fact that the pain relief outlasts the stimulation. It should not be overlooked, however, that the reduction of spasticity induced by posterior column stimulation or of torsion spasm appearing after thalamic stimulation may also last for hours following the stimulation. Furthermore, in some instances, pain may eventually disappear without further treatment. It has been objected [*Meyerson,* 1980] that rather large, unphysiologic amounts of naloxone are needed to counteract the pain-reducing stimulation and that the naloxone effect is quite irregular.

While an increase of beta-endorphin was found in the CSF of the third ventricle after stimulation of the periventricular or periaqueductal gray [*Richardson and Akil,* 1973] or of the border between it and the reticular formation at the rostral end of the mesencephalon [*Amano* et al., 1980a, b], *Andy* [1980] reported that in a patient in whom pain relief could be obtained by stimulation of the CM-parafascicular complex, preoperative application of high doses of morphine did not alleviate the pain and naloxone did not cancel the pain relief induced by the electrical stimulation. Apparently, in some instances, other mechanisms are responsible for the beneficial effect of electrical stimulation. *Terenius* [1978], pointing out that the pain relief induced by conventional high frequency stimulation is not naloxone reversible, calls attention to the possibility that pain modulating mechanisms other than endorphin activity may exist, for instance, analgesic effects of substance P and somatostatin.

Furthermore, *Zimmermann's* [1975] statement should be recalled that long-lasting, repetitive stimulation induces a pronounced *hyperpolarization* of neurons and nerve fibers in which they are rendered less excitable. Hyperpolarization is produced by the active transport of sodium ions out of the cell. Such a process could contribute to a long-lasting decrease of responsiveness to noxious stimulation. Further studies are necessary in order to clarify this problem. The question also arises as to whether stimulation of the posterior column may increase the production of endorphins. In this respect an analysis of afferent impulses to the hypothalamus [*Spiegel* et al., 1954a, b] may be mentioned. It was pointed out by these authors that collaterals of the medial lemniscus, the central continuation of the posterior columns, may reach cell groups of the reticular formation, and that fibers originating in the reticular formation may enter the hypothalamus. Here a neurovascular chain influences the pituitary gland, the main source of endorphins [*Guillemin* et al., 1977]. This circuit may explain how posterior column stimulation may induce increased endorphin secretion.

The experience that pain relief following stimulation of the posterior column may become diminished after some time has been explained by development of fibrosis around the electrode, and changing the electrode site over the posterior columns has been advised [*Ray,* 1975]. It has to be admitted, however, that the pain relief following such stimulation is rather unpredictable. It is, therefore, understandable that some authors, like *Siegfried* et al. [1980], are cautious in their recommendation. These latter authors restrict the indications to persons older than 60 or 65 years, if they suffer chronic pain of benign origin, preferably in the cephalic region, and to younger people only if they suffer from malignant disease with a limited life expectancy of only a few years.

Involuntary Movements, Disturbances of Muscle Tone and Posture

Clinical Indications

It is an old experience that conditions inducing extensive, although not exclusive, pallidal lesions such as CO poisoning are associated with hypokinesis. This experience induced *Spiegel and Wycis* [1950b] to attempt a control of *choreiform movements* by pallidal lesions. Of 9 cases with such movements, definite improvement was obtained in 4 (3 Huntington's chorea, 1 postencephalitic chorea) and a slight improvement in 2 patients with Huntington's chorea. There was no change in one senile and one electric chorea; a hemiplegia developed in 1 patient. *Riechert* [1980], evaluating late results, found that 50% of choreo-athetosis cases were improved.

Before operation is considered, *pharmacotherapy* of Huntington's chorea should be attempted of course. In this respect the following may be recalled: while in Parkinson's disease the ratio of cholinergic to dopaminergic activity is shifted in favor of the cholinergic system, due to the striatal dopamine reduction, the reverse is found in Huntington's disease, Gilles de la Tourette syndrome and tardive dyskinesia: a shift of the ratio to hyperdopaminergic versus hypocholinergic activity. Consequently, blocking or depleting of dopamine [*Barbeau* et al., 1980] or increasing brain ACh activity may reduce the choreic movements. *Davis* et al. [1980] attempted the latter approach by intravenous infusion of physostigmine (4.0 mg in 200 ml of saline over 60 min), thus inhibiting the acetylcholine esterase, or by oral administration of the ACh precursor choline chloride (0.5 g/ml water gradually increased to 20 g/day). They conclude that more potent cholinomimetics may be necessary for more consistent reduction of movements.

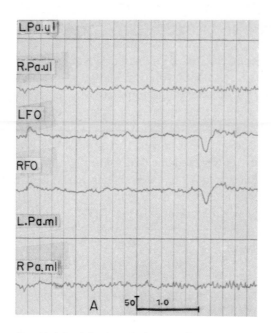

Fig. 15. After injection of 1 % tetracaine (pontocaine) HCl, 0.5 cm³ into the left pallidum (LPa) of an athetotic patient. RPa = Right pallidum; u, m, l = upper, middle, and lower depth electrodes; LFO and RFO = left and right frontooccipital scalp electrodes, respectively. From *Spiegel* et al. [1956b]; reproduced with permission.

Hemiballismus apparently is a manifestation of pallidal hyperactivity caused by a release of the pallidum from an inhibition originating in the corpus subthalamicum. It could be controlled or reduced by a combination of pallidoansotomy with a lesion of the zona incerta [*Talairach* et al., 1950], by coagulation of the pallidum internum and of the medial and posterior part of the internal capsule close to the pyramidal tract or of parts of the ventrolateral thalamus [*Riechert*, 1980], by procaine-alcohol injection into the pallidum [*Niemeyer*, 1955], pallidoansotomy [*Orthner and Roeder*, 1959; *Spiegel and Wycis*, 1962] or by a nigral lesion [*Spiegel and Wycis*, 1952]. Surgical treatment should be considered, of course, only after conservative methods (administration of haloperidol or of tetrabenazine) have failed.

In *athetotic* movements, one deals only in a certain group of cases with pallidal hyperactivity; in some instances a progressive atrophy of the pallidum exists. Before producing pallidal lesions, *Spiegel and Wycis* [1962]

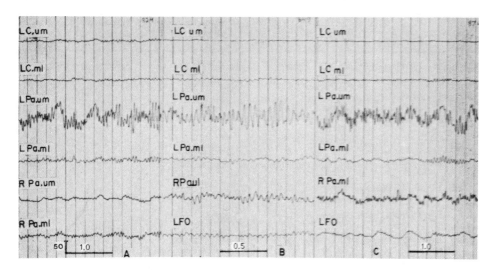

Fig. 16. Cerebral palsy patient with athetosis, awakening from barbiturate anesthesia. Frequent, high amplitude discharges from the left pallidum. Depth electrodes in left caudate nucleus (LC) and left and right pallida (LPa; RPa), three electrodes (u = upper, m = middle, l = lower) in each ganglion. LFO = Left frontooccipital scalp electrodes. Time: 1 s in *A* and *C;* 0.5 s in *B;* calibration: 50 μV. Same source as figure 10.

studied, therefore, the effect of temporary depression of the pallidal activity by injection of 0.25–0.50 cm^3 of a 0.5–1% procaine solution or 0.5 cm^3 of a 1% pontocaine solution (fig. 15). In some patients the electropallidogram was also recorded preceding the procaine injection (fig. 16). Of 12 patients in this group, the procaine injection suggested a possible favorable effect of a pallidotomy only in 9; 4 of these (1 with posthemiplegic athetosis, 3 with cerebral palsy) showed a definite diminution of the abnormal movements in the limbs opposite the pallidal lesion. In 5 of these pallidal lesions that were kept rather small in order not to interfere with the circulation of the internal capsule and thus with the patient's few voluntary movements, the operation had only a slight or no influence upon the athetotic movements; in 3 of these 5 patients a certain improvement was obtained in that the spasticity decreased in some muscle groups. In the first patient of the group of 12, the procaine test was not performed; a small pallidal lesion resulted in a transient improvement, but an enlargement of the pallidal lesion accentuated the hyperkinesis, and the patient died several weeks later. While *Bertrand* [according to *Lapras,* 1960] failed to find an effect of pallidotomy on athetotic hyperkinesis, *Klein* [1955] observed, following ansotomy, a

Table II. Pallidoansotomy in 71 cases of paralysis agitans and parkinsonism

	%
Tremor	
Influenced	77.1
Abolished or markedly reduced	45.7
Amplitude moderately reduced	31.4
Rigidity, definitely reduced	79.6
Speech disturbances improved (present in 41 patients)	23.8
Rehabilitation	45.0
Former occupation resumed	15.5
Partial rehabilitation	29.5
Walking improved	44.2
Ability to dress improved	48.8

slowing of the movements and disappearance of movements of large amplitude. *Riechert* [1957a] emphasized that bilateral operations should be performed in two stages, with an interval of several weeks between the operations on the two sides; he also recommended, at least in an early stage of his
work, asymmetry of the lesions. He felt that the double-sided disease has
worse prognosis and that relapses appear more frequently. He experienced
15.7% relapses. *Narabayashi* et al. [1960] reported marked improvement
after procaine-oil-wax pallidotomy in 21.2%, fairly good results in 41.2%
and slight improvement in 27.5% of 80 cases of double athetosis and spasticity in infantile cerebral palsy.

    Pallidoansotomy [*Wycis and Spiegel,* 1952], affecting chiefly the me-
dial part of the pallidum and the ansa lenticularis, was particularly practiced
in *paralysis agitans* and in parkinsonism. The experiences of *Spiegel and
Wycis* [1954, 1962] and *Spiegel* et al. [1958b] are summarized in table II for
postoperative observation periods of several months to 8 years. The
patients (aged 19–79 years, duration of disease 2–34 years) had responded
poorly to the medication used at that time.

    The effects upon *tremor* were mostly contralateral; homolaterally in
one instance a reduction and twice an increase of the tremor appeared.
Recurrence of tremor occurred in 7 cases within a few days to 20 months,
particularly if the lesions were limited to the anterior part of the pallidum.

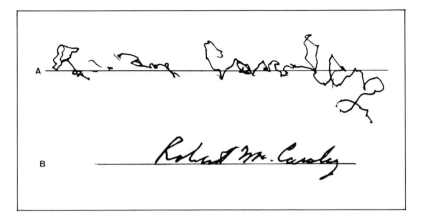

Fig. 17. Handwriting of parkinsonian patient before *(A)* and 2 years 10 months after *(B)* left-sided pallidoansotomy. From *Spiegel and Wycis* [1962]; reproduced with permission.

The *rigidity* was definitely diminished in the opposite limbs in 79.6%. In 2 patients it was slightly reduced also on the same side. The diminution of rigidity induced by moderate contralateral pallidal lesions improved not only voluntary but also associated movements, while extensive pallidal lesions interfered with associated movements, but did not prevent so-called willed movements. Relief of rigor and elimination of *muscle cramps,* one of the most important causes of pain suffered by these patients, was also noted.

The motor power that is often rather low without operation may drop further postoperatively, but usually only transitorily. Tremor and rigidity may be relieved without definite permanent decrease of motor power. Similar results were reported by other authors [*Meyers,* 1942; *Cooper and Pouloukhine,* 1955; *Riechert,* 1957b; *Walker,* 1957; *Orthner and Roeder,* 1959]. Even *contractures* that had lasted for years were relieved, e.g., a woman who could not write with the right hand for 30 years because of its contracture showed a legible handwriting 2 years after left pallidoansotomy. The handwriting of a Parkinson patient with tremor before and 2½ years after pallidotomy is shown in figure 17.

The increase in muscle activity on passive shortening of the muscle seen in the extensor muscles of the hand and in the flexor muscles of the foot is a sensitive sign of clinically latent rigidity. When the passive shortening of a rigid muscle does not evoke an increase of the electromyogram, the effect of a stereotactic lesion seems to be sufficient [*Struppler*, 1982]. *Speech* was improved only in about a quarter of our affected patients; mainly whispering speech became louder. In 5 patients, however, speech became less understandable.

Oculogyric crises could be abolished or reduced even after unilateral pallidotomy, according to *Hassler and Riechert* [1954], *Orthner and Roeder* [1959] and *Orthner* [1965]. *Spiegel and Wycis* [1962] found them unchanged in one case; the result was uncertain in view of the scarcity of the preoperative appearance in a second case. In the first few days postoperatively, the *gait* of the patients may be disturbed; a deviation to the operated side may be noted [*Selby*, 1967]. According to *Siegfried and Fisch* [1967], a lesion of the central vestibular system is one of the causes of postoperative lateropulsion.

Bradykinesia improved only in some instances. *Housepian and Pool's* [1960] statement that poverty of expression persists postoperatively is valid in many cases, and *Orthner and Roeder's* [1959] observation that the diminution of initiative may even be accentuated after bilateral pallidotomy can be confirmed. Occasionally *sialorrhea* was relieved. Transient hyperthermia was reported by *Guiot and Brion* [1953]. About half of the patients became euphoric [*Walker*, 1957] apparently due to their improved physical condition.

Hemiplegia was reported in 3–20% in the literature [*Walker*, 1957]. It was due to direct encroachment of the lesion upon the internal capsule, or to interference with its blood supply, to hemorrhage or edema. In *Spiegel and Wycis'* patients, permanent hemiplegia occurred in 5.6%, transient lasting up to several months in 12.7%.

Hemiballismus observed by some authors due to the encroaching of the lesion upon the corpus subthalamicum did not occur after their pallidotomies nor after lesions of Forel's field H. The *mortality* rate was 2%.

Relation of Medical Management to Stereotactic Intervention in Parkinson's Disease

In order to avoid the reproach that conservative treatment was not sufficiently applied before he decided to operate on a parkinsonian patient, it is advisable that the stereotactic surgeon should be familiar with the principles of the present drug treatment of the disease. In recent years, *L*-dopa (levodopa) is being administered in combination with a decarboxylase inhibitor, carbidopa (alpha-methyldopa hydrazine). This combination

(Sinemet) prevents or reduces the conversion of levodopa to dopamine by the decarboxylase in the periphery. As a consequence, a larger part of the administered L-dopa is available and can pass through the blood-brain barrier, and lower doses of levodopa are sufficient. One starts with Sinemet 25/100 containing 25 mg of carbidopa and 100 mg levodopa, t.i.d. This proportion of carbidopa to levodopa is more efficient in reducing or eliminating the nausea and vomiting than the previous initial ratio of 10 mg carbidopa to 100 mg levodopa. Gradually the dose is increased according to the clinical effect, with the patient being closely observed for side effects. The maximum daily dose is 8 tablets of Sinemet 25/250 containing 25 mg of carbidopa and 250 mg levodopa. The point of view of Krayenbühl's Zürich University Clinic expressed by *Siegfried* [1973] that in every Parkinson patient such a medication should be applied deserves hearty agreement. A stereotactic operation may still be warranted, if the tremor is very pronounced so that the patient is incapacitated. One has to deal not only with cases in which dopa medication fails to result in sufficient relief (about 15% of parkinsonian patients), but also with patients in whom the drug treatment has lost its efficiency or with clinical fluctuations, 'on-off effects' on prolonged medication. Furthermore, side effects may appear (orthostatic hypotension, cardiac arrhythmias, dyskinesia, myoclonia, dystonia, sleep disturbances, confusion, hallucinations). In such cases, 'drug holidays' may be tried, e.g., intermittent drug withdrawal for 5–7 days or weekly for 2 days. This may be effective in 70–80%, particularly regarding sleep disturbances and hallucinations [*Weiner,* 1981]. In some complications, e.g., severe dyskinesias, an alternative to levodopa or Sinemet, the rather expensive bromocriptine, an ergot derivative stimulating dopamine receptors, may be used [*Calne* 1981]. The dopa medication is gradually reduced, while the bromocriptine dose is increased in steps from an initial dose of 1.25 mg to a clinically effective dose (maximum daily 40–60 mg). In view of the side effects of this drug (particularly hypotension, hallucinations, delusions), a low dose bromocriptine therapy (weekly increases by 1.25 mg to a daily dose of about 12 mg [*Teychenne,* 1981]) may be preferable. Besides drug treatment, physiotherapy is an important part of the management of the Parkinson patient.

Stereotactic intervention should be considered only after all pharmacologic attempts have failed. It is prudent to advise the patient and his family, preceding operation, that surgical treatment as well as pharmacotherapy can only relieve signs and symptoms of parkinsonism, but are unable to stop the progression of the degenerative changes underlying the ailment.

Treatment with *L*-dopa or its combination with carbidopa, although representing a considerable advance in the pharmacotherapy of Parkinson's disease still suffers from undesirable side effects, particularly on long-term administration, such as the appearance of dyskinesias and psychotic manifestations. Among attempts to remedy this situation, the development of *metal chelates* of dopa is of great interest. In rat experiments by *Diamond* et al. [1980] *L*-dopa-zinc chelate produced less than 50% of the stereotypy induced by equivalent doses of *L*-dopa or of a *L*-dopa-carbidopa combination, the stereotyped behavior being used as a model for dyskinesias and psychoses. Both copper and zinc chelates of *L*-dopa produced significantly greater striatal dopamine levels than did *L*-dopa and also a fivefold rise in striatal norepinephrine content; due to this latter increase, stereotypy is inhibited. Further developments of these studies are eagerly awaited.

Muscular Hypertonicity

It has been mentioned that in some *cerebral palsy* patients in whom the pallidoansotomy had only an insignificant effect upon athetosis, a decrease of *spasticity* was observed in certain muscle groups opposite the lesion. Such muscle groups were, e.g., the flexors of the elbow and wrist, the triceps surae or the flexors of the fingers. Conversely, decrease of the involuntary movements could be associated with a failure to influence the spasticity.

Usually in hemiplegic adults the hypertonicity of the muscles could not be influenced; yet in one 29-year-old female suffering from a left-sided spastic hemiplegia, probably following an embolism of the middle cerebral artery, and in whom the phenomenon of *tonic perseveration of voluntary contraction* of the flexor and extensor muscles of the left forearm had existed for 7 years, right-sided pallidoansotomy markedly reduced not only the spasticity, but also the tonic perseveration, so that alternate flexion and extension of the hand and fingers could be performed quickly [*Spiegel and Wycis,* 1962]. These effects of pallidoansotomy upon spasticity were not regular occurrences, and later studies showed that pulvinar and dentate lesions are more efficient in relieving this form of muscular hypertonia [see p. 69 and 75].

If clinically a central paresis is suspected and no pyramidal signs or increased tendon reflexes are observed, *Struppler* [1982] recommends study of the *tonic vibratory reflex*. This reflex can be elicited by vibrating the muscle belly or tendon which excites chiefly muscle spindles. It is decreased in supraspinal paresis.

Torsion spasm (dystonia musculorum deformans) was slightly improved in 1 patient after unilateral pallidotomy; in a second patient the torsion and opisthotonus were permanently eliminated by *Spiegel and Wycis* [1962] after bilateral lesions of this region; associated athetoid movements of the extremities were greatly reduced and eventually disappeared. 4 years postoperatively the only disturbance noted was jerking movements of the trunk on walking. In a patient with opisthotonus without torsion, bilateral pallidal procaine injections were ineffective, so that lesions of these ganglia were not produced. Torticollis and retrocollis, which may be the initial manifestations of torsion spasm, are discussed on pages 123 and 124.

Anatomical Lesion Sites

Infrequently, lesions of the head of the *caudate nucleus* were performed in order to reduce the inhibitory influence of this nucleus and to counteract the bradykinesia of Parkinson's disease. A slight increase in the speed of flexor-extensor movements of the fingers of the opposite hand was observed in 3 of 4 patients [*Spiegel* et al., 1965c].

Heimburger [1975a] assumed an antagonism between the caudate nucleus and putamen; the marked atrophy of the caudate nucleus in advanced Huntington's chorea suggested a decreased motor inhibition permitting innervation of involuntary movements by the relatively intact putamen. Accordingly, he performed stereotactic *putamenotomy* for athetosis of cerebral palsy and other hyperkinetic states of the upper extremity (Huntington's chorea, intention tremor, dystonia musculorum deformans with choreiform and athetoid movements, action myoclonus, hemiballism). An improvement was observed after 8 of 10 operations, particularly in the opposite arm.

Lesions of Walker's *nucleus ventrolateralis* (VL), corresponding to Hassler's *nucleus ventralis oralis anterior and posterior* were proposed by the latter author in order to interrupt cerebellothalamocortical and pallidothalamocortical systems and thus to prevent abnormal, uncontrolled (ungesteuerte) cerebellofugal and pallidofugal impulses from reaching the precentral cortex. Lesions of this thalamic area were first successfully performed by *Riechert* [1952, reported by *Hassler and Riechert,* 1954], particularly in tremor and rigor of Parkinson's disease. *Riechert* [1980] and his group found ventrolateral thalamotomy (lesion of the nucleus ventralis oralis) preferable to pallidotomy in Parkinson's disease (e.g., regarding tremor) as well as in hyperkineses (effect longer lasting, less complications). There was, however, an improvement of rigidity in 85% after pallidotomy, in 64% after thalamotomy. Athetosis was ameliorated in 50% only. In the long-term observations of *Krayenbühl* et al. [1963] there was elimination or improvement of tremor in 85%, of rigor in 80% of Parkinson patients.

Since the pallidothalamic fibers end in the anterior part of the ventro-lateral complex, the *nucleus ventralis oralis anterior,* this nucleus, besides the pallidum, is the logical target for relief of parkinsonian rigidity.

It is interesting that *Krayenbühl* et al. [1961] succeeded in improving akinesia in 25% of their patients, a symptom rarely relieved by operative procedures. After bilateral thalamotomies, they observed complete relief of tremor and rigidity in 65%.

In some instances *Riechert's* [1957b] lesions included the nucleus ven-tralis anterior (*Hassler's* nucleus lateropolaris) and interrupted frontopetal fibers from the dorsomedial nucleus passing through this nucleus. This may explain that in one of the patients with such bilateral lesions a psychic syndrome developed, similar to that following bilateral section of the thal-amofrontal pathways. On an empirical basis, *Cooper and Bravo* [1958a] performed their chemothalamotomy in the ventrolateral region. *Spiegel and Wycis* [1962] observed in 2 cases of dystonia musculorum deformans (torsion spasm) a slow improvement after lesions of the ventrolateral nucleus.

Various parts of the *ventral nuclei* of the thalamus have been the target of lesions in patients afflicted by *tremor;* anterior parts of the nucleus ven-tralis caudalis externus (nucleus ventralis posterolateralis) were chosen by *Andrew* et al. [1974] in intention tremor and essential tremor[7], sometimes also the nucleus ventralis intermedius (Vim). The nucleus ventralis lateralis (VL) was selected by *Cooper and Bravo* [1958a, b] and by *Krayenbühl and Yasargil* [1961, 1962] in *intention tremor.* For the treatment of intention tremor in multiple sclerosis, *Riechert* [1980] found particularly effective

---

[7] While the *parkinsonian tremor* at rest appears when the involved muscles are relaxed, has frequencies between 4 and 6 Hz (average 5.5 Hz) [*Hoefer and Putnam,* 1940] and is suppressed or reduced in amplitude on active movements, the *postural tremor* appears when the patient holds the arms outstretched or the head upright and shows frequencies between 4 and 5 Hz. It is associated with 'lesions of the cerebellar hemisphere' [*Marshall,* 1968]. The inherited, benign *essential tremor* appears in some patients as juve-nile or adult tremor with frequencies of 8–10 Hz, in others as senile tremor with frequen-cies of 5–6 Hz; it occurs when the patient innervates the activity of some muscle groups. It is also considered a postural tremor, although it is increased during movements such as eating, drinking, or writing. There are no other neurological disturbances in these patients. The *intention tremor* occurs on movements directed toward a goal, as in the finger-nose test; it is increased in amplitude when the goal is approached. It occurs in multiple sclero-sis. The pathological changes affect the brachium conjunctivum system and result in a loss of inhibitory cerebellar impulses transmitted by the dentate nucleus-nucleus ruber-nucleus ventralis lateralis chain to the precentral cortex.

lesions of the nucleus ventralis oralis posterior, where cerebellofugal fibers end. *Van Manen* [1974] observed, 3 months or longer after placing VL lesions, good results in hereditary, essential tremor but less favorable results in multiple sclerosis and posttraumatic tremor[8].

In parkinsonian tremor and intention tremor, *Jasper and Bertrand* [1964, 1966] recorded bursts of unit discharges in the Vim synchronous with the tremor. Consequently they restricted lesions in parkinsonian tremor to this nucleus. According to *Narabayashi and Ohye* [1980], if cells with rhythmic burst discharges synchronous with the peripheral tremor can be identified within the Vim by microelectrode recording, small lesions, about 3 mm in diameter, may abolish the tremor. Yet, in patients relieved of parkinsonian tremor, histologic studies performed by *Hassler* et al. [1979] indicated that the Vim was intact or only slightly affected by the thalamotomy, so that for tremor at rest coagulation of the nucleus ventralis oralis posterior is recommended. *Dieckmann and Hassler* [1972] placed lesions in the nucleus ventralis oralis posterior in myoclonia.

Lesions of the *dorsomedial nuclei* of the thalamus chosen because of the connections of this nucleus with the pallidum had only a transient effect in Huntington's chorea [*Spiegel and Wycis, 1950b*].

Rand et al. [1962a, b] selected the CM as a target in dyskinesias. The rationale for this procedure apparently is to be sought in the projection of CM mainly to the basal ganglia. *Adams and Rutkins* [1965] applied CM lesions successfully in parkinsonian tremor and rigidity, and *Ramamurthi and Davidson* [1975] chiefly in cerebral palsy children and torsion dystonia. Lesions of the CM alone were insufficient in cerebral palsy. When spasticity predominated, the CM lesions were combined with dentatotomy; this combination increased the beneficial effect on muscle tone. In torsion dystonia the CM lesion was combined with that of 'other thalamic areas'.

Pulvinar lesions may serve as the first step or may be produced in combination with other lesions for the relief of hypertonus and/or dyskinesias [*Cooper* et al., 1971, 1973a; *Martin-Rodriguez and Obrador, 1975*; *Gillingham* et al., 1977; *Kanaka and Balasubramaniam, 1978*]. *Gillingham* et al. [1977] pointed out that there are no marked side effects; this is impor-

---

[8] Before considering surgery, propranolol (beta adrenoceptor blockade, 60 mg/day) should be tried in essential tremor [*Winkler and Young,* 1974; *Tolosa and Loewenson,* 1975]. As an alternative to propranolol, particularly in patients with essential tremor who also suffer bronchospasms, metoprolol tartrate (Lopressor, 25 mg twice a day gradually increased to 50 mg three times daily) has been recommended [*Newman and Jacobs,* 1980].

tant, if bilateral lesions are necessary. If the reduction of the hypertonus or involuntary movements was insufficient, lesions in the nuclei ventralis oralis posterior and anterior, and occasionally in the pallidum were added. *Chescotta* et al. [1977] combined lesions of the CM and the pulvinar in athetosis and torsion dystonia.

Narabayashi [1977] chiefly performed lesions at the ventral border of the *ventrolateral* and *ventral intermedius nucleus* in athetosis and hypertonicity of cerebral palsy. *Heimburger* [1975b] advocated sequential lesions of *multiple areas* in spastic cerebral diplegia without involuntary movements: bilateral simultaneous dentatotomy and bilateral posterior thalamotomy, including portions of the centrum medianum and pulvinar.

Mundinger and Ostertag [1977] placed lesions in cerebral palsy successively in the contralateral zona incerta, the ventrooral, intermediate and ventrocaudal nuclei, then in the pulvinar and, after at least 1 week, in the homolateral dentate nucleus. *Guidetti and Frajoli* [1977] also pointed out that in the treatment of *spasticity and dyskinesias* often a single operation is insufficient, while several operations are capable of reducing dystonia and athetosis.

Mundinger and Ostertag [1977] as well as *Narabayashi* [1977] emphasize the importance of proper selection of the cerebral palsy candidates for operation and postoperative physiotherapy. *Narabayashi* [1977] demands at least borderline intelligence and high motivation of the patients for recovery. He chooses children below early school age and excludes adults in whom secondary peripheral changes have occurred. The improvement in coordinated movements and fine finger movements develops in at least 3–6 months [*Mundinger and Ostertag,* 1977].

In the *subthalamus,* cerebellothalamic and rubrothalamic as well as pallidofugal and corticorubral fibers can be interrupted (fig. 18). *Spiegel and Wycis* [1962], *Spiegel* et al. [1963b], *Spiegel* [1965b], and *Wycis and Gildenberg* [1965] placed, therefore, lesions in *Forel's field H (campotomy)* in cases of Parkinson's disease, athetosis and myoclonia.[9] In 88.2% of Parkinson patients, rigor was abolished or diminished (fig. 19). Relapse occurred in

---

[9] A lesion of the medial part of the substantia nigra, interrupting also the mesencephalic part of Forel's field H relieved hemiballism [*Spiegel and Wycis,* 1950, reported in 1952]. Stimulation of H, similar to that of the pallidum, increased a tremor induced by stimulation of the mesencephalic tegmentum [*Spuler* et al., 1962] in cats. Tremor induced by Serpasil could be eliminated by a lesion including Forel's field H_2 [*Strassburger and French,* 1961]. *Meyers* [1958, 1962] chose as targets first the substantia nigra, then H_1, H_2 and H.

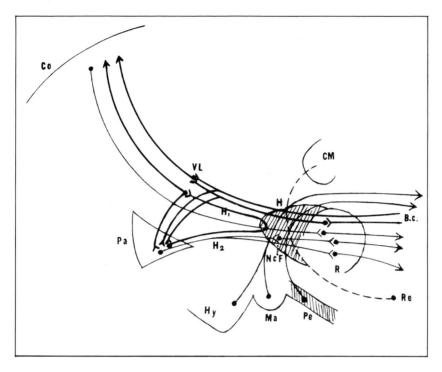

Fig. 18. Fiber systems forming, or passing through, Forel's field H. B.c. = Brachium conjunctivum; CM = centrum medianum; Co = cerebral cortex; H, H_1, H_2 = fields of Forel; Hy = hypothalamus; Ma = corpus mammillare; NcF = nucleus campi Foreli; Pa = pallidum; Pe = pedunculus cerebri; R = nucleus ruber; Re = formatio reticularis; VL = nucleus ventralis lateralis thalami. From *Spiegel* et al. [1963b]; reproduced with permission.

only 1 case. *Tremor* was initially improved in 88.8%; within 2 weeks to 10 months, the tremor returned in 15.5%, so that the improvement persisted in 73.3% (fig. 20).

Among 13 patients with cerebral palsy and *athetosis,* an improvement of the involuntary movements initially was obtained in 12 cases; this result was retained in 9 of the 13 cases (somewhat less than three-quarters of the patients). The decrease of the athetotic movements was ascribed, besides the lesion of pallidorubral and pallidotegmental fibers, to the interruption of corticorubral and corticotegmental fibers, particularly fibers originating in the frontal lobe. In 3 cases of *myoclonia* the jerking movements on the side opposite the campotomy totally subsided or were markedly reduced [*Wycis and Spiegel,* 1969] (fig. 21, 22). In one of these cases the involuntary

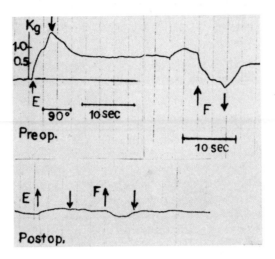

Fig. 19. Myotonogram showing resistance to passive extension (E) and flexion (F) in right elbow of a parkinsonian patient before and after left campotomy. Same source as figure 18.

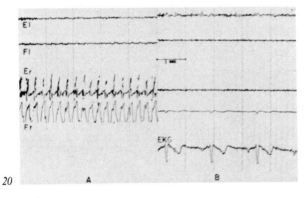

Fig. 20. Electromyogram of extensors (E) and flexors (F) of left (l) and right (r) forearm in a parkinsonian patient with right-sided tremor before *(A)* and after *(B)* left-sided campotomy. Same source as figure 18.

Fig. 21. Myoclonia. EMGs of muscles on the left side of the neck (1–5) and the left shoulder (1–3) before *(A)* and after *(B)* right-sided campotomy. Intervals between vertical lines correspond to 1 s. From *Spiegel* et al. [1963b]; reproduced with permission.

Fig. 22. Myoclonia. EMGs (same case as in figure 21) of right and left platysma muscles 6 years following a right-sided campotomy and 4 years after an additional left-sided campotomy. From *Wycis and Spiegel* [1969]; reproduced with permission.

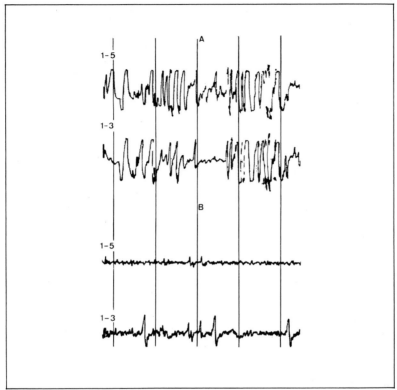

6 YRS POST-R. CAMPOTOMY (1962)
4 YRS POST-L. CAMPOTOMY (1964)

RIGHT PLATYSMA

(UNIPOLAR RECORDING)

LEFT PLATYSMA

1 SEC

jerks were also diminished on the homolateral side. Abnormal vocalization, causing grunting noises, was relieved after bilateral operation. The postoperative observation time was 6, 4 and 1/2 years, respectively. The beneficial effect of the operation was tentatively explained as due to elimination of facilitatory impulses from the ventrolateral thalamus passing through Forel's field to the reticular formation of the mesencephalon and rhombencephalon.

As to complications, in 45 Parkinson patients subjected to campotomy, there was no mortality in the first postoperative weeks. 2 patients with advanced parkinsonian tremor died several months after operation, but no certain connection with the operation was established. Partial oculomotor paresis lasting from several days to several months appeared in 5 patients in whom the lesion of Forel's field was performed at mesencephalic levels. In order to avoid or minimize this complication, the campotomy subsequently was located cranial to the oculomotor nucleus and roots at diencephalic levels; the protruding stylet of the electrode was shortened from 3 to 2 mm and directed anteromedially instead of medially. A transient contralateral hemiplegia lasting from 3 weeks to 1 month developed in 9 patients and an opposite analgesia lasted 1 week in 1 patient. There appeared no hemiballism and only slight, transient ataxic disturbances in 2 cases. The relative insignificance of the latter disturbances in lesions of cerebellothalamic and rubrothalamic fibers in front of the nucleus ruber is in agreement with negative findings of *Carrea and Mettler* [1955] in monkeys. Somnolence lasting from 1 day to 2 weeks was noticed in 10 of the 45 Parkinson patients and transient psychic disturbances, alone or combined with somnolence or following it in 12. Following bilateral campotomy in 9 cases, a dysarthria developed in only 1 patient, a cerebral palsy girl with bilateral athetosis. Incontinence of the bladder lasting several weeks developed in 2 cases.

Andy [1962] chose an area lateral to the corpus Luysi in hemiballism. Parkinsonian tremor was reduced in the experience of *Andy* et al. [1963] by lesions of Forel's field and of the zona incerta. *Mundinger* [1965] and *Mundinger* et al. [1972] selected the *zona incerta* with the lesions encroaching upon the adjacent fields H_1, H_2 and H in Parkinson's disease and spasmodic torticollis. Relief of severe action myoclonus and intention ataxia in multiple sclerosis could be obtained by coagulation of the dentatothalamic fibers and pallidothalamic fibers at the *base of the ventral oral nuclei* where they pass through the zona incerta [*Riechert* et al., 1975]. In *Riechert's* [1980] experience, subthalamotomy had a particularly good effect on oculogyric crises and wink spasms.

The *pallidofugal fibers* to the ventrolateral nucleus of the thalamus, at the point where they pass through the posterior limb of the internal capsule, were the target selected by *Guiot* et al. [1960] and by *Gillingham* [1962] in dyskinesias. Sometimes their lesions encroached upon the pallidum and/or the ventrolateral area of the thalamus. This procedure was also applied in oculogyric crises [*Gillingham and Kalyanaraman,* 1965] and in dystonia and athetosis [*Dierssen,* 1966]. The point of the posterior limb of the internal capsule from which threshold contralateral motor responses could be elicited was chosen by *Poblete* et al. [1977] as the site of the lesion in hemiballism. Occasionally mesencephalic areas were the target in extrapyramidal disorders. Only a transitory improvement was obtained by lesions of the *mesencephalic tegmentum* in parkinsonian tremor and rigor and in athetosis [*Spiegel* et al., 1960b]. In oculogyric crises, *Wycis and Spiegel* [1958] combined such operations with lesion of the periaqueductal gray. In a case of hemiballism, *Spiegel and Wycis* [1952] stopped the involuntary movements by lesions of the *substantia nigra. Meyers* et al. [1958] and *Rand* [1959] chose this target in various hyperkinetic and hypertonic disorders.

Lesions of deep cerebellar nuclei, especially *dentatotomy* have been initiated by *Delmas-Marsalet* [1935] and by *Tóth* [1961] for the relief of parkinsonian rigidity. The procedure has been applied, however, chiefly in the treatment of spasticity [*Heimburger and Whitlock,* 1965; *Zervas* et al., 1967; *Zervas,* 1970; *Krayenbühl and Siegfried,* 1969; *Nashold and Slaughter,* 1969; *Siegfried* et al., 1970]. Elimination of the *nucleus fastigii* combined with thalamic lesions proved also beneficial in spastic athetosis [*Hassler and Riechert,* 1961]. According to *Krayenbühl* [1975] bilateral dentatotomies combined with unilateral thalamotomy or subthalamotomy can give the best results in severe bilateral hyperkinesia. A combination of dentatotomy with lesion of the Vim of the thalamus was performed by *Kanaka and Balasubramaniam* [1975] for treatment of infantile hemiplegia with athetosis. While the lesion of the dentate nucleus reduced the hypertonus, the Vim lesion was supposed to diminish the involuntary movements.

In the evaluation of long-term effects of dentatotomy in cerebral palsy, particularly upon the spasticity, and in other disorders, *Siegfried and Verdie* [1977] and *Zervas* [1977] express similar views. There were no or only initial complications. According to *Siegfried,* the alleviation of spasticity is only moderate and decreases over the years. He considers dorsal column stimulation for the treatment of spasticity [*Cook and Weinstein,* 1973, in multiple sclerosis] as more promising. *Zervas* found in advanced cerebral palsy only initial improvement of the motor performance and considered the further use of dentatotomy in this condition unwarranted. The operation can help the dyskinesia in Parkinson's disease and dystonia musculorum deformans. In the latter disease it improved daily motor performances. However, he recommended thalamotomy as the initial procedure in most cases of dystonia musculorum deformans and reserved dentatotomy as a last resort for severe painful limb and axial posturing. Patients with multiple sclerosis, athetosis, or cerebral palsy with retrocollis were not benefitted. In *Siegfried's* experience, ventrolateral thalamotomy and subthalamotomy gave better results for treatment of involuntary movements than dentatotomy, but should be done only unilaterally, due to frequent complications of bilateral operations. More improvement of involuntary movements of the trunk may be obtained by dentatotomy.

Tóth and Vajda [1980] point out that the effects of different lesions have special main features. Pallidal lesions influence arrhythmic hyperkinesia, lesions of VL and Vim rhythmic hyperkinesia and rigidity, lesions of the dentate nucleus spasticity, rigidity and hypokinesia of fine movements. They practiced, therefore, a *multitarget technique* in Parkinson surgery and implanted chronic electrodes in various combinations (in the contralateral pallidum, VL and Vim and ipsilateral dentate nucleus). The small lesions caused by electrode insertion drastically reduced the Parkinson syndrome for 2–3 weeks.

Therapeutic Stimulations

Muscular hypertension may be reduced not only by elimination of cerebellofugal impulses but also by *cerebellar stimulation*. Experiences on decerebrate cats reported by *Moruzzi* [1950] showed that stimulation of the vermal anterior lobe with 1-ms pulses at low frequencies (2–10 Hz) increased, but at high frequencies (30–300 Hz) reduced decerebrate rigidity. These experiences have been applied to the treatment particularly of *spasticity of cerebral palsy* patients. Indeed, on stimulation of the cortex of the anterior lobe in spasticity [*Upton* et al., 1979; *Galanda* et al., 1980] or in spastic athetosis [*Vaernet,* 1977], as well as on stimulation of the dentate nucleus [*Schvarcz and Sica,* 1980] for relief of spasticity, high frequency currents (usually 100–200 Hz) have been used. Such stimulation, besides relieving spasticity, improved voluntary movements, balance, posture and speech. Intractable headache on cerebellar stimulation in cerebral palsy, requiring cessation of the treatment, was reported by *Reynolds and Hardy* [1980].

Stimulation of the *nucleus ventralis posterolateralis* of the thalamus for 1–3 min [*Mazars* et al., 1975, 1980] abolished sensory deafferentation pain as well as accompanying dyskinesias (jumping amputation stump, athetosis, thalamic hand, intention tremor). The effect lasted for several hours or days.

In *spasmodic torticollis, Mundinger* [1977a] implanted an electrode connected with a stimulation system into the nuclei ventrales orales anterior and posterior, the zona incerta including the H_1 and H_2 fascicles on the side opposite the spasm of the neck muscles shown in the electromyogram. The 7 patients could apply the stimulation themselves (optimum 5 pulses per second) intermittently; after stimulation lasting 30–40 min torticollis was definitely improved for 4–7 h.

Spinal Cord Procedures

Various therapeutic procedures have been carried out on the spinal cord, chiefly for treatment of spasticity. *Bischof's* [1951] *longitudinal myelotomy* for relief of spasticity in the legs has been successfully employed by *Laitinen* et al. [1971, 1974] in multiple sclerosis with spasticity of the legs. They performed the myelotomy through a T_{9-12} laminectomy. A midline incision was made between the posterior columns and extended laterally between the anterior and posterior horns, so that the reflex fibers maintaining the spasticity of the legs were interrupted. The diminution or abolition of the spasticity permitted a return of voluntary movements of the legs. It will be discussed on page 134 that spasticity in the legs could be reduced by chronic *dorsal column stimulation* in multiple sclerosis patients [*Cook and Weinstein,* 1973]. *Gildenberg* [1977] based his treatment of *spasmodic torticollis* on the assumption that this condition may be due to an aberration of tonic neck reflexes; he stimulated the posterior columns of the spinal cord at the level of C_2 using a high frequency current in an attempt to inhibit these reflexes. Of 6 patients who had dorsal column stimulators implanted, 4 had satisfactory relief during a follow-up period varying between 1 and 2½ years.

The advances of pharmacotherapy, particularly the introduction of *L*-dopa in the treatment of paralysis agitans and parkinsonism, have definitely decreased, but by no means eliminated the indications for guided operations in dyskinesias and dystonias.

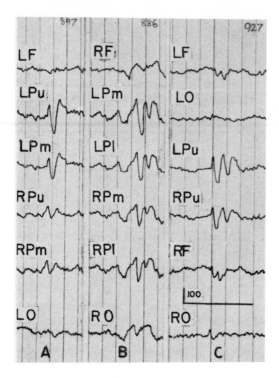

Fig. 23. Generalized tonic-clonic convulsions. High amplitude seizure discharges in the basal ganglia, but minimal changes in the scalp EEG. Depth electrodes in the left and right pallida (LP, RP) in a seizure-free interval. Scalp electrodes in the left and right frontal (LF, RF) and occipital (LO, RO) regions. u, m, and l = Upper, middle, and lower pallidal electrodes. Time: 1 s; calibration: 100 µV. From *Spiegel* et al. [1956b]; reproduced with permission.

Convulsive Disorders

Stereotactically implanted depth recording electrodes may be helpful in determining the focus of origin of seizures, particularly in instances in which the surface electroencephalogram is insufficient (fig. 23) as has again been pointed out by *Bancaud* et al. [1965] and *Rasmussen* [1980]. *Bancaud* et al. [1966] emphasized the value of *stereoelectroencephalography* obtained by several depth probes not only in the surgical management of subcortical tumors but also of epilepsy: localization, shape and extent of an excision can be 'tailored individually', also in open surgery, instead of use of standard procedures.

Stereotactic lesions produced in patients suffering from convulsive disorders that were unrelieved by medication were devised in order to eliminate the convulsive foci and/or to interrupt pathways carrying epileptogenic impulses. The electrographic findings in *petit mal* were inconsistent. In some cases seizure discharges were limited to the thalamus or propagated from there to the cortex [*Wycis* et al., 1949; *Spiegel* et al., 1951a, b]; in others, the discharges were found primarily in the cortex and white matter [*Hayne* et al., 1949; *Meyers* et al., 1950]. *Bickford* et al. [1955] assumed the existence of an abnormally facilitated diffuse thalamic system. While attempts to prevent petit mal attacks by lesions of thalamic areas, e.g., of the lamina medullaris interna [*Spiegel* et al., 1951a, b; *Hassler and Riechert*, 1954], were only occasionally and transitorily effective, destruction of a calcified focus in the caudate nucleus plus pallidotomy in a case of tuberous sclerosis [*Baird* et al., 1956a, b] practically stopped the seizures.

The *pallidum* seemed a suitable target because it receives descending impulses not only from the striatum, but also from the frontal cortex. The *amygdala* is a nodal point where corticofugal impulses from the tip of the temporal lobe, the pyriform lobe and the insula may be interrupted [the related literature is quoted by *Spiegel* et al., 1958a, b]. A propagation into deep temporal lobe structures occurs from distant, not only ipsilateral, but also contralateral, epileptogenic foci [*Engel* et al., 1980]. The effect of *pallidoansotomy* alone or combined with *amygdalotomy* was studied by *Spiegel* et al. [1958a, b; 1962] in epileptics refractory to medication in whom seizure discharges were demonstrable in the basal ganglia, particularly in the pallidum or in this ganglion and in the amygdala on repeated examination (fig. 24). The changes induced by 5 pallidotomies and 9 pallidoamygdalotomies were followed up in 13 cases for from 2 to 4½ years and in 1 case for only 6 months. In 4 of the 5 pallidotomies and in 6 of the 9 pallidoamygdalotomies the operation was performed unilaterally only, the side being determined by the severity of the pathologic discharges revealed by the depth electrograms. The seizures were controlled or their frequency markedly diminished in 9 of the 14 patients (64.2%) despite a marked reduction of the medication. There were 9 cases with *salaam convulsions*. They were considered as a form of myoclonic epilepsy by *Penfield and Jasper* [1954]. Of these 9 cases with salaam seizures (up to 100 or more per day) 1 was uninfluenced; after 2–4½ years 7 were completely controlled by pallidotomy or pallidoamygdalotomy; in 1 case 2–3 rudimentary seizures

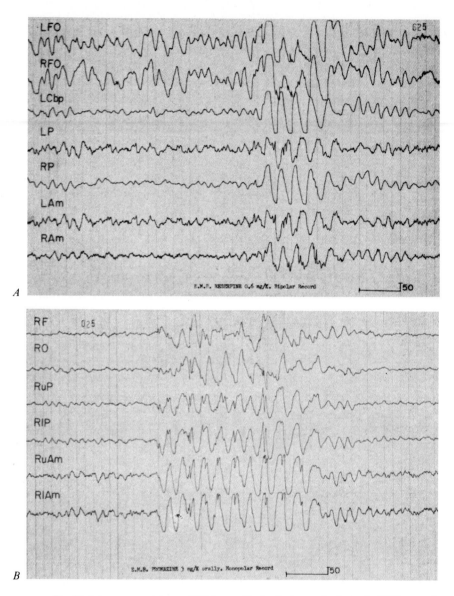

Fig. 24. Salaam convulsions. *A* High amplitude discharges in the scalp EEG precede those in the striopallidum and in the amygdala. Reserpin sedation. Bipolar record. *B* High amplitude discharges in the amygdala precede those in the scalp EEG. Promazine sedation. Monopolar record. Am = Amygdala (u = upper, l = lower lead); Cbp = bipolar caudate; F = frontal lead, O = occipital lead; P = pallidum. From *Spiegel* et al. [1958a]; reproduced with permission.

appeared per day. These seizures responded well also to CM lesions [*Kalya-naraman and Ramamurthi*, 1970].

Gillingham et al. [1976] and *Gillingham and Campbell* [1980] found lesions involving the pallidum conducive to particularly favorable long-term results for the control of intractable epilepsy. Lesions were placed in the posterior limb of the internal capsule *(capsulotomy)* in epilepsia partialis continua [*Walker,* 1958; *Jelsma* et al., 1973], also in generalized epilepsy, even bilaterally [*Kalyanaraman and Ramamurthi,* 1970], of course with paralysis of the respective limbs. In cases with a frontal focus, *Bertrand* [1979] found marked improvement after interruption of the *corticospinal tracts.* Based upon animal experiments, *Jinnai and Nishimoto* [1963] placed bilateral lesions in Forel's field H in order to interrupt epileptogenic impulses originating in the cortex and basal ganglia. There were initially favorable results; however, in *Bertrand's* [1979] experience, these successes were only transient. Bilateral stereotactic Forel field surgery was found partially successful in generalized tonic-clonic seizures by *Ramani* et al. [1980]. There was, however, a mild to moderate decline in cognitive functions, particularly memory, visual-spatial and constructional tasks. The authors consider, therefore, the bilateral operation justified only in patients with severe preoperative cognitive deficits in whom the benefits of seizure control outweigh the risk of further cognitive decline.

Thalamic lesions for the control of epilepsy were produced unilaterally by *Mullan* et al. [1967] using a strontium needle. 2 of 9 patients became seizure free, 4 were improved. It could not be decided, however, which lesions were responsible for the clinical improvement. This paper contains interesting thoughts suggesting that a lesion of the unspecific diffuse thalamocortical projection system might influence the spread of generalized epileptic seizures. Since *Hanberry and Jasper* [1953] presumed that the path of the unspecific, diffuse thalamic projection system passes through the region of the nucleus ventralis anterior, the suggestion by *Mullan* et al. [1967] that lesions of this nucleus should be produced is plausible; this idea was followed by *Bouchard* [1976] and *Bouchard* et al. [1975]. Lesion of the n. ventralis anterior in grand mal led to 'fairly encouraging results', but the number of cases was not sufficient to draw any definite conclusions [*Pertuiset* et al., 1966].

In *temporal lobe epilepsy* replacement of ablation of the temporal lobe by stereotactic procedures makes it possible to eliminate foci and interrupt the conduction of epileptogenous impulses, while undesirable side effects of the extirpation, amnesia, pareses, aphasia, hemianopsia, or development of a Klüver-Bucy[10] syndrome are avoided or minimized. The importance of the amygdala, the periamygdaloid region (mesial temporal region) and the hippocampus in the mechanism of temporal lobe epilepsy was demonstrated by electrographic studies and by electric stimulation. *Walker and Marshall* [1961] pointed out that *psychomotor attacks* are usually initiated by spike discharges in the amygdala and the hippocampus [similarly *Angeleri* et al., 1964]. *Feindel* [1961], an associate of *Penfield,* observed on stimulation of the periamygdaloid area behavior automatisms, complex automatic movements, mastication, and blocking of memory recording. On stimulation of this region, *Chapman* [1958] induced temporal lobe seizures, a behavior suggesting that the subjects were startled or experienced fear, depersonalization, or visual hallucinations. *Bancaud* et al. [1966] elicited chewing, swallowing and autonomic responses by amygdaloid stimulation. The experiences of *Horowitz and Adams* [1970], as well as those of *Weingarten* et al. [1977], indicated that the bodily sensations, alimentary sensations, sense of fear, déjà vu feelings and psychic illusions and hallucinations elicited by *Penfield and Perot* [1963] on electric stimulation of the temporal cortex in temporal lobe epilepsy, could be reproduced by electric stimulation of the deep structures of the temporal lobe.

Narabayashi et al. [1963] and *Narabayashi and Mizutani* [1970] originally performed stereotactic amygdalotomy in order to influence hyperactive, destructive children. There appeared, however, a definite initial improvement of psychomotor seizures (automatisms, dreamy state, visceral or psychic seizures) that lasted only for about 6 months to 1 year. Diminution of the frequency and severity of grand mal attacks also occurred, but gradually. There was an impressive EEG improvement; even the centrencephalic type of EEG could be favorably influenced. Similar experiences were reported by *Balasubramaniam and Ramamurthi* [1970] and by *Laitinen and Toivakka* [1980]. The latter observed on electrical stimulation of the amygdala, besides epileptiform fits and after-discharges, an ipsi- or bilateral slowing of the EEG. Lobectomy and even hemispherectomy often may be avoided by amygdalotomy [*Balasubramaniam and Kanaka,* 1975a].

---

[10] Following bilateral temporal lobectomy in rhesus monkeys involving particularly the amygdala and the pyriform cortex, *Klüver and Bucy* [1939] observed a peculiar syndrome of abnormal docility, fearlessness, lack of aggressive behavior, passivity combined with compulsive exploratory, chiefly olfactory behavior, excessive oral activity (sucking, biting), sexual hyperactivity toward the opposite and the same sex. Visual agnosia was an additional symptom unrelated to the temporal lobe cortex or deep ganglia.

Medial lesions of the amygdala were considered by *Narabayashi* [1980] more beneficial than lateral ones. Emotional and behavioral normalization and abolition or lessening of seizures went parallel in his experience. Memory defects or the Klüver-Bucy syndrome did not appear after medial lesions of the ganglion.

The *hippocampus* is an important target in view of its low threshold for eliciting convulsions. Instead of the usual hippocampectomy, *Nádvornik* et al. [1975] eliminated the temporal segment of the gyrus hippocampi by introducing the electrode in the longitudinal axis of this gyrus, as recommended by *Talairach* et al. [1958]; the results were similar to those of the classical technique. Hippocampotomy in temporal lobe epilepsy was replaced by *section of the fornix* [*Hassler and Riechert, 1957; Umbach and Riechert, 1959*], so that hippocampofugal fibers were interrupted. In order to avoid spread to the opposite side from a focus, *anterior commissurotomy* and interruption of hippocampal commissures were added [*Bouchard* et al., 1975]. Restriction of hippocampotomy to one side prevents amnesia.

Since not infrequently several epileptogenic foci are found and multiple pathways propagating impulses from such foci exist, single subcortical lesions usually relieved seizures only transitorily, and it became necessary to devise various *combinations of subcortical, stereotactic lesions.* Therapeutic lesions of the amygdala were combined by *Talairach and Bancaud* [1973] with hippocampal lesions using implantation of radioactive ^{90}Y. *Mempel* et al. [1980] performed chiefly medial amygdalotomies and also some anterior hippocampotomies in their epileptics. Besides a beneficial effect on the frequency and severity of the seizures, there was definite reduction of psychomotor excitation, anger, aggressiveness, disappearance of states of fear and flight. Combination of fornicotomy with amygdalotomy seemed indicated particularly in patients exhibiting aggressiveness [*Bouchard* et al., 1975]. Combined fornicotomy, anterior commissurotomy and amygdalotomy in temporal lobe epilepsy occasionally may only improve mood and social behavior, while the seizures may be only temporarily improved [*Schaltenbrand* et al., 1966]. *Mundinger* et al. [1976], however, regarded the combination of amygdalotomy and fornicotomy as effective in both generalized epileptic and psychomotor attacks. Stimulated by *Mullan's* above-mentioned considerations, *Bouchard* [1976] combined fornicotomy with *ventralis anterior thalamotomy,* preferably in patients with centrencephalic traits, or produced such thalamic lesions plus amygdalotomy in generalized forms of epilepsy [*Bouchard,* 1974].

A further route of propagation of limbic seizures to other brain structures, namely by way of the *medial thalamic (dorsomedial) nucleus,* was demonstrated by *Brazier* [1972]. Accordingly, *Ganglberger* [1976] produced lesions at the rostroventral margin of this nucleus in 6 cases with psychomotor and grand mal seizures who had been only temporarily relieved by fornico-anterior commissurotomy. 3 of these 6 patients became free of seizures, and in 2 the seizures appeared less frequently and were of shorter duration.

In epileptics in whom the clinical picture and/or the EEG suggested a focus in one hemisphere only, *Schaltenbrand* et al. [1966, 1970] coagulated the *corpus callosum* and other commissures in order to prevent the development of a mirror focus; the paresis and hemianopsia caused by hemispherectomy could be avoided. For the treatment of the psychic disturbances, particularly outbursts of violence appearing in epileptics, *Le Beau* [1952], and *Choppy* et al. [1973] performed lesions of the *anterior gyrus cinguli or cingulotomy.* A stereotactic approach to this area was chosen by *Diemath* et al. [1966].

In animal experiments it was found [*Snider and Cooke,* 1953] that electrically induced cerebral seizures were blocked by *stimulation of the cerebellar cortex* or of the fastigial nuclei. Analogous clinical experiences were reported on chronic stimulation of the lobus anterior cerebelli [*Cooper* et al., 1973b, 1974] or of the dentate nucleus [*Šramka* et al., 1976, 1980] in patients, mostly with grand mal, often combined with psychomotor seizures, and in petit mal. There was at least a temporary improvement [see also *Nashold* et al., 1975]. The effect upon muscular hypertonia in cerebral palsy patients, some of them also with athetosis, was already mentioned [see p. 6]. Follow-up studies by *Manrique* et al. [1980] for 15 months to 3 years showed no long-term changes in a patient with intractable epilepsy, but in 3 patients with involuntary movements there was slight improvement. Decerebration seizures developed in 1 case after chronic stimulation for 3 months; in another patient tremor and violent jerks of the extremities appeared after 6 months. While *Davis* et al. [1980] regard chronic cerebellar stimulation a valuable aid in improving the capacities of spastic patients and suppressing seizure, *Ivan* et al. [1981] consider the risk of this procedure hardly justifiable, because its efficiency is rather low. Placebo effects may account for the contradictory reports.

An attempt to analyze the effects of chronic stimulation of the cerebellar cortex in epileptic patients showed, even without electric stimulation, loss and degeneration of Purkinje cells [*Salcman* et al., 1976]. Following implantation of platinum electrodes over the cerebellar arachnoid and still

more marked after chronic electric stimulation, the loss of Purkinje cells
became more severe, in addition to development of marked meningeal pro-
liferation and gliofibrillar reaction [*Gilman* et al., 1975; *Manrique* et al.,
1980; experimental studies by *Babb* et al., in rhesus monkeys, 1979]. The
latter authors state that there may be no long-term benefit on seizure rate or
severity. *Gilman* [discussion of *Salcman's* paper, 1976] stated that one has
to seek another mechanism than Purkinje cell stimulation by which cerebellar stimulation affects epilepsy. Alternative mechanisms are suggested by
Bantli et al. [1976]. According to these authors, cerebellar cortical stimulation induces antidromic activation of cerebellar afferents, activation of neurons of the dentate nuclei and transsynaptic activation of neurons of the
ascending reticular formation.

Subcortical Tumors

The importance of the histologic determination of the nature of a subcortical lesion preceding radiation treatment is emphasized by *Mundinger*
et al. [1980]; the material is obtained by *stereotactic biopsy*. Similarly *Norén
and Collins* [1980] employ such a procedure for cerebellopontine angle
lesions, particularly when radiology is inconclusive.

In the treatment of subcortical tumors, extensive operative procedures
can be avoided by implantation or injection of radioisotopes. Treatment of
5 inoperable brain tumors by stereotactic implantation of radioactive gold
was attempted by *Talairach* et al. [1955]. A pinealoma regressed so that the
obstructed aqueduct became patent and the hydrocephalus diminished. A
decrease of the intracranial pressure was obtained in 2 inoperable tumors
and the 'general toxic effects' of the tumors disappeared. 2 patients died a
few days postoperatively. In 44 stereotactic tumor operations, *Riechert*
[1957a] used this approach not only for the primary treatment of tumors,
but also for secondary treatment of malignant tumors in which there was a
danger of relapse. In small tumors he injected a suspension of radioactive
gold absorbed to graphite that does not enter the general circulation as
easily as colloidal gold, or Plexiglas capsules filled with radioactive P were
inserted into the tumor. Cobalt needles (70–150 mCi) were stereotactically
implanted in large tumors, particularly for destruction of their borders. This
was sometimes combined with infiltration of the tumor mass with radioactive gold. It is interesting to note that insertion of radioactive isotopes
increased the survival time of patients with malignant gliomas 2–3 times.

Regarding complications, the necrosis of tumor tissue may lead to cyst formation or increased intracranial pressure, necessitating a puncture or a reopening of the wound.

More recently, *Mundinger* [1974] found ^{192}Ir more efficient than ^{198}Au or ^{90}Y in the treatment of *pituitary adenomas*. 89% of the patients with eosinophilic adenoma survived up to 8 years postoperatively, 79% of the chromophobic adenoma patients survived up to 16 years. In a further study [*Mundinger and Busam,* 1979], a life expectancy of 84.7% of patients with suprasellar adenomas and of 87% with intrasellar adenomas was recorded after 12 years. Visual function improved in 55% of the chromophobic adenomas and in 24% of the eosinophilic adenomas. Acromegalic signs disappeared in 64%. 85% of the patients were fully or partially able to work again. *Schaub* et al. [1979b] pointed out that stereotactic implantation in growth hormone (GH) secreting adenomas showed an advantage of interstitial gamma therapy with ^{198}Au compared with beta emitter (^{90}Y) hypophysectomy. The ^{198}Au implantation inhibits GH release without interfering with other pituitary hormones. ACTH producing microadenomas could be selectively destroyed by radiosurgery [*Rähn* et al., 1979], using *Leksell's* gamma irradiation technique in 17 cases of Cushing's disease. The ACTH production was increased during the first hours, giving rise to a peak in cortisol excretion. A lasting reduction of the cortisol level occurred within 6 months after irradiation. 6 out of 7 patients with Cushing's disease observed for more than 1 year became normalized, and the seventh improved.

Long-term irradiation with ^{129}Ir observed by *Mundinger and Hoefer* [1974] for up to 6 years proved an effective palliative method of treatment for *supratentorial semimalignant gliomas* of the midline that are otherwise inoperable and resistant to conventional irradiation technique. CT permitted *Ostertag* et al. [1979] to observe the effects of interstitial ^{192}Ir irradiation of cerebral gliomas. There developed a ring formation around the implant corresponding to a demarcation zone of radionecrosis. Low density areas in the white matter can mimic recurrence of the neoplasm. There are delayed effects appearing first after 4 months and becoming fully developed after 6 months. In cerebral tumors, *Mundinger and Schildge* [1979] apply stereotactic curietherapy with the ^{192}Ir gamma contact irradiation apparatus. This irradiation is combined with permanent implantation of ^{192}Ir wires or ^{125}I seeds. Tumors of the hemispheres are resected and immediately afterwards grade III and IV gliomas are irradiated. This curietherapy is intensified by bromdesoxyuridine and methotrexate. *Mundinger* et al. [1980] recently favor ^{125}I, since it requires less radiation protection due to its soft radiation. It has a half-life of 60 days.

The following *life expectancy* of inoperable gliomas was found by *Mundinger* et al. [1979] after permanent interstitial ^{192}Ir implantation: after 5 years, pilocytic astrocytomas of the midline 63.4%, fibrillary astrocytomas 36.8%, hemispheric gliomas grade I and II 38.7%. Objectively and subjectively, one-fifth of the patients were freed of their pathologic symptoms. In tumors of the *pineal region* ^{192}Ir or ^{125}I were implanted [*Weigel and Mundinger,* 1979]. Germinomas reacted well, but reimplantations were sometimes necessary. Five French stereotactic groups (Paris-St. Anne, Bordeaux, Grenoble, Marseille and Rennes) reported on results of interstitial implantation of ^{192}Ir for several days combined with external radiation treatment of inoperable hemispheric gliomas; they found the following: among 24 astrocytomas followed for 1 year and over, tumor growth was controlled in 17 cases and recurrence occurred in 7 patients. 11 malignant gliomas were observed for 3–47 months after irradiation. Their treatment was followed by remission and/or stabilization in comfortable condition (mean 10.4 months) before the final recurrence [*Szikla* et al., 1979b].

When glioma cysts were treated with intracystic injection of colloidal beta emitters, ^{90}Y or ^{186}Re, severe white matter edema was observed after application of yttrium but was absent or slight after use of rhenium [*Schaub* et al., 1979a]. A practical and efficient method of treatment for small- and medium-sized acoustic neurinomas, namely radiosurgery (use of a gamma unit) was described by *Norén and Leksell* [1979]. 7 patients with tumors 9–24 mm in diameter were treated with radiosurgery exclusively. They were observed for 4–9 years. In all cases the tumor was arrested; in all but one the size of the tumor has gradually decreased, and all patients have returned to their work.

In *cystic craniopharyngiomas,* radioactive isotopes were injected by the stereotactic approach, first by *Leksell and Lidén* [1953] and by *Wycis* et al. [1954] (fig. 25). In a recent survey of 85 cases observed at *Leksell's* department at the Karolinska Hospital, *Backlund* [1979] and *Backlund* et al. [1979] found injection of colloidal ^{90}Y solution in craniopharyngioma cysts rewarding. In solid craniopharyngiomas the author has attempted crossfiring of the target by narrow beams of ^{60}Co gamma radiation. A pronounced tumor shrinkage was verified by X-ray in a number of cases.

Cyst fluids obtained from brain tumors by stereotactic puncture contain not only nucleic acid, but also enzymes able to break down these acids. An increase of the enzymatic action was associated with deterioration of the

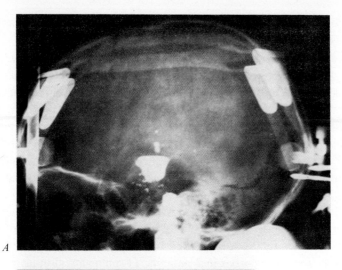

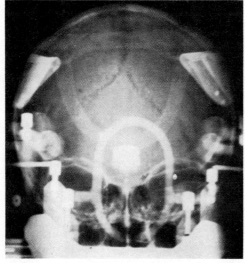

Fig. 25. Craniopharyngioma. Cystic cavity filled with Pantopaque. *A* Lateral view. *B* Anteroposterior view. Subsequently injection of colloidal chromic ³²P. From *Wycis* et al. [1954].

clinical picture. Injection of radioactive phosphorus into a cystic tumor is able to produce at least a marked involution of the tumor accompanied by a pronounced decrease of the enzymatic action of the cyst fluid [*Spiegel-Adolf and Wycis,* 1954, 1957].

A new, promising method for treatment of formerly inoperable deep seated tumors is the use of *laser beams. Kelly and Alker* [1980] couple a CO_2 laser system to a modified Zeiss operating microscope and a stereotactic guide. First the localization and tridimensional extension of the tumor is determined by CT scanning. The center of the tumor is placed in the focal point of the stereotactic guide. The incision is produced by the laser beam and is extended towards this focal point; the tumor is then vaporized by the laser beam. The resulting cavity is monitored by lateral and AP roentgeno-grams, and the vaporization is repeated until the cavity corresponds to the preoperatively determined extension of the neoplasm. The authors state that, theoretically, all of the tumor visualized by the CT scan could be eliminated and that the damage surrounding the laser-generated incision is limited to 1–2 cell layers.

Since tumor-specific lymphocytes were found circulating in patients with glioma, *Jacques* et al. [1980] attempted, besides tumor removal, *adjuvant immunotherapy.* In order to increase the effect of the lymphocytes upon a glioma, he applied lymphocytes obtained from the thoracic duct directly to the tumor site. A stereotactic approach to the neoplasm was calculated by a computer; the stereotactic guide was combined with a micromanipulator.

Functional Pituitary Surgery

The main indications for ablation of a normal pituitary gland are car-cinomas of the mammary gland and of the prostate with metastases, and diabetic retinopathy. In the sex-linked carcinomas, the stimulating in-fluence of estrogens and androgens, besides that of GH, upon the tumor growth is decreased or eliminated. *Riechert* [1980] points out that hypophy-sectomy can again induce a remission in patients who had shown temporary improvement of a *mammary carcinoma* after oophorectomy and adrenal-ectomy. In cases of *carcinoma of the prostate* he prefers conservative hor-monal treatment, since he observed only minimal effects of hypophysec-tomy upon the objective symptoms, although alleviation of pain occurred in about 90%.

In *diabetic retinopathy* the depression of the GH apparently is important [*Schaub* et al., 1979b]. In this condition, *Riechert* [1980] estimates an improvement rate of nearly 75% after hypophysectomy. He cautions, however, that the increased sensitivity to insulin requires a close postoperative watch for hypoglycemia. Renal, cerebral and ocular complications (retinal detachment, massive hemorrhage into the vitreous body) are contraindications.

In *malignant exophthalmus* hypophysectomy has been only occasionally practiced. Its use in *malignant hypertension* has been abandoned by *Mundinger and Riechert* [1967], since these patients are too debilitated, and since a similar depression of blood pressure could be obtained by pharmaca, e.g., alpha-methyldopa. (Acromegaly, see under Subcortical Tumors.)

Mundinger and Riechert [1967] point out that the operative *mortality* of the open surgical hypophysectomy with transcranial approach was 17.6 ± 10.6%, while none of their patients died within the first 2 months after stereotactic implantation of radioisotopes from any operative complications. They compute an operative mortality of 1.5–2.1% for the stereotactic implantation technique (apparently from the reports in the literature). The visual disturbances or oculomotor nerve paralyses also appeared less frequently (in 1.2% after the stereotactic radiosurgery) than after the open operations (4%). Furthermore, it is important, particularly in the treatment of cachectic, debilitated patients, that the pituitary gland can be reached stereotactically with the patient under local anesthesia. The pituitary gland can be punctured by guided instruments by a transfrontal [*Mundinger and Riechert*, 1967; *Poblete and Zamboni*, 1974] or by a transnasal, or transmaxillary transsphenoidal route [*Talairach and Tournoux*, 1955; *Talairach* et al., 1956].

The *transsphenoidal approach* avoids possible cerebral lesions and injury of the optic nerve or chiasma. *Riechert* [1980] developed a combination of open operation and stereotactic approach using the advantage of the good visualization offered by the former method and the accuracy of reaching the target inherent in the latter. By this combined method the pituitary gland was reached through the maxillary and the sphenoid sinus, with the guided electrode determining the direction and the depth of penetration.

Radioisotopes have been implanted into the pituitary gland by *Riechert and Mundinger* since 1953 [according to *Mundinger and Riechert*, 1967]. They used first Plexiglas capsules filled with ^{32}P-molybdenum, but were later more satisfied by ^{198}Au seeds, ^{198}Au absorbed to graphite, and ^{90}Y pellets. In their monograph [*Mundinger and Riechert*, 1967], they considered the latter the radioisotope of choice for hypophysectomy, while in recent publications, *Mundinger* [1974, 1975] preferred ^{192}Ir for protracted long-term tumor irradiation. *Talairach* et al. [1962, 1970] applied radioactive ^{90}Y and ^{198}Au in functional pituitary surgery. *Forrest* et al. [1958], who found pituitary necrosis produced by radon insufficient, and *Rank* et al. [1962b], likewise employed ^{90}Y.

None of the possible complications of *transfrontal approach* to the pituitary gland (meningeal and intracerebral hemorrhages, injury of the optic nerve or of the chiasma, puncture of the carotid artery) was experienced by *Mundinger and Riechert* [1967] in the cases in which guided cannulas were used. The only complication after transfrontal hypophysectomy for relief of pain due to prostatic carcinoma which was observed by *Moser* et al. [1980] was an asymptomatic quadrantanopsia.

A serious complication of hypophysectomy by the transnasal, transsphenoidal route is *CSF rhinorrhea* and the subsequent *meningitis.* In its genesis two factors play a role: necrosis of the diaphragma sellae, occurring particularly if radioisotopes are placed too closely to this structure, and the defect of the anterior wall of the sella turcica caused by its puncture. The lesion of the diaphragma could be avoided if implantation of isotopes were replaced by stereotactic RF current [*Zervas,* 1965, thermal hypophysectomy]. As pointed out by *Zervas and Hamlin* [1974], this method avoids necrosis of the diaphragma sellae, since the heat reaching it is dissipated by the flow of the blood in the cavernous sinus and by the suprasellar CSF. Cryosurgery of the pituitary [*Rand* et al., 1964] and ultrasound [*Hickey* et al., 1961] may also be substitutes for implantation of radioactive isotopes. Attempts have been made to close the defect in the *anterior wall of the sella turcica* by metallic screws and by injection of fluid that later becomes solid. Recently, *Zervas and Hamlin* [1974] reduced this complication to less than 1% by packing the electrode track in the pituitary gland with small pieces of bovine fascia lata and plugging the sellar defect with a silicone rubber dowel impregnated with silver.

Pituitary irradiation with *proton beams* can be mentioned here only briefly, since it is beyond the scope of this review. It has been applied to the treatment of mammary carcinoma with metastases by *Tobias* et al. [1955]. In recent years proton radiosurgery has been applied by *Kjellberg* et al. [1979] in the treatment of various tumors such as adenomas, acoustic neurinomas, meningiomas, and craniopharyngiomas; it also may be palliative for glioblastomas. Two techniques have been used. In one the center of the tumor may be necrosed. The inert central mass and the capsule have to be excised. In the second, low proton doses avoid necrosis and induce arrest of growth and sometimes reduction of the size of the tumor.

An unexpected beneficial effect of hypophysectomy in the carcinoma cases, besides the remission of the hormone-dependent tumors or their metastases is the *relief of the apparently intractable cancer pain.* For this latter indication, the pituitary gland was destroyed by injection of alcohol [*Moricca,* 1974; *Corssen,* 1977; *Katz and Levin,* 1977; *Lipton* et al., 1978] or by cryosurgery (introduction of liquid nitrogen (–20 °C), *Gye* et al. [1979]; see also review by *Check* [1979]). The latter method is preferable because complications caused by the spread of alcohol (damage to the oculomotor and/or abducens nerve, hypothalamic lesions) are avoided. Complete pain relief is frequently [in 40%, *Lipton* et al., 1978] obtained after the first injection; sometimes several injections are required. Diabetes insipidus due to the pituitary ablation can be controlled with prednisolone [*Lipton* et al., 1978] and hypothyroidism with thyroxine preparations. The mechanism of this pain relief is not clear. The relief was observed even if the tumor no longer reacted to the hormonal changes. An interruption of central pain-conducting pathways is excluded because the beneficial effect was obtained after cryohypophysectomy, a procedure which is limited to the gland. Endorphins are not increased after the pituitary ablation [*Lipton* et al., 1978].

Vascular Anomalies, Hematomas, Abscesses, Vegetative Disorders, Hydrocephalus, and Foreign Bodies

In order to produce thrombosis in an *intracranial aneurysm,* carbonyl iron powder was injected into its lumen and held there by a magnet [*Alksne* et al., 1967]. For the same purpose, a copper, beryllium or cadmium wire was stereotactically inserted, and a DC current passed through it [*Mullan,* 1969]. *Riechert* [1962a] reached *arteriovenous angiomas* using a combined open and stereotactic approach. Proton irradiation [*Kjellberg* et al., 1979] may induce narrowing and obliteration of the vascular lumen in arteriovenous malformations by producing an endotheliitis, deposition of hyaline amyloid substances beneath the endothelium. In intracranial arteriovenous malformations, stereotactically directed narrow beams of ^{60}Co gamma radiation were applied to obtain obliteration [*Steiner* et al., 1974]. A drawback of the method is the latency of 1–2 years between the radiation and the assessment of the obliteration. This is an argument against radiation of those arteriovenous malformations in which total surgical excision is feasible [*Steiner* et al., 1979] Stereotactic clipping of arterial and arteriovenous cerebral aneurysms [*Kandel and Peresedov*, 1980] resulted in elimination or significant reduction of the aneurysm in all 23 cases. Successful radiation of a stereotactically located carotic-cavernous fistula was reported by *Barcia-Salorio* et al. [1979].

Intracerebral hematomas could be evacuated [*Backlund and van Holst*, 1978; *Higgins and Nashold*, 1980] by stereotactic introduction of a cannula following localization by CT. Similarly, multiple deep intracerebral *abscesses* were aspirated stereotactically after about 0.05 cm³ of Pantopaque was instilled into an abscess cavity under CT guidance [*Walsh* et al., 1980]. The latter authors point out that depth targets that cannot be localized by angiography, ventricular contrast or neurophysiological methods may be approached by conventional stereotactic technique after CT-directed labeling.

Narabayashi [1962], demonstrating a vasomotor influence of the pallidum, relieved a patient's suffering from *Raynaud's disease* by pallidotomy. In paraplegics with *paralysis of the urinary bladder, Nashold* et al. [1972] produced micturition by stimulating the intermediolateral gray matter at the level of the first sacral segment. In some cases of *hydrocephalus, Riechert* [1957a] inserted a tube stereotactically into the third ventricle and connected it with the cisterna ambiens. He also used the stereotactic approach for removal of *foreign bodies*.

Physiological Foundations, Observations and Implications

Observations regarding the function of subcortical structures in man could be made not only after their elimination for therapeutic purposes, but also on electrographic recording and stimulation, which served as a refinement of the localization of the electrode tip prior to the destruction of the target area. Occasional autopsies permitted observation of the electrode position, of intended and unintended lesions, and of secondary degenerations.[11]

Internal Capsule and Corpus callosum

Frontothalamic fibers form a discrete bundle in the *anterior limb* of the internal capsule. To this the success of *anterior capsulotomy* in obsessive-compulsive states [*Herner,* 1961] is related.

The view regarding the position of the *motor fibers* in the internal capsule needs a certain revision. *Guiot* et al. [1959] located these fibers posterolaterally in the posterior limb of the internal capsule, and *Smith* [1969] placed them at the level of the posterior part of the corpus Luysi and the anterior part of the nucleus ruber in histopathologic studies of stereotactic lesions. In agreement with these findings, the corticofugal fibers of the pyramidal tract to the extremities were located by *Hassler and Riechert* [1961] in the posterior limb of the internal capsule at the frontal plane of the ventral caudal sensory thalamic nuclei. Pallidothalamic fibers transversing the internal capsule were found in the frontal plane of the nucleus ventralis oralis posterior, and *transcapsular lesions* could be performed by *Gillingham* [1962] in paralysis agitans without significant motor, sensory or speech disturbances.

---

[11] The physiology and pathophysiology of various subcortical structures are here discussed only in relation to the experiences during or after stereotactic operations.

After *capsular lesions of afferent fibers*, proprioception and spatial dis-crimination were less involved than after cortical or thalamic lesions; this suggested the existence of extracapsular pathways [*Obrador and Dierssen*, 1966]. In the *cerebral peduncle, Martinez* et al. [1967] found corticofugal fibers to the face most anteriorly and to the leg most posteriorly. In the central part of the *corpus callosum, Schaltenbrand* et al. [1970] found trans-verse fibers connecting cortical sensory areas most caudally, more anteri-orly the fibers connecting the leg areas, and then those for the arms and the face. Stimulation of the most anterior fibers inhibited speech. *Motor arrest* could be induced by stimulation of the corpus callosum, white matter of the frontal lobe, caudate nucleus, or nucleus reticularis oralis thalami [*Kwak* et al., 1978].

Striatum (Caudate Nucleus and Putamen) and Pallidum[12]

Connections of the Striatum and Pallidum
Afferent connections of the striatum (partly shown in figure 26) are sup-plied by collaterals of fibers of the internal capsule. It is not certain to what extent these are collaterals of corticopetal or corticofugal fibers.

Corticostriatal conduction is mediated also by the fasciculus subcallo-sus [*Kodama*, 1929] connecting the frontal lobe with the caudate nucleus. Epileptic discharges may spread from the precentral gyri to the putamen [*Walker* et al., 1956]. Differences in functional disturbances of these ganglia may be related to the differences of their connections. Pathways from the hypothetical cortical strip areas have become rather doubtful.

Further striatopetal fibers derive from the rostral tegmentum mesence-phali [*Nauta and Kuypers*, 1958], the substantia nigra [*Rosegay*, 1944; *Mettler*, 1957], the nuclei of the *nonspecific thalamic projection system* [see p. 148] and the anterior nuclei of the thalamus. *Nashold* et al. [1955] failed to find degenerative changes in the thalamus following striatal lesions and concluded that the thalamic projections to the striatum are either not exten-sive or formed by collaterals. Electrographically, an influence of the nonspe-cific system, of the dorsomedial thalamic nucleus (DM) and the nuclei ven-trales posteriores could be demonstrated [*Spiegel* et al., 1957a]. According

---

[12] In order to keep the number of references reasonable, only the most important are here quoted. An extensive list related to the striopallidum is found in *Spiegel* [1964].

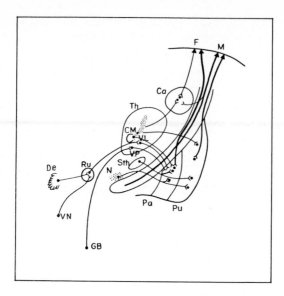

Fig. 26. Chief afferent connections of the striatum and pallidum. Ca = Caudate nucleus; CM = centrum medianum; De = dentate nucleus; F = frontal lobe; GB = Goll's and Burdach's nuclei; M = motor cortex; N = substantia nigra; Pa = pallidum; Pu = putamen; Ru = nucleus ruber; Sth = corpus subthalamicum; Th = thalamus; V.L = nucleus ventralis lateralis; VN = vestibular nuclei; V.P = nuclei ventrales posteriores. Punctuate area dorsolateral from CM = intralaminar nuclei.

to microelectrode studies [*Albe-Fessard* et al., 1960], heterogeneous afferent impulses (corticofugal, somatic, visual, auditory impulses) converge on one and the same striatal neuron. They may have been integrated, at least partly, in the reticular formation of the brain stem and in the CM [*Albe-Fessard and Gillett,* 1961].

The main *striatofugal fibers* (fig. 27) end in the pallidum, particularly its external part [*Wilson,* 1914; *Vogt and Vogt,* 1920; *Papez,* 1942], although some end in the related nucleus entopeduncularis. *Strionigral fibers* pass through the pallidum and the cerebral peduncle and terminate in the pars reticularis of the substantia nigra [*Papez,* 1942]. Further *pallidopetal impulses* are carried by corticofugal fibers chiefly from the frontal lobe [*Minkowski,* 1923/24] and, to some extent, from the motor and temporal cortex. This explains extrapyramidal conduction of corticofugal impulses that is important for motility, particularly in the subhuman brain, and for the innervation of some abnormal movements in patients, e.g., in chorea,

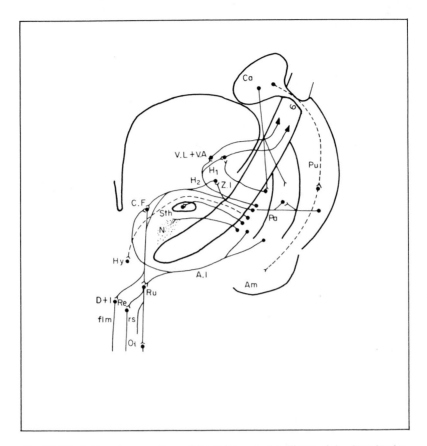

Fig. 27. Chief efferent connections of the striatum and pallidum. A.l = Ansa lenticularis; Am = amygdala; C.F = campus Foreli; D+I = nuclei Darkschewitch and interstitialis; flm = fasciculus longitudinalis medialis; H_1 = fasciculus thalamicus; H_2 = fasciculus lenticularis; Hy = hypothalamus; Oi = oliva inferior; Re = reticular formation; V.A = nucleus ventralis anterior, ZI = zona incerta; 6 = to area 6. Other abbreviations are the same as in figure 26.

athetosis and epileptic seizures. Additional impulses to the pallidum originate in the thalamus, chiefly in the nuclei of the nonspecific projection system, some few in the dorsomedial nucleus and the nuclei ventrales posteriores [*Spiegel* et al., 1957a]. Afferent impulses from the cerebellum, the substantia nigra and the corpus subthalamicum (mainly the latter) are of pathologic interest in view of their relation to hemiballism. An entrance of lemniscal impulses was described by *Bechterew* [1908–1911]. An effect of stimulation of the peripheral labyrinth [*Segundo and Machne,* 1956] and the triangular vestibular nucleus [unpublished experiments with *Szekely and Flanagan*] on pallidal unit discharges could be demonstrated by microelectrode studies. The importance of the pallidum for righting reflexes in primates was emphasized by *Denny-Brown* [1962].

Pallidofugal fibers terminate in (1) the nuclei of the so-called extrapyramidal system, the nucleus ruber, substantia nigra, corpus Luysi, mesencephalic tegmentum and the nuclei of the medial longitudinal fascicle [*Spiegel,* 1919; *Papez,* 1942], (2) the hypothalamus, and (3) the nuclei ventralis lateralis (VL) and ventralis anterior (VA) via the fasciculus lenticularis (H_2) and the fasciculus thalamicus (H_1) [*Ranson and Ranson,* 1939], but direct striothalamic fibers could not be demonstrated. The catatonia observed after chemical striatal stimulation (local injection of alumina cream into the head of the caudate nucleus of cats) is not prevented by extensive, more or less complete destruction of the pallidum and frontal lobectomy including the sigmoid gyri. This catatonia fails to appear after extensive lesions of the homolateral amygdala [*Spiegel and Szekely,* 1961]. We studied, therefore, the possibility of an extrapallidal conduction of caudatofugal impulses.

A conduction from the caudate nucleus to the putamen has been demonstrated by *Lévy* et al. [1959]. Using a Mnemotron computer that averages the potentials evoked by repeated stimulation, a conduction of impulses originating in the caudatum to the putamen and further to the amygdala could be recorded (fig. 28, 29). This was not prevented by extensive pallidal destruction [*Spiegel* et al., 1965b]. From the amygdala connections to the preoptic area, hypothalamus, subthalamus, thalamic nuclei and mesencephalic tegmentum are known [*Gloor,* 1960]. Since stimulation not only of the caudatum, but also of the amygdala can produce catatonia [*Kaada,* 1951], these experiments suggested that, in addition to the generally accepted striatofugal fibers to the pallidum, the conduction to the amygdala by way of the putamen is functionally important. It should be emphasized that a participation of the amygdala in the mechanism of catatonia was demonstrated in animal experiments, and on the other hand, amygdalotomy relieved some forms of hyperactive behavior [*Narabayashi,* 1980]. This problem seems to deserve further study. The solution may perhaps be sought in the functional differences between the medial and the lateral part of the amygdala [*Kaada,* 1972; *Narabayashi,* 1980].

Striatopallidal fibers, continued by pallidothalamic fibers, carry impulses that reach (1) the premotor cortex via the anterior part of the VL (*Hassler's* nucleus ventralis oralis anterior), (2) the prefrontal cortex via the

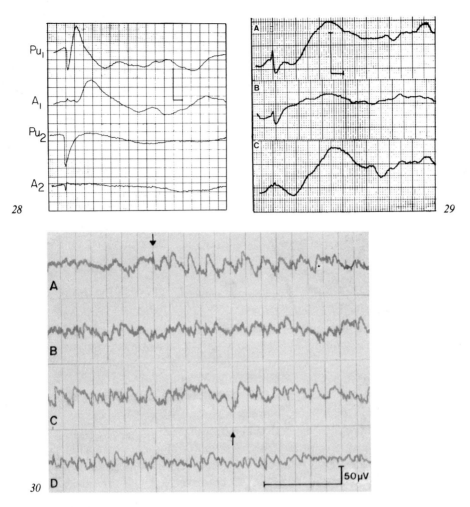

Fig. 28. Responses evoked in the left putamen (Pu) and amygdala (A) on 100 stimulations of the left caudate nucleus of a cat (0.2-ms pulses, 4 Hz, 3 V). Pu_1 and A_1 before,
Pu_2 and A_2 after production of an electrolytic lesion around the stimulating electrode in the
caudate nucleus. All records are bipolar. Calibration: 100 µV and 12.5 ms; sweep: 250 ms.
From *Spiegel* et al. [1965b]; reproduced with permission.

Fig. 29. Responses evoked in the left amygdala of a cat by 100 stimulations of the left
caudate nucleus (pulses of 0.2 ms duration, 4 Hz, 3.5 V) before *(A)* and after *(B)* electrolytic
lesion around the tip of the stimulating electrode in the caudate nucleus. *C* shows B sub-
tracted from A. Same source as figure 28.

Fig. 30. Effect of stimulation of the pallidum at a low frequency (5 Hz, 1-ms pulses,
10 V) upon the frontooccipital parts of the scalp EEG of an epileptic patient. Continuous
record from *A* to *D*. From *Spiegel* et al. [1960a].

hypothalamus-periventricular fibers – dorsomedial nucleus, (3) the diffuse, nonspecific thalamic projection system and the supplementary motor cortex via the nucleus ventralis anterior. The motor area (area 4) apparently does not receive impulses from the striopallidum by a direct pallidothalamocortical pathway; the premotor cortex (area 6), however, receives impulses by way of the nucleus ventralis oralis anterior, and its efferent fibers enter area 4 and then the pyramidal tract.

Due to the striopallidothalamic connections, stimulation of the striatum or pallidum may induce cortical recruitment [see p. 99] (fig. 30: effect of pallidal stimulation on the EEG). Stimulation of corticopetal fibers de passage may also play a role, while direct caudatocorticopetal fibers and the development of degeneration of caudate cells after cortical ablations are doubtful. A projection also exists to the thalamic nonspecific system by way of the above described conduction from the putamen to the amygdala, which latter ganglion partly sends impulses to the nucleus ventralis anterior [Gloor, 1960].

Striatopallidal Relationships

The conventional view assumes that the striatum exerts an inhibitory effect upon the pallidum. *Vogt and Vogt* [1920] assumed that chorea and athetosis are caused by a release of the pallidum from caudate inhibition. The thesis of inhibition of the pallidum by the striatum has been accepted also by other authors, e.g., by *Mettler* [1957] in his report at the First International Congress of the Neurological Sciences. On closer study, however, this doctrine meets with difficulties. It was found in cats that prolonged stimulation of the caudate nucleus, for instance, by injection of alumina cream, induced an increase of the amplitude of the electrical discharges of the pallidum recorded by macroelectrodes (fig. 31) [*Spiegel and Szekely*, 1961]. The pallidal unit discharges recorded by microelectrodes showed an increase in frequency on acute stimulation of the caudate nucleus with carbachol or camphor powder (fig. 32) [*Spiegel and Szekely*, 1962]. Large lesions of the head of the caudate nucleus induced by anodal electrolysis either failed to change the electrical activity in the acute stage or were followed by a depression of the electropallidogram demonstrable by macro- or microelectrodes, except in single instances in which transient spikes appeared. Several weeks following the production of the striatal lesion (fig. 33), the amplitude of the pallidal discharges gradually returned to the preoperative level or even exceeded it, at least for a while. The occasional transient spikes were interpreted as an irritation phenomenon due to the mechanical, stimulating effect of the oper-

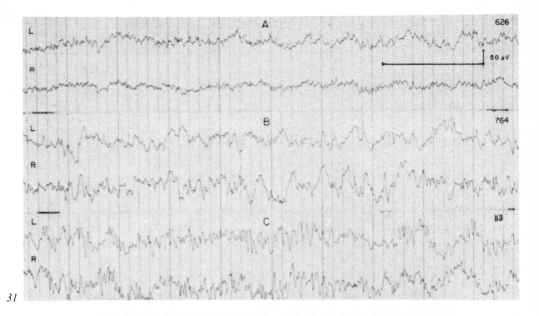

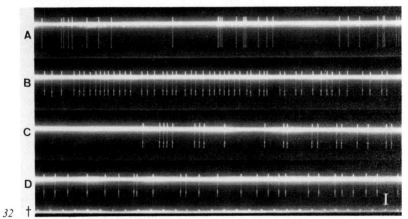

Fig. 31. Effect of stimulation of the left caudate nucleus by local injection of alumina cream upon the left (L) and right (R) pallidum. *A* Before injection. *B* 2 days after injection. *C* 7 days after injection (bipolar recordings). *A, B* In bulbocapnine catalepsy. *C* Without medication. From *Spiegel and Szekely* [1961]; reproduced with permission.

Fig. 32. Effect of stimulation of the head of the left caudate nucleus upon unit discharges of the left pallidum. *A* Before stimulation. *B* 3 min after insertion of powdered camphor 0.06 mg in the left caudate nucleus. *C* 10 min after the insertion. *D* 20 min after the insertion. t = Time; calibration: 100 μV. Experiments by *Szekely, Baird, Flanagan* and *Spiegel*, in *Spiegel and Wycis* [1962, p. 392]; reproduced with permission.

ation. The chief acute effect of the elimination of the striatal impulses to the pallidum, however, was a depression of its activity. The *increased pallidal discharges* appearing gradually after some weeks were regarded as an *isolation phenomenon* similar to the isolation phenomena noted on the spinal reflexes following elimination of impulses from higher centers [*Munk*, 1909]. The phenomenon was called by *Cannon and Rosenblueth* [1949] and by *Stavraky* [1961] supersensitivity of denervated structures. The existence of some inhibitory impulses appearing under certain conditions should not be denied, but their activity or the consequences of their elimination are more difficult to prove. On application of paired stimuli to the caudatum and to the pallidum [*Buchwald* et al., 1950] a preceding caudate stimulus inhibited the pallidal response to stimulation with intervals of less than 100 ms, but facilitated it with larger intervals. Following large lesions of the head of the caudate nucleus, the pallidal reaction to thalamic stimulation was only slightly increased, if at all.

Summing up, it seems that the effects of striatal elimination should be regarded as a manifestation of pallidal supersensitivity due to its partial denervation rather than a consequence of release from striatal inhibition.

Stimulation of the Striatum and of the Globus pallidus

Most of the kinetic effects observed on *electrical caudate stimulation* are due to spread to the internal capsule and are prevented by its degeneration, as was shown particularly by *Laursen* [1962a, b] in cats. Only the contraversive turning and circling [*Delmas-Marsalet*, 1925; *Akert and Andersson*, 1951] were not affected by lesions of the internal capsule and could also be elicited by chemical stimulation of the caudatum (acetylcholine, diisopropylfluorophosphate, *White and Himwich* [1957]; *Stevens* et al. [1961]; alumina cream, *Spiegel and Szekely* [1961] in cats). Similar effects were observed on electrical *stimulation of the pallidum* and nucleus entopeduncularis, the equivalent of its inner part [*Montanelli and Hassler*, 1962]. It would be desirable to have these latter stimulations repeated after degeneration of the internal capsule. On *stimulation of the putamen*, circling to the side of stimulation was observed (opposite to the pallidal effect). It seems tempting to draw the conclusion from these latter observations that there is an inhibitory influence of the striatum upon the pallidum. Such a conclusion, however, is hardly justified, since on caudate stimulation running to the opposite side occurs (in the same direction as on pallidal stimulation); this suggests a synergism between the caudate nucleus and the pallidum. The conclusion that the striatum inhibits the pallidum based on

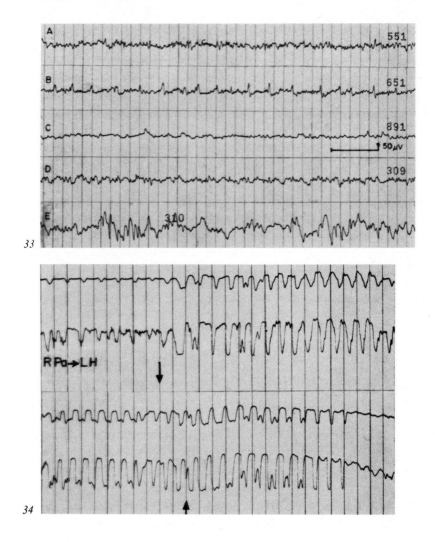

Fig. 33. Effect of lesion of the left caudate nucleus upon the electropallidogram. Spontaneous discharges of the left pallidum. *A* Before operation. *B* 30 min after operation. *C* 2 days after operation. *D* 10 days after operation. *E* 42 days after operation. Same source as figure 30.

Fig. 34. Effect of pallidal stimulation upon parkinsonian tremor of the left hand. Increase of amplitude of parkinsonian tremor by stimulation of contralateral pallidum. (Harvard stimulator, exponential pulses, 50 μs at half amplitude, 25 Hz, peak current 19 mA.) The tremor is recorded at two amplifications. ↓ = Stimulation on; ↑ = stimulation off. Same source as figure 30.

the stimulation of the putamen disregards the synergistic activity of the caudatum and the pallidum despite the fact that, in many species, the caudate nucleus represents the major part of the striatum.

Pallidal stimulation in patients without involuntary movements failed to produce tremor. In parkinsonian patients the amplitude (fig. 34) or, more rarely, the frequency of the *tremor* could be *increased* or a latent tremor could be activated [*Spiegel and Wycis,* 1962] by stimulation of this ganglion. Only occasionally an inhibiting effect upon the tremor was observed. The influence of the strength of the stimulus, type of the stimulating electrode (mono- or bipolar), and degree of the sedation of the patient was stressed. Similarly, *Schaltenbrand* [1965], stimulating the ansa lenticularis or the nucleus ventralis oralis, could produce tremor in parkinsonian patients only. Since pallidothalamic fibers (fasciculus lenticularis) pass through *Forel's field H* (FH) [see fig. 18], it is understandable that stimulation of FH [*French* et al., 1962; *Obrador,* 1962; *Spiegel* et al., 1963b] could evoke or influence parkinsonian tremor (fig. 35, 36).

Spindle formation and recruiting observed in the electrocorticogram on stimulation of the caudatum in cats apparently are also due to spread to the internal capsule. These reactions could not be elicited from the head of the caudate nucleus in monkeys, in which species this ganglion is more distant from the internal capsule than in cats [*Goldring* et al., 1963]. In man, *Housepian and Purpura* [1963] also failed to find spindle formation on caudate stimulation. In cats, *Spiegel and Szekely* [unpublished] could still produce spindle formation by caudate electric stimulation despite extensive lesions of the pallidum and amygdala, interrupting the caudatofugal fibers; this is in agreement with the view that these cortical electrical reactions are caused by a spread to the capsula interna.

Epileptic seizures could be elicited experimentally not only by electrical [*Jung and Toennies,* 1950], but also by chemical stimulation (alumina cream application) [*Spiegel and Szekely,* 1961] of the caudatum. After elimination of a tuberous sclerosis nodule located in the caudate nucleus [*Baird* et al., 1956a, b; *Macagnani and Vizioli,* 1958], the convulsions ceased in the affected patients.

Inhibition of cortically induced movements [*Mettler* et al., 1939] and of spontaneous movements [*Akert and Andersson,* 1951] may be induced by electrical stimulation of the caudatum. The latter authors considered these effects as a state of partial sleep. Inhibitory effects observed in monkeys and in man were also interpreted as sleep-like conditions [*Heath and Hodes,* 1952]. Speech arrest and confusion were produced by stimulation not only

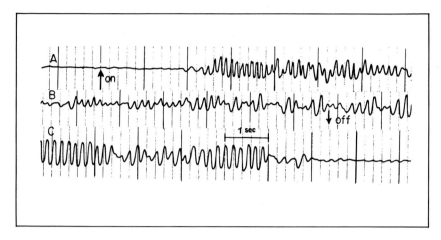

Fig. 35. Parkinsonian tremor evoked by stimulation of Forel's field H. Photoelectric record of movements of right index finger. (Small bulb attached to finger; its light falls on photocell connected to electroencephalograph.) Stylet of electrode is inserted in front of the left red nucleus, between 1 mm above and 1 mm below the intercommissural line. DC, 10 mA flowing from (↑) on to (↓) off. After a latent period of about 2 s, a tremor develops that first attains a frequency of 9 Hz; then the rate drops to 6 Hz. The tremor outlasts the flow of current and eventually has a frequency of 4 Hz. From *Spiegel* et al. [1964b]; reproduced with permission.

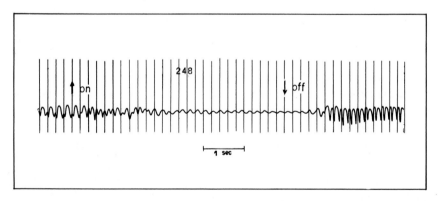

Fig. 36. Parkinsonian tremor in right index finger; decrease of its amplitude on stimulation of left Forel's field H (2-ms pulses, 100 Hz, 5 V on Grass stimulator, 2 V on the CRO, 1 mA as measured by a current probe). The frequency of tremor (4–5 Hz) is not changed. (Its doubling in part of the record is an artifact appearing when movements of the light beam exceeded borders of the photo cell.) From *Spiegel* et al. [1964b]; reproduced with permission.

of the caudatum, but also of the adjacent white matter of the frontal lobe and anterior limb of the internal capsule [*Van Buren*, 1962]. It has been suspected that these inhibitory effects are also due to spread to the internal capsule [*Peacock*, 1954].

The difficulties encountered on electrical stimulation due to spread of the current to the internal capsule can be avoided by use of *chemical stimulation*. Injection of acetylcholine into the head of the caudate nucleus produces a rather slight and short-lived inhibition [*Stevens* et al., 1961], while application of alumina cream has a prolonged effect [*Spiegel and Szekely*, 1961]. Within a week after unilateral injection, the cat's movements become slower; then its spontaneous movements, including eating and drinking, reactions to painful or other stimuli (confrontation to a mouse – fig. 37), become markedly reduced. So-called active catalepsy develops, so that the animal placed with the forepaws on one support and with the hindlegs on another remains suspended between these supports (fig. 38). It has been pointed out that this inhibitory effect of caudate stimulation is mediated by conduction of the caudate impulses to the amygdala via the putamen. Alumina cream injection into the internal capsule did not produce this effect, so that a role of stimulation of corticofugal or of corticopetal, e.g., thalamocortical fibers could be excluded.

An inhibitory influence of the striatum upon kinetic innervation is also indicated by the differences in the behavior of *chronic striatal and thalamic cats* [*Wang and Akert*, 1962]. Striatal cats (without neocortex and rhinencephalon, but with the striatum preserved) are very inactive, while thalamic cats (striatum also removed) are very active. Thus, the striatum has an inhibitory effect on the lower kinetic centers also when the neocortex is absent and its descending pathways are degenerated. This is in agreement with earlier experiments [*Spiegel and Szekely*, 1961] showing that catatonia induced by alumina cream injection into the caudatum is not prevented by preceding frontal lobotomy.

An *inhibitory influence of the striatum* not only on lower centers, but also on the *cerebral cortex* exists; the latter was demonstrated by *Denny-Brown* [1962]. Following bilateral caudate lesions in monkeys, visual compulsions were noted. He concluded that such lesions released visually determined cortical automatisms. *Parkinsonian bradykinesia* is caused by decrease or loss of the inhibitory dopamine effect upon the speed-reducing influence of the striatum. It can be counteracted by administration of *L*-dopa, the precursor of dopamine, by surgical lesions of the caudate nucleus [*Spiegel* et al., 1965a, b], or by stimulation of Forel's field [*Spiegel*, 1966],

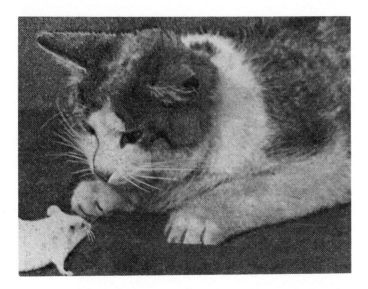

Fig. 37. Catatonia induced in a cat by injection of alumina cream into the head of the caudate nucleus. Akinetic cat staring at a mouse. From *Spiegel and Szekely* [1961]; reproduced with permission.

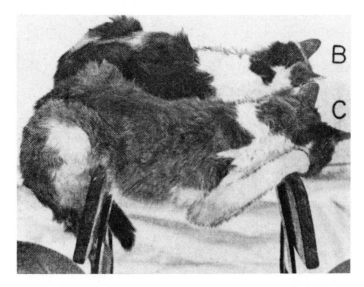

Fig. 38. Cat in striatal catatonia induced by intracaudate injection of alumina cream (C) and one in bulbocapnine catatonia (B). Both are suspended between two chairs. Same source as figure 37.

probably due to stimulation of reticulothalamic fibers. Slowing of movements can be obtained by stimulation of fibers passing from the pallidum to the nucleus ventralis oralis anterior [*Hassler* et al., 1965].

The pathogenesis of akinesia is complex. This symptom is frequently a consequence of parkinsonian rigidity; this component can be relieved if the hypertonicity is reduced by pallidotomy or ventrolateral thalamotomy. The poverty of movements is chiefly due to lack of striatal dopamine. Improvement of this deficiency is the main goal of *L*-dopa administration. A third factor, impairment of starting movements (freezing) and of performing repetitive movements at frequencies above 2/s has recently been studied by *Narabayashi* [1980]. One is reminded of that form of cerebellar adiadochokinesis that is caused by a disturbance of the innervation of the single flexions or extensions; there apparently a specific cerebellar function is impaired, namely its influence upon the successive induction that is regulated by proprioceptive reflexes [*Goldstein*, 1927].

Some Observations Related to the Pharmacology of the Striatum

The importance of *dopamine* for the function of the striatum was demonstrated by the finding that in Parkinson patients the content of the caudate nucleus of this agent is very low [*Ehringer and Hornykiewicz*, 1960; *Hornykiewicz*, 1966] and that application of its precursor, *L*-dopa, is able to improve the akinesia [*Birkmayer and Hornykiewicz*, 1962].[13] Thus a lack or decrease of the dopamine content, particularly of the striatum, is associated with akinesia, and replacement of the dopamine may abolish this symptom. As a consequence of the dopamine deficiency there is an imbalance of the dopaminergic and the cholinergic systems in paralysis agitans in that the latter prevail.[14] Two types of dopamine receptors have been distinguished in the striatum, one associated with and the other independent of adenyl cyclase [*Kebabian and Calne*, 1979].

Since the main therapeutic effect of *L*-dopa, the precursor of dopamine, consists in relief of akinesia, and since the above-mentioned experiments of chemical stimulation of the caudate nucleus demonstrated an inhibitory effect of the striatum upon spontaneous movements, it seemed of

---

[13] A detailed account of the development of the use of *L*-dopa in extrapyramidal diseases is beyond the scope of this monograph.

[14] A number of antiparkinson agents used chiefly in the pre-dopa era, e.g., trihexyphenidyl HCl (Artane HCl) and cycrimine HCl (Pagitane HCl) exhibit anticholinergic effects.

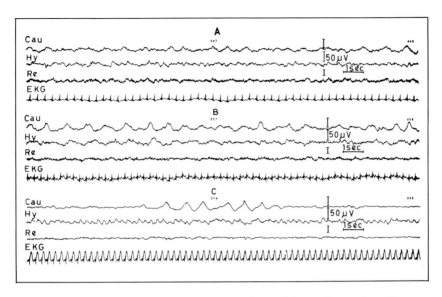

Fig. 39. Effect of *L*-dopa upon the electric activity of the caudate nucleus. Cat paralyzed by Flaxedil. Artificial respiration. Electrogram of the caudate nucleus (Cau), hypothalamus (Hy), reticular formation (Re), and EKG before injection *(A),* after intravenous
injection of *L*-dopa, 4 mg/kg *(B),* and after application of *L*-dopa (300 mg/kg, partly intravenously and partly intraperitoneally) *(C).* From *Spiegel* et al. [1965c].

interest to examine the effect of *L*-dopa upon the striatum. Two groups of
experiments were performed. In one the electrograms of the caudate
nucleus were recorded in cats after application of *L*-dopa [*Spiegel* et al.,
1965c]. Large doses of *L*-dopa (300 mg/kg injected partly intraperitoneally,
partly intravenously) that are in, or close to, the range producing hyperactivity in experimental animals, have a depressor effect upon the electrical
activity of the caudate nucleus. High amplitude slow waves appeared in the
electrocaudatogram, preexisting slow waves became more pronounced, or
long periods of flattening were observed indicating a depression of the electrical activity (fig. 39) of this ganglion. In microelectrode studies [*Bloom* et
al., 1965], the predominant effect of dopamine upon the cat's caudate
nucleus was a depression of spontaneous unit discharges, although some
units were facilitated. An inhibitory effect of dopamine upon discharges of
neurons of the rabbit's striatum induced by thalamic stimulation was also
described [*Herz and Zieglgänsberger,* 1966].

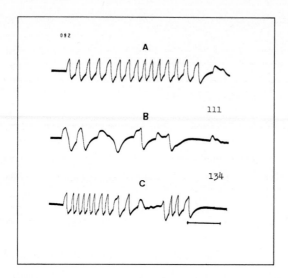

Fig. 40. Effect of intracaudate injection of *L*-dopa upon experimental bradykinesia (produced by injection of tungstic acid gel into the head of the caudate nucleus). Record of spontaneous running of rat. (Each deflection corresponds to a locomotion of 8.5 cm). *A* Before injection. *B* 12 min after injection of 4 µl tungstic acid gel into the left caudate nucleus. *C* 2 min after injection of *L*-dopa solution into left caudate nucleus (4 µl = 0.08 mg). Time (horizontal line at bottom of figure): 1 s. From *Spiegel* et al. [1967].

In a second series of experiments the caudate nucleus of rats was stimulated by local injection of tungstic acid gel [*Spiegel* et al., 1967] which produced slowing of locomotion. When this slowing had become definite, a solution of *L*-dopa was injected into the caudatum. The speed of running was significantly increased within a few minutes (fig. 40). In some animals the dopa injection resulted in a transient increase of speed beyond the initial value. In animals in which the tungstic acid injection resulted in complete akinesia, a catatonic state, the dopa injection produced only short-lived incoordinated movements or jumping, but normal locomotion did not reappear.

In control experiments intracaudate injection of corresponding amounts of dopa solvent or of physiological saline solution failed to change significantly the bradykinesia produced by the tungstic acid injection, so that the effect of the dopa injection cannot be explained by the mechanical injury caused by the injected dopa solution. It was inferred that the inhibitory action of striatal impulses upon spontaneous movements is diminished by the effect of dopamine upon the caudate nucleus. Thus, the therapeutic action of L-dopa in parkinsonian bradykinesia and akinesia can, at least partly, be explained by the diminution of the striatal inhibition of spontaneous movements.

An increase of dopamine receptors could be found in the brain of about two-thirds of cases of schizophrenia [Rees, 1981]. Neuroleptic drugs that alleviate signs of this psychosis, such as chlorpromazine, increase the turnover of dopamine [Carlsson and Lindquist, 1963]. According to these authors, this effect may be secondary to blockade of the dopamine receptors. A high, but not perfect, correlation between the blockade of dopamine receptors by neuroleptics producing extrapyramidal side effects and their antipsychotic actions has been observed [Rees, 1981]. Particularly the nucleus accumbens septi of the caudatum may be regarded as the possible site of action of neuroleptic drugs [Crow et al., 1978].

The striatum contains rather high concentrations of enkephalin [Bloom et al., 1978]. Microiontophoretic application of this agent or of endorphin to cells of the striatum induced chiefly an inhibition of the unit discharges of these cells (ratio of inhibitions to excitations about 4:1 [Nicoll et al., 1977]. Bloom et al. [1976] injected α-, β-, or γ-endorphins or met^5-enkephalin into the cisterna magna or the lateral ventricles of rats. β-endorphin was the most potent of these substances. Following injection of 7.4–14.9 $\times$ 10^{-9} mol, a pronounced catatonia with muscular rigidity appeared. These doses were about 1/100–1/400 of those at which met^5-enkephalin transitorily inhibited responses to noxious agents. These experiments, however, hardly permit one to answer the question as to which ganglia were stimulated in these experiments.

In this respect, studies performed by Hill et al. [1978] are of interest. These authors administered FK 33-824, a synthetic analogue to met^5-enkephalin to mouse, rat, rabbit and rhesus monkey and found it a potent, long-lasting analgesic agent. Injection of slightly higher than analgesic doses into the 4th ventricle of rabbits caused pronounced akinesia with muscular rigidity similar to that observed by Bloom et al. [1976] in the rat. In order to learn the possible site of the analgesic action of FK 33-824, this agent was injected into the 3rd or 4th ventricle or into the aqueduct of Sylvius of rabbits, while diffusion of the drug was restricted by injection of eucerine cream into certain points of the ventricular system. While blockade of the 3rd ventricle or of the aqueduct had no effect on the analgesic potency of the agent, blocking of the 4th ventricle abolished the analgesic effect. It was concluded that this analgesia depends, at least partly, on the drug's action upon structures easily reached from the 4th ventricle. Since akinesia was obtained on injection of somewhat higher doses by the same route, it may be surmised that a similar conclusion is justified regarding the localization of the catatonic action of the substance. An effect upon the substantia nigra may be suspected, since bilateral stimulation of that area, e.g., by picrotoxin [*Olianas* et al., 1978] results in catalepsy with marked muscular rigidity. The experiments quoted hardly permit one to draw conclusions regarding the functional equivalent of the depressor effect of microiontophoretically administered enkephalins or endorphins upon striatal unit discharges.

Clinically, in 8 patients tardive dyskinesia was slightly reduced by FK 33-824 (intramuscular injection of 1–3 mg), while a preexisting bradykinesia was increased [*Bjorndal* et al., 1980]. A possible interaction of enkephalin with dopamine was suggested. Regarding the negative effects of des-tyrosine-γ-endorphin in tardive dyskinesia [*Casey* et al., 1981], the authors admit that larger doses than used (16 mg), and prolonged observation after injection, may be necessary; other endorphins, e.g., β-endorphin, apparently have not been studied as yet in extrapyramidal disorders. As to the experiences of *Diamond and Borison* [1978] showing that 40 mg/kg of naloxone reversed the reserpine-induced parkinsonism in rats, *Castellanos* [1979] objected that their observations may be due to alterations of GABA activity. Apparently one faces rather contradictory reports, so that one has to await further experimental studies that may clarify the role of endogenous opiates in the functional activity of the striatum.

An approach to these problems was initiated by *Diamond and Borison* [1980]. They pointed out that opiates fail to have a significant effect upon extrapyramidal functions in man, while opiate addicts display a definite sensitization to drugs producing extrapyramidal side effects. Consequently they suggested that enkephalins may play a modulatory rather than a primary role in the control of extrapyramidal system functions and considered the possibility that the enkephalins may play a more central role in striatal diseases.

In the following animal models, they made observations summarized here in simplified form. The brain histopathology of Huntington's chorea was imitated in rats by bilateral striatal injection of kainic acid producing cell loss and decrease in ACh with intact dopamine levels. In these animals stereotyped behavior induced by *d*-amphetamine was potentiated by methionine-enkephalin. In contrast, in rats pretreated with haloperidol and showing hypersensitive striatal dopamine receptors similar to tardive dyskinesia methionine-enkephalin antagonized stereotyped behavior. Finally in rats with unilateral destruction of the nigrostriatal pathway due to unilateral injection of 6-hydroxydopamine into the substantia nigra a denervation hypersensitivity of the striatum to dopamine developed. Contralateral rotation produced by the direct agonist *L*-dopa was antagonized by methionin-enkephalin, while ipsilateral rotation induced by the indirect agonist *d*-amphetamine was potentiated by metenkephalin.

The authors interpreted the experiments as providing evidence for a presynaptic and a postsynaptic enkephalinergic neuron. After destruction of the striatal enkephalinergic interneurons by kainic acid enkephalin potentiates stereotyped behavior suggesting a facilitatory presynaptic enkephalin neuron. In the animals with postsynaptic hypersensitivity (pretreated with haloperidol) metenkephalin antagonized stereotyped behavior, indicating an inhibitory postsynaptic enkephalin neuron.

Regarding the interaction between the enkephalinergic and other neurons of the striatum, the following hypothetical concept has been developed particularly by *Schwartz* et al. [1978]. The endings of the afferent, dopaminergic nigrostriatal systems inhibit the cholinergic cells of the striatum. Blocking the dopaminergic transmission increases the activity of the cholinergic neurons. The amount of dopamine released by nigrocaudate terminals is regulated by axons of enkephalinergic cells which impinge on the nigrocaudate axons. The cholinergic cells of the striatum exert a double action. On the one hand they inhibit the enkephalinergic neurons, producing a feedback action. Blocking this influence induces an accumulation of met⁵-enkephalin. On the other hand they regulate the cells of origin of the strionigral pathway (apparently chiefly inhibition). This pathway influences the nigral cells which emit the dopaminergic nigrocaudate system. This influence is partly inhibitory by means of GABA release and partly excitatory by production of substance P. Partly similar to the hypothetical scheme outlined by *Schwartz* et al. [1978] is that developed by *Tagliamonte* and his associates [*Olianas* et al., 1978]. They also state that dopaminergic striatal receptors inhibit cholinergic cells (for further details of their views see the chapter Substantia nigra).

Narabayashi suggested that freezing, disturbance of initiating movements, might be due to decrease of norepinephrine in the CNS. Accordingly, he and his co-workers [*Narabayashi* et al., 1981] administered *L*-threo-3,4-dihydroxyphenylserine (*L*-threo-DOPS 1,200 mg in 2,400 mg *DL*-threo-DOPS) combined with a peripheral decarboxylase inhibitor (carbidopa or benserazide 100 mg). Dramatic improvement of freezing symptoms was obtained in 5 of 9 cases, moderate improvement in 2 and slight improvement in 1. There were some side effects: slight irritability, dizziness, and hypomania in 1 patient.

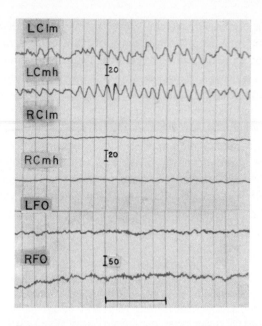

Fig. 41. Depression of the electrical activity of the right caudate nucleus in post-hemiplegic athetosis of the left hand. C = Caudate nucleus; h = upper, l = lower, m = middle electrode; LFO, RFO = left and right frontal and occipital leads. Time 1 s. From *Spiegel* et al. [1956b]; reproduced with permission.

Elimination of the Striatum

Elimination of the inhibitory striatal influence by lesions of the cauda-tum or putamen results in hyperkinesia in animals [in cats and monkeys; *Mettler,* 1942] and in man. In cats, the major part of the striatum is formed by the caudate nucleus, while in primates, one finds a shift of tissue to the putamen; consequently bilateral caudate lesions produce hyperkinesia in cats, but only in some monkeys [*Harman and Carpenter,* 1950]. There are few experiences of circumscribed striatal lesions in man. Hemichorea asso-ciated with a circumscribed lesion of the opposite caudatum was reported by *Austrogesilo and Gallotti* [1924] and *Austrogesilo and Borges-Fortes* [1937]. In Huntington's chorea, atrophy of the caudate nucleus, as well as of the putamen, was noted. Significant differences in the atrophy of these two ganglia were not mentioned by some authors [*Bruyn,* 1968]; yet *Heimburger* [1975a] emphasized the marked atrophy of the caudatum, while the puta-men is relatively intact. *Spatz* [1927] pointed out that foci in the anterior part of the caudate nucleus in some instances produced contralateral chorea, in others contralateral hemiathetosis. His statement still holds true that an explanation of these symptomatological differences with similar location of the pathological process is as yet impossible. *Spiegel and Wycis* [1962] found that in a hemiplegic woman, with athetotic movements on the left hemiplegic side, electrical discharges of the contralateral (right) caudate nucleus were definitely reduced compared with those on the left side (fig. 41). There exists one observation of cystic lesions of the *putamen* associated with choreiform movements of the other side [*Davison and Goodhart,* 1940], while in *Steck's* [1921] case of involvement of the putamen the involuntary movements were slower and described as athetotic. In the majority of cases of athétose double, chiefly the putamen showed bilaterally *Vogt's* [1911] status marmoratus, hypermyelinization and loss or degeneration of the small and large cells in the marbled areas.

In the genesis of involuntary movements following striatal lesions, three factors seem to play a part: (1) the loss of striatofugal inhibitory impulses to the cerebral cortex as well as to lower centers by way of the above outlined pathways; (2) corticofugal impulses mediated to the periphery by means of corticopallidal tracts, and (3) hyperactivity of the pallidum due to its partial isolation after striatal lesions.

Role of the Pallidum in Kinetic and Static Innervation (Muscle Tone)
Following CO intoxication, rigidity of the skeletal muscles combined with hypo- or akinesia was repeatedly observed, and anatomical examination revealed bilateral softening of the pallidum. It is, of course, tempting to deduce from these observations a role of the pallidum in the kinetic innervation and in the maintenance of muscle tone. It should not be overlooked, however, that the lesions caused by CO poisoning are by no means limited to the pallidum. They extend to the internal capsule, the putamen, and the cornu ammonis; the thalamus and cerebellum may also be affected. Necrosis of cerebral cortical areas and softening in the white matter of the cerebrum have also been found [*Peters,* 1951]. The lesions produced by chronic carbon disulfide poisoning in monkeys [*Richter,* 1945] are also not limited to the pallidum.

It seems important, therefore, to study as far as possible the relationship of the pallidum to the innervation of so-called *willed* movements and associated movements in patients in whom extensive pallidal lesions limited to this ganglion had been produced surgically. Such lesions, at least in some patients with athetosis, could diminish the overflow of innervation to muscle groups beyond those which the patient intends to innervate. If one considers such pathologic movements as an exaggeration of normal associated movements, these observations seem to suggest that the pallidum plays a role in the innervation of some associated movements. It may be objected that, after pallidoansotomy in parkinsonian patients, associated movements, e.g., of the arms in walking, may return. This may be seen after relatively small pallidal lesions that relieve the rigidity; they restore the associated movements as far as they are prevented by the rigidity. Extensive pallidal lesions, however, interfere with associated movements. In this connection, *Mettler's* [1945] view should be recalled that the pallidum mediates particularly associated movements induced by proprioceptive stimuli.

In some types of choreatic movements [*Spiegel and Wycis,* 1950b; *Riechert,* 1957a], hemiballism [*Roeder and Orthner,* 1957], and the experimentally produced choreoid hyperkinesia of monkeys [*Mettler and Carpenter,* 1949; *Carpenter* et al., 1950], the involuntary movements may be decreased or abolished by pallidal lesions. If one considers choreic movements in man caused by hyperactivity of released cortical mechanisms, these observations are in agreement with the view that some corticofugal impulses inducing complex movements are conducted via the pallidum. For hemiballism it is assumed that the pallidum is released by a lesion of the corpus subthalamicum [*Martin,* 1959, 1960], so that pallidal hyperactivity is an important factor in the genesis of these involuntary movements.[15] Extensive bilateral pallidal lesions or interruption of the outflow of the pallida may induce a *decrease of initiative, hypokinesia* and sometimes a *slowing of the movements* [in monkeys, *Ranson and Ranson,* 1939; in man, *Spiegel* et al., 1958a, b; *Hassler,* 1959; *Hassler* et al., 1960, 1979; *Hartmann-von Monakow,* 1959]. In these disturbances, involvement of the hypothalamus may participate [*Ranson and Ranson,* 1939; *Orthner and Roeder,* 1959].

Denny-Brown [1962] made the interesting statement that the pyramidal tract is 'useless to the organism without the extrapyramidal system'. This statement is based on bilateral pallidal lesions in monkeys. His lesions, however, were by no means limited to the pallida. His figures 50c and d show that the lesions destroyed a considerable part of the cross section of the internal capsule, and his conclusions are based on combined pallidocap-

---

[15] *Dierssen* et al. [1961] described a case which they diagnosed as hemiballism, and in which autopsy revealed an intact corpus subthalamicum. It is doubtful, however, whether the movements shown in the selected frames from a motion picture should be regarded as typical ballistic movements.

sular lesions. In our experience in man, extensive bilateral pallidal lesions did not prevent so-called willed movements.

The importance of the pallidum in the mechanism of some *labyrinthine reactions* has been recognized in recent decades. *Mettler* [1957] pointed out that bilateral pallidal lesions induce a 'degradation' in the adjustment to vestibular stimulation. His monkeys with bilateral pallidal lesions retained abnormal postures in which they were placed, due to impairment of the proprioceptive vestibular reflexes. *Denny-Brown's* [1962] careful analysis of monkeys with bilateral pallidal lesions revealed loss of all placing reactions, labyrinthine and optic righting reactions. The tonic body contact response, however, was very intense. The disturbance of postural regulation in pallidal lesions may play an important role in the production of disorders of locomotion observed in diseases affecting the pallidum, as pointed out by *Martin and Hurwitz* [1962].

Regarding the relationship of the pallidum to so-called *muscle tone* (the passive resistance of the skeletal muscles to stretch), until recently one found *Foerster's* [1921] doctrine of pallidum rigor ('Starre') produced by destruction of this ganglion the dominant teaching. This theory was caused by ignorance or disregard or underestimation of the nigral cell degeneration in Parkinson's disease and overestimation of the pallidal alterations that are chiefly senile changes found also in persons of the same age without parkinsonian signs. The experience that circumscribed stereotactic lesions of the pallidum and ansa lenticularis (pallidoansotomy) [*Wycis and Spiegel,* 1952; *Spiegel and Wycis,* 1954], with only minimal injury to adjacent regions, could reduce or abolish parkinsonian rigor, definitely refuted the concept of pallidal rigor.

Somatotopic Localization in the Striatum and Pallidum

A somatotopic localization in the striatum and pallidum was postulated over half a century ago, based on pathological findings, particularly by *Vogt and Vogt* [1920]. *Hassler* et al. [1960] concluded from stimulation and coagulation in man that the head, mouth, pharynx and larynx are localized in the rostral part of the pallidum, the arm in the middle part and the lower extremity in the caudal part. Since there is a definite arrangement of the striatofugal fibers to the pallidum, one may expect that the striatum also may have a corresponding somatotopic localization. *Denny-Brown* [1962] denies such a localization. He believes that topographic selectivity reflects some relative localization of optic and contactual reactions. Visual responses appear more prominent in lesions of the anterior putamen. He also states, however, that any well-defined lesion of the putamen involves the hand more than the mouth and the foot least of all. This apparently is an analogy to the cortical representation that also shows a predominance of the hand area in the motor, as well as in the somesthetic, cortex.

Substantia nigra

The substantia nigra consists of two areas, a zona compacta with cells showing melanin pigment in the adult human and, ventral to it, between it and the cerebral peduncle, a zona reticularis with cells rich in iron. It receives afferent fibers from the cerebral cortex, chiefly from the motor area and from the striatum. Due to the difficulty to demonstrate the latter, their existence was controversial for a long time. The silver staining technique demonstrated efferent fibers from the caudate nucleus [*Voneida*, 1960] as well as from the putamen [*Nauta and Mehler*, 1961] to the substantia nigra.

Efferent projections were described from the substantia nigra to the mesencephalic tegmentum, pallidum and striatum. The scarcity of degenerations to the striatum from nigral lesions in the monkey was noted by *Carpenter and McMasters* [1964]. But the existence of nigrostriatal projections cannot be doubted in view of the findings of *Rosegay* [1944], *Llamas and Reinoso-Suarez* [1969], *Moore* et al. [1971] and *Usunoff* et al. [1974]. For the visualization of the degeneration products of these thin fibers the Nauta method proved useful.

The anatomical findings were supplemented by biochemical and histochemical studies. Catecholamines were demonstrated in the striatum [*Bertler and Rosengren*, 1959] and in the substantia nigra [*Hornykiewicz*, 1966]. Monoamine containing neurons could also be demonstrated in the striatum and the substantia nigra histochemically by fluorescence microscopy [*Dahlström and Fuxe*, 1964]. The melanotic pigment of the substantia nigra apparently is a metabolic product of its catecholamines. An incision between the substantia nigra and the caudatum induced a decrease in striatal catecholamines [*Poirier*, 1964; *Poirier and Sourkes*, 1965]. In the substantia nigra, an interruption of the striatonigral connections produced a drop of gamma-aminobutyric acid (GABA) [*Hassler*, 1974]. Thus, the nigrostriatal neurons were considered dopaminergic and the inhibitory striatonigral paths at least partly GABA-ergic. The latter are also partly cholinergic.

Olianas et al. [1978] described in rats a nigral nondopaminergic neural system in the pars reticularis. Bilateral stimulation of these neurons by picrotoxin, a GABA antagonist, produces catalepsy with rigidity; their bilateral inhibition by GABA or muscimol or destruction by kainic acid induces hyperactivity, stereotyped sniffing and gnawing of rats. These effects are independent of the integrity of the nigrostriatal dopaminergic pathway. The nigral system that is sensitive to kainic acid is antagonistic to striatal dopamine in the control of posture. Inhibition or destruction of the nigral nondopaminergic neural system produces effects similar to those observed following stimulation of striatal dopamine receptors. The nigro-striatal dopamine system inhibits the kainic acid sensitive nigral neurons by activating a strionigral GABA-ergic pathway.

Descending pathways from the substantia nigra have been described to the rhombencephalic reticular formation and the spinal cord [*Hassler*, 1966]. They are probably dopaminergic. They inhibit a rise of muscle tone and activate the gamma fibers, effects similar to those noted on systemic application of *L*-dopa, the precursor of dopamine. Reserpine, which depletes the nigra cells of dopamine, induces rigidity of the skeletal muscles; this is comparable to the result of degeneration of the nigra cells. In parkinsonian patients with degeneration of the nigral cells, the catecholamine and serotonin content of the substantia nigra was found markedly diminished [*Hornykiewicz*, 1966].

Cerebellar Nuclei

A *relaxation* of hypertonic muscles could be produced, particularly in spasticity, by lesions of the dentate nucleus, while the tonus of normal muscles apparently was not significantly reduced [*Delmas-Marsalet*, 1935; *Tóth*, 1961; *Heimburger*, 1965; *Nashold*, 1969; *Krayenbühl and Siegfried*, 1969; *Zervas* et al., 1967; *Zervas*, 1970; *Siegfried* et al., 1970]. Unexpectedly, the classical signs of cerebellar deficit, dysmetria, ataxia, tremor, and decomposition of movements, were mostly not manifest, perhaps due to the incompleteness of the nuclear lesion (chiefly in the ventrolateral part). Extensive lesions of the dentatorubrothalamic fibers in Forel's field H [*Spiegel* et al., 1963b] also produced ataxia only occasionally. If the lesion of the cerebellar nuclei was placed less than 10 mm from the midline, temporary appendicular ataxia, asthenia, ocular disturbances, and torticollis were observed [*Nashold and Slaughter*, 1969]. Ablation of the nucleus interpositus encroaching upon the fastigial nucleus may induce appendicular ataxia [*Zervas* et al., 1967]. It may be astonishing that dentate lesions influenced the axial muscles favorably, although it is generally recognized that the cerebellar hemispheres, which send impulses to the dentate nuclei, innervate the extremities. The observation that such lesions had a favorable effect on the patient's control of trunk stability [*Heimburger,* 1967], while cerebellar impairment usually produces disturbances of balance, may perhaps be explained by the experience that in a pathologically altered brain the effects of lesions may differ from those in a normal brain. While *Heimburger* observed the most pronounced relaxation in contralateral extremities after lateral lesions, other workers in this field noted ipsilateral effects in agreement with conventional views. It may be hoped that future histopathologic examinations will clarify the controversial observations.

Speech

Bilateral lesions of the most anterior part of the posterior limb of the internal capsule or the rostral part of the cerebral peduncle induced dysarthria [*Hassler* et al., 1965]. In one instance aphonia appeared after coagulation of the most anterior part of the left cerebral peduncle. Speech disturbances observed on stimulation in the vicinity of the caudate nucleus [*Van Buren,* 1963] might have been due to an influence on this ganglion or on the white matter. Confusion of the patient might also have played a role.

On stimulation of various points of the ventrolateral area of the thalamus, the speech was accelerated in some instances and arrested in others [*Guiot* et al., 1961; *Hassler,* 1967]. Factors similar to those regarding various effects of thalamic stimulation on tremor probably played a role. Lesions of this area or of the pallidum increased dysarthria and dysphasia or reduced the voice volume [*Hermann* et al., 1966]. *Krayenbühl* et al. [1965] pointed out that speech disturbances appeared chiefly after thalamic lesions in the dominant hemisphere. This was confirmed by *Hermann* et al. [1966] and *Choppy* [1973], while *Meyers* [1966] and *Riklan and Levita* [1969] defended a bilateral subcortical dependence of the speech mechanisms. *Schaltenbrand's* [1965] experience that compulsory speech was elicited by stimulation of the nucleus ventralis oralis anterior on the dominant side only further supports *Krayenbühl's* thesis [see also *Blumetti and Modesti,* 1980, and chapter on Memory and Cognitive Processes, p. 177].

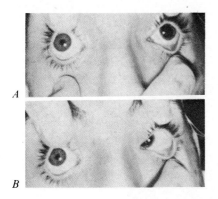

Fig. 42. Adduction of homolateral eye on stimulation of Forel's field. *A* Before stimulation: eyes divergent, left pupil dilated. *B* During stimulation (DC, 5 mA): adduction of left eye due to stimulation of oculomotor innervation of left internal rectus muscle. From *Spiegel* et al. [1964b]; reproduced with permission.

Meyers [1966] studied the effect of subcortical lesions on three speech qualities: force (volume), arthria and prosody, i.e. variations in stress, pitch and rhythm. Impairment of prosody causes monotony of speech. He found disturbances of these three qualities after lesions of the intermediate three-fifths of the peduncles, of Forel's fields H, H_1 and H_2, and of the dorso-medial margin of the substantia nigra and the adjacent midbrain tegmentum, but not after lesions of the ventrolateral areas of the thalamus, contrary to *Hermann* et al. [1966]. In our experience these disturbances appeared infrequently after Forel's field H lesions. *Meyers* explains these disturbances by interference with corticospinal, corticobulbar and dentato-rubrothalamic tracts [see also chapter on Memory and Cognitive Functions, p. 176].

Ocular Movements

The posterior part of Forel's field H (FH) is adjacent to the most anterior roots of the *oculomotor nerve*. Therefore, stimulation of this region frequently produces adduction of the homolateral eye [*Spiegel* et al., 1964] (fig. 42) and coagulation produces weakness of the ipsilateral internal rectus muscle [*Spiegel* et al., 1963b]. This is in agreement with *Warwick's* [1964]

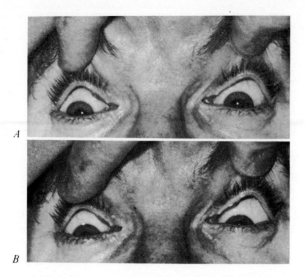

Fig. 43. Induction of conjugate eye movements downward by stimulation of Forel's field. Stimulating electrode lateral to left nucleus ruber at level of intercommissural line (2-ms pulses, 100 Hz, 15 V). Before *(A)* and during *(B)* stimulation. Same source as figure 35.

experiments in monkeys localizing the innervation of this muscle in the anterior pole of the oculomotor nucleus.

Conjugate eye movements, mostly horizontally to the opposite side, but sometimes in a vertical direction, upward or downward (fig. 43) could also be elicited from FH [*Spiegel* et al., 1964b; *Johansson and Laitinen,* 1965]. Similar effects were observed by *Hassler* et al. [1960] on stimulation of the internal capsule and of the pallidum externum. More caudally, the pathway for conjugate eye movements enters the midbrain tegmentum [*Nashold,* 1967]. *Nystagmus* was observed in some cases on stimulation of the thalamic-subthalamic area [*Johansson and Laitinen,* 1965], of FH [*Spiegel* et al., 1964b], and the stratum lemnisci of the superior colliculus [*Takebayashi and Komai,* 1966].

Regarding the innervation of the *eyelids,* blepharospasm, as well as opening of the eyes, was observed, the former on stimulation of the thalamic-subthalamic area [*Johansson and Laitinen,* 1965; *Johansson,* 1969], the latter on stimulation of the nucleus ventralis oralis anterior [*Hassler* et al., 1960].

Neck Muscles

Retroflexion of the neck in a case of cerebral palsy with athetotic movements could be abolished almost completely by unilateral campotomy (lesion of FH) [*Spiegel* et al., 1963b]. This effect may be due to a lesion of pallidofugal fibers to the interstitial nucleus passing through the FH or to encroaching of the lesion upon the interstitial nucleus; this question cannot be definitely answered without histologic examination. According to *Sano* et al. [1970b], retroflexion of the neck appeared on stimulation of the region of Cajal's *interstitial nucleus*[16] of the medial longitudinal fasciculus; relief of retrocollis was obtained by elimination of this area. Stimulation of points adjacent to the interstitial nucleus elicited ventroflexion of head and neck.

While *Sano* reported improvement of the position of the head without side effects involving ocular movements, *Nittner and Petrovici* [1974] experienced vertical gaze paralysis (Parinaud's syndrome) and paralysis of convergence following bilateral stereotactic lesions of the interstitial nucleus region, with only slight improvement of the patient's retrocollis. A concomitant lesion of the pretectal area, however, could not be excluded. *Hassler and Dieckmann* [1970], based on *Hassler's* previous animal experiments, state that the interstitial nucleus is responsible for rotating movements of the body, especially of the head around its longitudinal axis, and that turning movements to the contralateral side have their main center in the pallidum and nucleus entopeduncularis. Interruption of the pallidothalamic fibers in Forel's H_1 bundle (fasciculus thalamicus) results in a posture of the head turned to the side of the lesion. In previous stereotactic operations with *Riechert,* coagulation of the inner part of the nucleus ventrooralis (Voi, nucleus ventrooralis internus) had been effective against torsion dystonia, movements of the extremities and trunk, but had only a transient effect on spasmodic torticollis.

In *spasmodic torticollis,* the abnormal posture of the head and neck is caused chiefly by contraction of the sternocleidomastoid muscle on the side opposite the direction of the deviation of the chin and of the trapezius and deep neck muscles (splenii) homolateral to this direction. Since the muscles involved vary, it has been emphasized [*Bertrand* et al., 1978] that it is

---

[16] This nucleus and its efferent fibers in the medial longitudinal fasciculus transmit pallidofugal impulses to motor cells in the brain stem and spinal cord.

important to ascertain, by simultaneous bilateral electromyography of all possibly involved muscles, which muscles are the most active. The stereotactic operation on the thalamus must be performed on the side homolateral to the contracting sternocleidomastoid muscle (contralateral to the hyperactive deep neck muscles). In a typical case with the chin deviated to the left side, the sternocleidomastoid muscle contracting on the right side, and the electromyography of the deep neck muscles showing increased discharges on the left side, the guided electrode is inserted into the right thalamus.

Since coagulation of the Voi alone did not have a permanent effect, *Hassler and Dieckmann* [1970] combined its elimination with interruption of the interstitiothalamic fibers, if the head was tilted; or they combined Voi lesions with coagulation of Forel's H_1 bundle against turning of the head to the opposite side. When lesions of the nucleus ventralis oralis extending to interstitiothalamic fibers were insufficient, denervation of the sternocleidomastoid muscle had to be added. Voi thalamotomy was performed by *von Essen* et al. [1980] in patients with mainly horizontal spasmodic torticollis contralateral to the side to which the face had been turning. The improvement appeared very slowly during 6–12 months postoperatively. In cases of spasmodic torticollis, *Bertrand* et al. [1978] combined lesions of the Voi and the pallidum with avulsion of the spinal accessory nerve and/or section of the first cervical nerve and the posterior rami of C2, C3 and C4. Since the Voi lies close to the corticobulbar fibers, the authors avoid bilateral Voi lesions with their danger of pseudobulbar paralysis. *Riechert* [1980] combines resection of the accessory nerve with partial resection of the hypertrophied sternocleidomastoid muscle in spasmodic torticollis patients in poor general condition; a stereotactic procedure is performed only if this does not produce long-lasting results. Intradural section of the anterior roots of the three first cervical nerves is reserved as a last resort.

On stimulation of the *central tegmental tract* [17] homolateral neck muscles contracted [*Sano* et al., 1967a]. Elimination of the inferior olive was performed by *Sano* et al. [1967a] in torticollis. In view of the proximity of the accessory nerve roots, it is not certain that the effect of this *olivotomy* should be related to elimination of this ganglion only.

[17] Fibers descending to the inferior olive chiefly from the pallidum, the zona incerta, the periaqueductal gray, and the nucleus ruber.

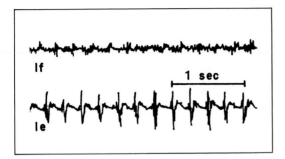

Fig. 44. Electromyograms of antagonistic muscles in paralysis agitans. le, lf = EMGs of left extensor and flexor muscles of fingers. Alternate contractions of antagonists. From *Spiegel and Wycis* [1954]; reproduced with permission.

Mechanisms of Rigidity and Tremor at Rest

The parkinsonian tremor at rest persists after deafferentation of a shaking extremity, while rigidity is reduced or abolished [*Pollock and Davis, 1930*]. Consequently, a central origin of this tremor has to be assumed. Different frequencies were recorded in the face, arm and leg muscles. Apparently, different spinal cord segments have their own different rates of discharge [*Jung, 1941*]. This suggests that the *basic mechanism of the tremor rate* is located in the *spinal cord,* a view shared by *Walker* [1958a, b] and *Hassler* et al. [1979].

Electromyographic studies revealed [particularly *Hoefer and Putnam,* 1940] a *synchronization* of the motor unit discharges innervating a certain muscle group. *Antagonistic* muscle groups, e.g., extensors and flexors, are mostly *alternately innervated* (fig. 44). Apparently the spinal mechanism of reciprocal inhibition of antagonists is also involved, although prolonged recording may show periods with simultaneous contractions of antagonistic muscles [*Spiegel and Wycis,* 1954] (fig. 45).

Furthermore, the *gamma motor fiber-muscle spindle loop* plays a role. The muscle spindle is arranged in parallel with the fibers of the main muscle. In its central part it contains sensory annulospiral and flower spray endings; its polar parts are contractile. If the muscle is passively stretched, these sensory endings are stimulated. The same is accomplished by impulses conducted by the thin, efferent gamma fibers [*Leksell,* 1945] that originate in the small gamma motoneurons and are part of the anterior root. The impulses mediated by the gamma fibers induce contraction of the polar

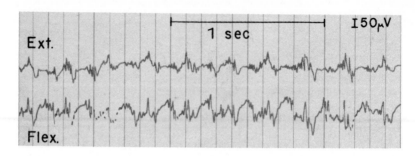

Fig. 45. Electrograms of antagonistic muscles in paralysis agitans. Ext. = Extensors; Flex. = flexors of left forearm. Simultaneous discharges in extensors and flexors. From *Spiegel and Wycis* [1954]; reproduced with permission.

parts of the muscle spindle, which results in stretching of its central part and activation of the sensory endings. Their discharges are conducted to the spinal cord. The afferent fibers synapse partly on the large phasic alpha motoneurons, and partly on the smaller tonic alpha motoneurons [*Granit,* 1957], causing reflex contraction of the muscle (stretch reflex, myotatic reflex). Collaterals terminate on intermediate neurons that inhibit the motoneurons of antagonistic muscles. It seems that these impulses which serve innervation of the posture of various parts of the body inhibit the amplitude of the static tremor, since *deafferentation increases its amplitude.* It should be emphasized that the gamma loop, although important for modifying the tremor, is not essential for the tremor genesis, since the *Parkinson tremor persists after interruption* of the *gamma loop* by section of the posterior roots [*Pollock and Davis, 1930*].

The spinal cord motoneurons are controlled by dopamine, either by the circulating catecholamine or by the substance released by fibers originating in the substantia nigra and descending to the spinal cord. If this inhibitory mechanism is depleted of dopamine by degeneration of the nigra cells or by application of reserpine, the motoneurons of the anterior horn discharge rhythmically, causing the resting tremor. The ability of ganglion cells to emit rhythmic discharges can be found already in invertebrates, e.g., in the ganglion cells of crustacea [*Walter,* 1959]. The gamma loop mechanism is influenced by *supraspinal* centers. A facilitating as well as an inhibitory effect of the motor cortex [*Granit and Kaada,* 1952] and the pyramidal tract [*Kato,* 1964] was recorded. On stimulation of the substantia nigra, *Wagner* [1964] and *Hassler* [1972] reported acceleration of the activity of the gamma fibers on stimulation of the caudal half and inhibition on stimulation of the anterior third of the substantia nigra. Stimulation of the ventro-lateral area of the thalamus inhibited the discharges of the gamma muscle spindle system in cats, according to *Stern and Ward* [1960]. *Langfitt* et al. [1963], however, demonstrated inhibition as well as facilitation of gamma motoneuron activity on stimulation of the thalamus (chiefly ventrolateral area) and of the globus pallidus in cats. Small doses of pentobarbital abolished the spontaneous gamma activity in some experiments.

In these cases inhibition from thalamic stimulation was often converted to facilitation. The level of spontaneous activity was more important than the level of anesthesia in determining the qualitative response obtained (facilitation when the spontaneous activity was depressed). Another factor determining the type of response is the frequency of the stimuli applied [*Narabayashi,* 1963; *Hongo* et al., 1963]. While low frequency of stimulation inhibited the spindle mechanism, the inhibition gradually changed to facilitation on increase of the stimulus frequency.

Stern and Ward [1960] failed to obtain an influence of thalamic stimulation on the gamma spindle system after ablation of the motor cortex in acute experiments in cats. *Langfitt* et al. [1963], however, found such reactions preserved after degeneration of the internal capsule in chronically decorticated cats. This is in agreement with the experiences of *Spuler* et al. [1962] regarding the persistence of the modifying effect of stimulation of the ventrolateral thalamus upon the mesencephalic tegmental tremor despite degeneration of the fibers descending from the sigmoid gyri, the frontal lobe and the pallidum.

Resting tremor apparently is a pathological modification of the normal static innervation. It could be shown [*Folkerts and Spiegel,* 1953] that on prolonged stimulation of the mesencephalic tegmentum a tonic reaction, e.g. the extension of a forelimb changed into a tremor. In mammals, the spinal cord is not sufficient to sustain the static innervation, and additional circuits in the reticular formation of the brain stem participate in its maintenance. In cats it was shown by *Bernis and Spiegel* [1925] that the rigor of decerebrate rigidity, the highest degree of pathological increase of the static innervation, is not abolished by lesions of the vestibular nuclei. A complete relaxation of the skeletal muscles could be obtained only if the lesion encroached upon the rhombencephalic reticular formation. It was concluded by *Bernis and Spiegel* [1925] and *Spiegel* [1927] and similarly over two decades later, by *Magoun and Rhines* [1948] that, besides the spinal myotatic reflexes, the *reflex activity of the reticular formation plus that of the vestibular nuclei* maintain the static innervation.

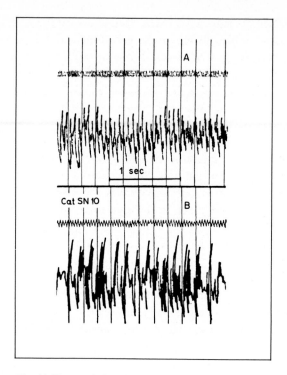

Fig. 46. Tremor induced by stimulation of the mesencephalic tegmentum of a cat. Electromyogram of the right triceps on stimulation of the center of the right substantia reticularis (level of the posterior part of the colliculus inferior). The experiment shows the influence of the frequency of stimulation on the frequency of the tremor. *A* At stimulus frequency of 50 Hz, tremor frequency 16 Hz. *B* At stimulus frequency of 30 Hz, tremor frequency 7 Hz. Pulse duration: 1 ms, voltage: 10 V, equal in *A* and *B*. From *Folkerts and Spiegel* [1953].

One may suspect, therefore, that, in addition to the spinal cord, the reticular formation of the brain stem participates in the innervation of resting tremor. On stimulation of the *mesencephalic tegmentum* of cats, a tremor was observed by *Spiegel* et al. [1953], studied in more detail by *Folkerts and Spiegel* [1953; presented at the Amsterdam Neurological Association on June 15, 1953] and noted independently by *Jenkner and Ward* [1953] in monkeys. The frequency of this 'tegmental tremor' often lagged behind that of the stimuli (fig. 46). Up to frequencies of 18 Hz it was usually equal to or half of the simulation frequency. At higher frequencies, it corresponded to half the stimulus frequency or showed still lower values [*Alexander* et al., 1960].

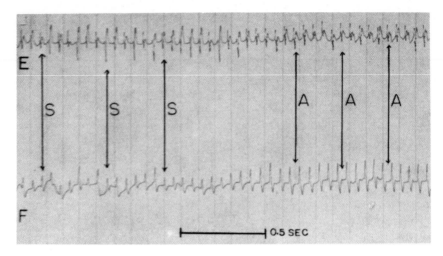

Fig. 47. Stimulation of the left mesencephalic tegmentum of a cat whose left bra-chium conjunctivum had been destroyed electrolytically 3 weeks previously. Stimuli: 5-ms pulses, at 6 V, 20 Hz. Left brachium conjunctivum found completely degenerated on his-tologic examination. Electromyogram of extensor carpi ulnaris (E) and of flexor carpi radialis (F) of left forearm; note simultaneous (S) as well as alternate (A) discharges of antagonistic muscles. From *Wycis* et al. [1957].

Frequencies higher than 5–6 Hz, of course, are not related to parkinso-nian tremor at rest; but one of the characteristics of that tremor, *alternate contractions* of agonistic and antagonistic muscles, can be found in mesen-cephalic tremor [*Wycis* et al., 1957] (fig. 47) between periods of simulta-neous contraction that are demonstrable in some cases of parkinsonian tre-mor also [documented by *Spiegel and Wycis,* 1954]. Tremor with synchro-nization of reciprocal motor unit discharges resulting from stimulation of the pontine reticular formation was also observed by *Aronson* et al. [1962] in monkeys. Such a tremor could no longer be induced after decerebrate rigidity had been produced by bilateral coagulation of the midbrain and ventral thalamus. A similarity between the mesencephalic tegmental tremor and the parkinsonian tremor can be found in the reaction of both types to pallidal stimulation or stimulation of the ventrolateral area of the thala-mus.

Degeneration of the brachium conjunctivum [*Wycis* et al., 1957] (fig. 47), of fibers descending from the pallidum and from the frontal lobe including the motor cortex also did not prevent the mesencephalic tegmen-tal tremor. It seems, therefore, probable that this tremor is due to stimula-

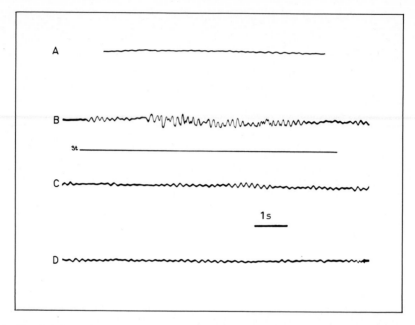

Fig. 48. Stimulation of the right mesencephalic tegmentum (dorsomedial area) of a parkinsonian patient. Photoelectric record of the movements of the left index finger. *A–D* Continuous record; St = stimulation (Harvard stimulator, exponential pulses 0.05 ms, 60 Hz, 10 V. From *Spiegel and Wycis* [1958]; reproduced with permission.

tion of cells of the reticular formation. The finding that the mesencephalic tremor can be evoked despite degeneration of the descending pallidofugal fibers does not exclude that one may consider the mesencephalic reticular formation and its descending axons, at least partly, as belonging to the pallidofugal, tremor facilitating system. Figure 48 shows a tremor of 6 Hz induced by stimulation of the dorsomedial part of the mesencephalic tegmentum in a Parkinson patient.

In monkeys with tremor at rest similar to the parkinsonian tremor produced by experimental lesions in the ventromedial part of the mesencephalic tegmentum [*Ward* et al., 1948; *Cordeau* et al., 1960; *Gybels,* 1963] unit discharges synchronous with the tremor could be recorded from various parts of the cerebrum. These regions were: the motor and somatosensory area [*Gybels,* 1963], preponderantly of the opposite cortex [*Cordeau* et al., 1960], the lenticular nucleus (probably pallidum and putamen) [*Cordeau,* 1961], the posterior limb of the internal capsule, and the nucleus ventralis posterolateralis of the thalamus [*Lamarre and Cordeau,* 1962]. In interpreting these observations one has to bear in mind that passive movements of a limb, e.g. of the forepaw of a cat, may induce unit discharges in various parts of the central nervous system, for instance in the pallidum [unpublished experiments with *Szekely*]. *Lamarre and Cordeau* [1962] found that some units in the contralateral sensorimotor cortex, internal capsule and lentiform body kept on firing in the lull periods between the tremor episodes in the absence of visible tremor. These interesting observations, however, do not prove with certainty the existence of a pacemaker for the tremor in one or another of the above-mentioned areas, because in these experiments electromyograms were not recorded. Our observations in Parkinson patients have shown that rhythmic discharges in some muscles may still be recorded in the absence of visible tremor. Thus, it cannot be excluded that in some of these experiments the rhythmic unit discharges observed in various central areas were caused by afferent impulses from rhythmically contracting muscles fibers which did not induce a visible tremor.

It is important, therefore, that rhythmic activity could also be recorded from the motor cortex of shaking monkeys after they were paralyzed by Flaxedil [*Lamarre and Cordeau,* 1962, 1964]. Thus, some central rhythms can persist in the absence of afferent impulses from shaking muscles, and this possibility should not be denied for those ventral thalamic nuclei from which a 4–5 Hz rhythm was recorded in Parkinson patients [*Albe-Fessard* et al., 1963; *Jasper and Bertrand,* 1964]. *Albe-Fessard* et al. [1966] assume that the latter nuclei play an important, if not a major, role in the control of muscular tremors.

It is difficult, however, to accept the view that this area represents a pacemaker for the rate of discharges of the tremor producing neurons for all parts of the body, since different tremor rates were observed, e.g., in the arms and in the legs of Parkinson patients [*Jung,* 1941]. This objection to the concept of a pacemaker of the tremor rate in all parts of the body does not mean, however, that supramedullary centers are not important in triggering or modulating (facilitating or inhibiting) the rhythmic discharges of the spinal motoneurons maintaining the static tremor. In order to clarify the concepts of tremor production, it may be useful to distinguish (1) basic tremorogenic mechanisms located in various spinal segments and serving as their own pacemakers from supramedullary (2) triggering or facilitating or (3) inhibiting centers.

In the spinal mechanism three components can be differentiated: the rhythmic discharges of the motoneurons, the reciprocal inhibition of antagonists responsible for alternate contraction of antagonistic muscle groups, and the modulating influence of the gamma loop.

The main facilitating cell groups and tracts are the pallidum, parts of the ventrolateral nucleus (nucleus ventralis oralis) and the premotor cortex which discharges, at least partly, through the motor cortex (area 4) and the pyramidal tract. On stimulation of the pallidum a latent parkinsonian tremor may become manifest or an existing parkinsonian or an experimental tremor may become augmented. Since pallidofugal impulses reach the mesencephalic tegmentum, the reticular formation of the mesencephalic tegmentum may be part of the facilitating pallidofugal system. Interestingly, interruption of the *pyramidal tract* usually abolishes the Parkinson tremor, while volitional innervation suppresses it. Perhaps an explanation of this paradox may be found in the fact that, on volitional innervation, the cerebellum becomes activated by way of the brachia pontis, and that an inhibitory influence of the cerebellum upon tremor mechanisms is rather probable. It should be emphasized that the facilitating *pyramidal impulses* are *dispensable* for tremor maintenance, at least in some instances. There are reports of persistence of static tremor despite lesions of the posterior part of the internal capsule inducing hemiplegia [*Dierssen* et al., 1962], of the pyramidal tract [*Davison*, 1942], or destruction of the cerebral peduncle [*Mettler* et al., 1947].

An *inhibitory function* of the *substantia nigra* is indicated by the experience that degeneration of its cells in paralysis agitans [*Trétiakoff*, 1919] and parkinsonism [particularly *Hassler*, 1972] or interruption of its efferent fibers by lesions in the ventromedial part of the mesencephalic tegmentum [see chapter on Substantia nigra, p. 118] is associated with appearance of tremor and rigor, which are apparently release phenomena. The experience that application of *L*-dopa, the product of the nigra cells, reduces or suppresses an existing tremor in Parkinson patients, points in the same direction.

A relation of the *cerebellum* to the tremor mechanism is suggested by experimental experiences. Coagulation of the dentate and interposed nuclei could produce ataxic and static tremor in the primate [*Carrea and Mettler*, 1941], and a lesion of the ventral, crossed, ascending limb of the brachium conjunctivum induced tremor without ataxia [*Carrea and Mettler*, 1955]. Stimulation of the ventrolateral nucleus of the thalamus with 60-Hz pulses in monkeys was able to produce tremor only if the animals were stimulated after cerebellectomy [*Narabayashi* et al., 1974]. These observations point to an *inhibitory cerebellar influence* upon tremorogenic circuits. It may be objected that dentate stimulation in cats induced an increase of the amplitude of a tegmental tremor, while the effect on tremor frequency was variable. The frequency of the dentate stimulation usually was 24 Hz and occasionally up to 60 Hz [*Alexander* et al., 1959]. It would be interesting to ascertain whether higher frequencies applied to the dentate nucleus would have an inhibitory effect, in view of the reversal of the effect of cerebellar stimulation on muscular hypertension observed in decerebrate cats on alteration of the stimulus frequencies from low to high rates. Since opposite effects (facilitation or inhibition) may be observed on stimulation of various areas depending on the stimulus frequency applied, it seems that, in many instances, a more definite concept of the normal function of an area can be obtained by the study of its elimination than by stimulation experiments.

In contrast to the *parkinsonian* tremor, its *rigidity* is a reflex phenomenon. As already mentioned, it is reduced or abolished by deafferentation of a rigid extremity. A very high gamma activity in the rigidity of decerebration induced by intercollicular midbrain section of cats has been demonstrated by *Granit* [1957]. The hyperactive gamma loop maintains an excessive reflex excitation of the tonic motoneurons, so that increased tonic stretch reflexes result. It was pointed out in the discussion of the tremor mechanism that the maintenance of the static innervation of higher mammals and of man requires supraspinal reflex arcs, activation of reticulospinal neurons [*Bernis and Spiegel*, 1925] by collaterals of the ventral spinocerebellar tract, and of vestibulospinal neurons by the labyrinth. According to *Granit* [1957] the reticular formation of the brain stem has a particularly strong effect upon the gamma loop.

Since cocainization of peripheral nerves selectively eliminates the activity of the gamma fibers [*Leksell,* 1945] and abolishes the stretch reflex of decerebrate cats as well as the rigidity of paralysis agitans [*Matthews and Rushworth,* 1957], it has been assumed that this rigidity depends on the activity of the *gamma loop.* Furthermore, since pallidoansotomy reduces or abolishes parkinsonian rigidity [*Spiegel and Wycis,* 1954], it is tempting to postulate that the pallidum maintains the rigor by sending efferent impulses to the gamma loop by way of the reticular formation of the brain stem. Thus, a *pallidorubroreticulospinal system* induces the increased activity of the gamma loop that results in rigidity.

The experience that the parkinsonian rigidity can be abolished not only by pallidotomy, but also by *ventrolateral thalamotomy,* was explained by

Hassler et al. [1979] by interruption of a pallidothalamocortical system facilitating the gamma loop that maintains the muscular hypertension. A system was demonstrated, however, that apparently originates in the ventrolateral area of the thalamus and can facilitate the activity of the mesencephalic and oral pontine reticular formation despite degeneration of the corticofugal fibers descending from the frontal lobe including the motor area [*Spuler* et al., 1962] (fig. 63). Furthermore, facilitation of the gamma loop by ventrolateral thalamic stimulation [*Langfitt* et al., 1963] was obtained despite degeneration of these corticofugal fibers, suggesting that an interpretation of the favorable effects of ventrolateral thalamotomy upon parkinsonian rigidity should also consider a *pallidothalamoreticulospinal system* descending to the gamma loop and functioning independently of the motor cortex.

Circuits Possibly Related to Relief of Pain and Spasticity by Posterior Column Stimulation

The relief obtained in spasticity and pain by posterior column stimulation (PCS) is poorly understood. (The problem has been discussed in detail by *Spiegel* [1982]; here it is outlined, in a modified form, with permission of the American Medical Association, copyright owner.)

Regarding *spasticity,* there are a number of observations indicating an effect upon spinal activity. In decerebrate cats an inhibition of monosynaptic reflexes of lumbar muscles was obtained on spinal stimulation [*Krainick* et al., 1977; *Siegfried* et al., 1978]. In such preparations PCS decreased the firing frequency of lumbar motoneurons and increased that of Renshaw cells [*Siegfried* et al., 1978]. An activation of pathways in dorsal and ventral quadrants of the cord was recorded by *Bantli* et al. [1975]. In patients in whom PCS was performed, a decrease of the H reflex was recorded [*Krainick* et al., 1977].

Although an influence of PCS on spinal cord activity has been established, one has to bear in mind that the maintenance of the postural innervation in mammals, which is increased in human spasticity, depends not only on spinal myotatic reflexes, but also on supraspinal mechanisms, particularly vestibular reflexes and rhombencephalic reflexes transmitted by collaterals of the ventral spinocerebellar tract to reticulospinal fibers [*Bernis and Spiegel*, 1925; *Spiegel,* 1927]. In their discussion of dorsal cord stimulation in spastic movement disorders, *Siegfried* et al. [1978] arrived at a

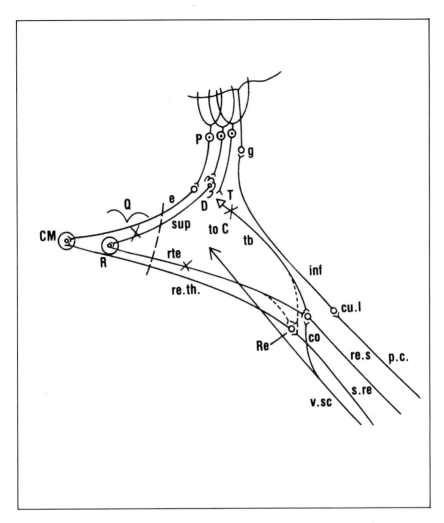

Fig. 49. Circuits possibly involved in the relief of pain and of muscular hypertension in spasticity on posterior column stimulation. C = Cerebellum; CM = centrum medianum (as representative of the thalamic endings of the spinoreticulothalamic system); co = collateral; cu.l = lateral cuneate nucleus; D = dentate nucleus; e = fibers from nucleus emboliformis to CM; g = granular cell; inf = inferior cerebellar peduncle; P = Purkinje cell; p.c. = posterior column; Q = corpora quadrigemina; R = nucleus ruber; Re = reticular formation; re.s = reticulospinal fibers; rte = rubrotegmental tract; re.th. = reticulothalamic tract; s.re = spinoreticular tract; sup = superior cerebellar peduncle; T = nucleus tecti; tb = tectobulbar tract, v.sc = ventral spinocerebellar tract; - - - - = hypothetical collaterals; – – – = decerebrating cut; × = partially or chiefly crossing fibers. From *Spiegel* [1982]; reproduced (with modifications) with permission.

similar conclusion. Despite their findings of the above-mentioned effects of PCS, they state that the mechanisms of dorsal cord stimulation on spasticity are not yet elucidated; 'it seems that a supraspinal mechanism must be involved'.

The stimulating electrodes were placed at the midthoracic or higher levels on PCS, so that chiefly the cuneate fasciculus was stimulated. It is attempted here to outline circuits that may serve as the anatomical basis of this supraspinal mechanism.

As shown by figure 49, impulses that relieve *spasticity* may use fibers of the posterior column carrying A beta fibers and synapsing in the nucleus cuneatus lateralis; axons of this nucleus (dorsal superficial arcuate fibers) joining the inferior peduncle of the cerebellum reach the granular cells of the cerebellar cortex. In its anterior lobe, impulses inhibiting the static innervation are activated [*Loewenthal and Horsley,* 1897; *Sherrington,* 1898]. The further path is represented by axons of the Purkinje cells that reach the deep cerebellar nuclei; from here impulses are conducted partly by the superior cerebellar peduncle to the nucleus ruber and thence to the reticular formation of the rhombencephalon by rubrotegmental fibers, partly by the fastigio-(tecto-)bulbar tract that is adjacent to the inner aspect of the restiform body to the same area. The existence of this second pathway is indicated by the experience that stimulation of the anterior lobe of the cerebellum induces inhibition of the extensor tone of the arm (flexion) in decerebrate cats, even if the superior cerebellar peduncles are interrupted by a cut behind the posterior colliculi, and that this inhibitory effect is abolished by section of the inferior cerebellar peduncle [*Spiegel,* 1927]. The rubrotegmental and the tecto-(fastigio-)tegmental (bulbar) tract modify the above-mentioned reflex arc centered in the reticular formation. There is an activation or inhibition according to the frequency of the stimuli [*Moruzzi,* 1950] applied to the anterior lobe.

The *relief of chronic pain* obtained on stimulation of the posterior column [*Shealy* et al., 1967; *Nashold and Friedman,* 1972] was explained by *Hillman and Wall* [1969] by assuming that such stimulation induces impulses that are antidromically conducted and enter the dorsal horn of the spinal cord using collaterals of the posterior column fibers. It was postulated that these impulses inhibit cells of the dorsal horn receiving pain impulses by means of C fibers. This theory cannot explain, however, the observation [*Friedman* et al., 1974] that the perception of stimuli such as pin pricks is preserved during posterior column stimulation, since the descending impulses would block all pain impulses entering the posterior horn. It seemed necessary, therefore, to consider other possible explanations. The possibility that endorphins may be released by impulses ascending in the posterior columns and reaching the hypothalamus is discussed on page 58. The action of endorphins, however, would not be restricted to alleviation of chronic pain.

Experiences in multiple sclerosis have shown that stimulation of the posterior column may have a triple effect: it may ameliorate chronic pain and spasticity and improve the cerebellar ataxia [*Cook and Weinstein,* 1973]. Another possible mechanism explaining the beneficial effect of posterior column stimulation, therefore, may deserve consideration; it explains by one ascending path the effects on spasticity, pain and cerebellar ataxia: relief of pain by impulses ascending in the posterior column in the conventional way and reaching the cerebellar cortex as outlined above. These ascending fibers apparently are identical with those that may reduce muscular hypertonus in spasticity.

Cerebellofugal fibers originating in the Purkinje cells again reach the deep cerebellar nuclei. The latter send impulses by way of the superior cerebellar peduncle not only to the midbrain, but also to the diencephalon. Particularly the CM, where the paleospinoreticulothalamic pain system partly ends, receives fibers from the nucleus emboliformis [*Hassler,* 1950]. Thus, ascending impulses generated by stimulation of the posterior columns could activate not only cerebellofugal fibers modifying the static innervation, but also cerebellofugal tracts influencing the endings of the spinoreticulothalamic pain system. This would be an analogy to the striatum that is able not only to inhibit motor activity but also potentials evoked in the CM by peripheral pain receptors [see p. 56]. Cerebellar inhibition reaching the CM-intralaminar nuclei-nucleus parafascicularis complex would not interfere with the perception of stimuli such as pin pricks, since it is known that elimination of this nuclear group [*Mark* et al., 1963] relieves chronic pain, but does not prevent the perception of acute sensory stimuli.

There is a second possibility for transmission of inhibitory cerebellar impulses to the pain conducting spinoreticulothalamic system: collaterals of the rubrotegmental tract and of the tecto-(fastigio-)bulbar tract that inhibit or modulate the tonus-maintaining reflex arc in the reticular formation may also reach the synapses between the spinoreticular and the reticulothalamic pain tracts. The existence of these collaterals, however, is hypothetical. Evoked potential studies will have to ascertain whether such a second system exists. The final proof of a cerebellar pain-inhibiting system also will depend on such studies. At present, at least the above-mentioned observation can be offered in support of the cerebellar system outlined herein: posterior column stimulation not only relieved pain as well as spasticity, but also improved the patient's cerebellar ataxia.

Vegetative Effects

Apparently due to the fiber connections of the *dorsomedial nuclei* with the hypothalamus, lesions of the former nuclei produce some vegetative effects [*Spiegel and Wycis,* 1962]: hyperphagia (marked in 10% of the cases) inducing increase in weight, variable, transient changes in basal metabolism (decrease or increase), occasional transitory drop of blood pressure; there appeared in a few cases a transient decrease of postprandial hyperglycemia [*Shay,* 1962], occasionally transient impairment of the eosinophil response to stress [*Perloff* et al., 1952], transient hypertonicity [*Conger,* 1962] and incontinence of the urinary bladder in about 25% of the cases.

Stimulation of the efferent fibers of the *hypothalamus* passing through the prerubral region [*Spiegel* et al., 1964b] produced mydriasis, vasomotor reactions (vasodilatation from some points, vasoconstriction from others (fig. 50); the vasomotor reactions as well as the heart rate varied with the stimulus frequency; occasionally there appeared arrhythmia, ECG changes (fig. 51), and a galvanic skin reaction (fig. 52). Similar observations were reported by *French* et al. [1962] on stimulation of subthalamic areas and by *Sano* et al. [1967b]. They were related by the latter author to stimulation of the posterior hypothalamus, but his figures suggest that they were obtained from FH. Lesions of FH [*Carmel,* 1968] induced homolateral miosis, ptosis, hemianhidrosis. Pupillary dilatation could be obtained on stimulation of parts of the thalamus, subthalamus and also of the mesencephalic tegmentum [*Nashold,* 1967].

Inhibition of *respiration* was elicited on stimulation of the anterior nucleus [*Spiegel and Wycis,* 1962], of the ventrolateral nucleus [*Siegfried and Wiesendanger,* 1967], of the internal capsule and rostral cerebral peduncle [*Hassler* et al., 1965], while stimulation of the subthalamus [*French* et al., 1962] produced shallow respiration. Suppression of *perspiration* and of *oiliness* of the skin resulted from implantation of crystals of atropine sulfate into the *ventrolateral nucleus* [*Velasco-Suarez* and *Escobedo,* 1967]. Stimulation of the *nucleus ventralis oralis internus* [*Hassler* et al., 1965] induced vasodilatation in the face.

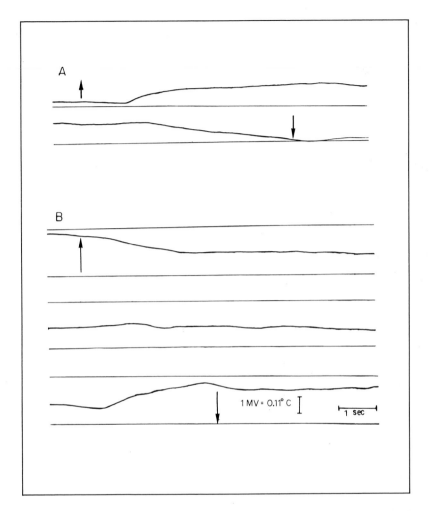

Fig. 50. Parkinson patient. *A* Vasodilatation. Stimulating electrode in front of left nucleus ruber (zero level, anteromedial direction of the stimulating stylet). Stimulation (DC, 10 mA) between arrows. Top and lower records are continuous. (These records are from patients with extrapyramidal disorders.) *B* Vasoconstriction. Electrode 2 mm deeper than in *A*. Same stimulation parameters (between arrows). The three records are continuous. For recording changes of the blood flow in the extremities, a thermistor (Fenwal GB 32P8) is placed lightly on the finger, hand or foot. The thermistor forms one part of a Wheatstone bridge that is supplied by a 1.5 V dry cell; the output of the bridge is connected to the polygraph (Grass). When room and body temperatures are constant, changes in skin temperature vary with the blood flow. The circuit was calibrated at temperatures between 36 and 37 °C. Upward (downward) deflection by 1 mV indicate increase (decrease) of skin temperature by 0.11 °C. From *Spiegel* et al. [1964b]; reproduced with permission.

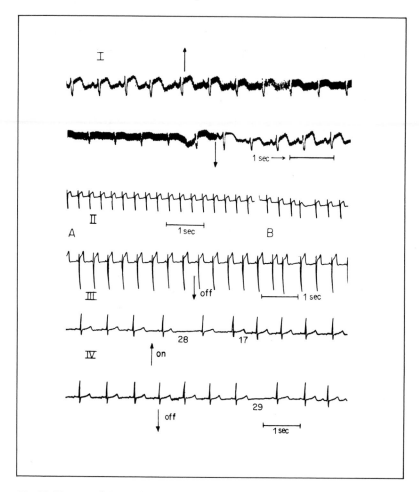

Fig. 51. Changes of the EKG of a Parkinson patient. I: Stimulation (between arrows) of the left Forel field, level of intercommissural line (2-ms pulses, 100 Hz, 8 V). Recording electrodes in this and following records: 5th left intercostal space to right arm. Depression of QRS complex and of T wave. The two records are continuous. II: Appearance of extrasystole. A = EKG before, B = 10 s after production of lesion of the right Forel field at 4 mm below intercommissural line, lateral to nucleus ruber. III: Appearance of extrasystole 2 s after stimulation (5-ms pulses, 4 Hz, 1.5 mA) of the left Forel field (2 mm above intercommissural line in front of nucleus ruber). IV: Appearance of wandering pacemaker during stimulation. Arrows indicate onset and end of stimulation (2-ms pulses, 100 Hz, 10 V) of Forel's field (level of intercommissural line, lateral to nucleus ruber). Note varying distances between QRS complexes during and following stimulation. These intervals are indicated, in several places, in millimeters (28, 17, 29) as measured in the original tracing. Same source as figure 50.

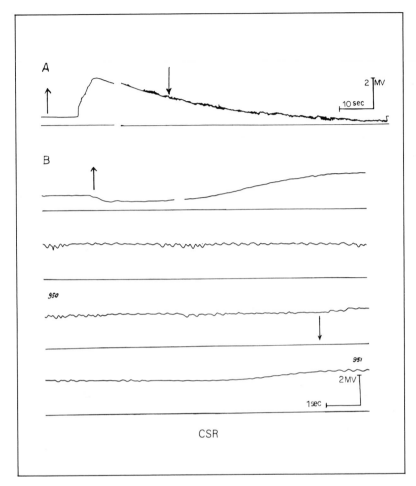

Fig. 52. Galvanic skin reaction recorded from palmar and dorsal aspect of left foot of a Parkinson patient. *A* Stimulating electrode in front of right nucleus ruber, level of inter-commissural line. Note that the reaction terminates during flow of current (DC, 10 mA, between arrows). *B* Stimulating electrode in front of nucleus ruber, 4 mm below intercom-missural line. Reaction persists after cessation of flow of current (DC, 10 mA, between arrows). The four records are continuous. Same source as figure 50.

Other vegetative symptoms observed on *thalamic stimulation* (no spe-cial localization given) were similar to those noted for *pallidal stimulation* (dilatation of the pupils, respiratory changes, anxiety, feeling of constric-tion) [*Riechert*, 1980]. After introduction of an electrode into the *nucleus ventrolateralis, Bechterewa* [1969] observed a slowing of the pulse, decrease of arterial pressure and hyperhidrosis. On electric stimulation with pulse frequencies of 25–50 Hz, there were fluctuations of the blood pressure (apparently sometimes increase of pressure) and increase of the skin temperature, chiefly on the contralateral cheek and thorax.

As to an influence of the *caudate nucleus* upon the vegetative nervous system, we have to depend on animal experiments. The effects of electrical stimulation of the caudate nucleus reported in the older literature were mostly due to spread to the internal capsule. Following degeneration of this structure, effects upon smooth muscle organs such as the pupil or the blood vessels, on caudate stimulation in cats, were no longer observed [*Spiegel and Takano,* 1929]. One also has to exclude the possibility of a spread of the stimulating current to the septum [*Laursen,* 1961a, b, 1962a, b]. If lesions of the caudate nucleus are produced, involvement of the septum may also be a complicating factor. *Heath* et al. [1954] observed metabolic and gastrointestinal disorders following lesions at the base of the septum (initial increase, then drop of the blood sugar, drop of the serum Na^+, increase of the serum K^+, rapid loss of weight, refusal to eat, appearance of hemorrhages and ulcerations in the duodenum and colon, drop of the red and white blood count, and development of adrenocortical hyperplasia). The lesions, however, were not limited to the septum, but involved more or less the medioventral aspect of the caudate nucleus. The combination of caudate and septal lesions induced effects different from those of punctures limited to the striatum. In *Heath's* cats poikilothermia and drop of the body temperature were observed, while fever appears after puncture of the caudate nucleus.

An effect of caudate stimulation upon the *liver* (increase of its positive potentials) was noted in cats (fig. 53); it could still be observed after degeneration of the fibers of the internal capsule descending from the sigmoid gyri and the frontal lobe [*Spiegel* et al., 1963a]. Furthermore, these effects could still be elicited even though large lesions had been placed in the septal area preceding the stimulation. These effects are conducted to the liver by way of the hypothalamus and the splanchnic nerves. They seem to be in close relationship to the mechanism of *temperature regulation.* It may be recalled that the increase of body temperature due to puncture of the caudate nucleus [*Aronsohn and Sachs,* 1885; *Richet,* 1884] or due to infection largely depends on an increase of the liver temperature [*Hirsch and Müller,* 1903]. The experiments of *Spiegel* et al. [1963a] showed that the increase of liver potentials on striatal stimulation is accompanied by an increase of liver temperature (fig. 54). These liver reactions were preserved after lesions of

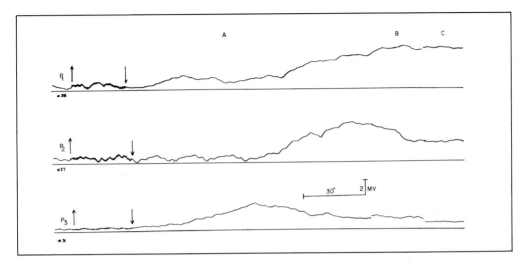

Fig. 53. Effect of caudate stimulation upon liver potentials of a cat. Various types of changes of DC potentials (P_1–P_3) of the liver on stimulation of the caudate nucleus. Stimuli: 10-ms pulses, 30 Hz, 15 V. Time interval between *A* and *B:* 40 s; same interval between *B* and *C*. Upward deflection in all graphs means positive. From *Spiegel* et al. [1963a]; reproduced with permission.

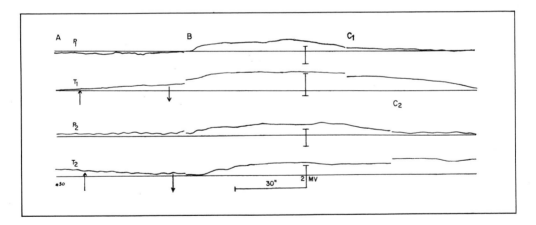

Fig. 54. Effect of stimulation of the left caudate nucleus of a cat upon the liver potentials (P_1, P_2) and the liver temperature (T_1, T_2) before (P_1, T_1) and after (P_2, T_2) extensive lesion of the left amygdala. Stimuli parameters: 10-ms pulses, 30 Hz, 15 V. The temperature was recorded by thermistors inserted into the liver close to the potential recording unpolarizable electrodes. Time intervals between *A* and *B*, 22 s; between *B* and *C1*, 64 s; between *B* and *C2*, 48 s; calibration: 2 mV = 0.4 °C. Same source as figure 53.

the pallidum or of the amygdala; they were prevented by combined lesions of these two ganglia.

Inhibition of sweat secretion [*Freeman and Krasno,* 1940] and the related inhibition of the galvanic skin reaction [*Wang and Brown,* 1956] probably are also part of the influence of the caudatum upon temperature regulation. The inhibitory effect of the striatum upon the galvanic skin reaction is further illustrated by the finding that this reaction is very marked in thalamic cats but weak in striatal cats [*Wang and Akert,* 1962].

Further vegetative effects of caudate puncture are *polyuria* [*Spiegel and Reynolds,* 1930] and increased output of salt in the urine [*Tokay,* 1931, upon my suggestion]. Retching, vomiting and refusal to eat observed for several days after coagulation of the caudatum or putamen [*Rosvold and Delgado,* 1956] probably are irritation phenomena, since on prolonged stimulation of the caudate nucleus by injection of alumina cream the cats also ceased to eat and drink [*Spiegel and Szekely,* 1961]. There appeared also inhibition of bladder contraction on caudate stimulation [*Freeman and Krasno,* 1940].

Pallidotomy induced vasodilatation in the skin, according to *Narabayashi* [1962]. *Bechterewa* [1969, p. 129] failed to find definite changes of skin temperature on stimulation of the globus pallidus or after placing electrolytic lesions in this ganglion. In the same monograph [p. 140], however, she reported that in one patient electrolysis of the left medial pallidum was followed by hyperemia of the opposite, later also of the homolateral cheek. Furthermore, after introduction of the electrode into the pallidum there appeared an increase of arterial pressure, extrasystoles, hyperhidrosis (more contralaterally than homolaterally, most marked on the 6th and 7th postoperative day). Electric stimulation at a frequency of 50 Hz induced decrease of the arterial pressure, chiefly on the same side. In *Riechert's* [1980] experience, besides mydriasis and inhibition of respiration, alert patients had a feeling of *constriction in the chest* and *anxiety* on pallidal stimulation; a few complained of a feeling of impending death.

The effect of basal ganglia operations in *Parkinson patients upon the vegetative system,* particularly respiration, the vascular system, the cerebral circulation and oxygenation was demonstrated by *Schmidt* [1966]. The vegetative symptoms induced by excitation or lesions of the ventrolateral thalamic nucleus and of the internal pallidum seem to be only partly due to an influence upon efferent fibers from these ganglia, since an edema of the oral hypothalamus was described after introduction of the electrodes into the pallidum or ventrolateral nucleus. Following extensive *hypothalamic lesions, Bechterewa* [1969] experienced irreversible vegetative signs and symptoms (loss of appetite, increased thirst, tachycardia, hypotonia, leukopenia, decubitus, cachexia). *Spiegel and Wycis* [1953] avoided such complications by placing only small lesions into the hypothalamus.

The anatomic basis for vegetative effects appearing on stimulation of the *amygdala* is the existence of amygdalohypothalamic fibers, chiefly in the stria terminalis, in ventral amygdalohypothalamic connections and connections with the fornix by way of the hippocampus. Stimulation of the amygdala [*Chapman,* 1960] elicited bilateral mydriasis, tachycardia, pallor, increase of blood pressure, respiratory changes, chiefly apnea, and occasional hyperhidrosis. Apparently these effects are, at least partly, humorally transmitted, since the rise of the blood pressure outlasts the stimulation. In *Kim and Umbach's* [1973] experience, visceromotor effects could be elicited from most parts of the amygdala, but the central part was the most reactive. The plasma cortisol level increased markedly.

A significant increase of total gastric secretion was observed by *Rama-murthi* et al. [1977] on stimulation of the amygdala and chiefly of the lateral hypothalamus. 2 h after lesion of these areas the gastric acid secretion fell below the initial value. Plasma corticosteroids were increased on stimulation of the amygdala and decreased on hippocampal stimulation [*Rubin* et al., 1966]. Confusion, fright or euphoria, amnesia and fumbling movements accompanied the vegetative changes. The finding of after-discharges not only in the amygdala, but also in the scalp [*Chatrian and Chapman,* 1960] suggested a spread of the excitation to other areas, particularly the cortex.

The hypothalamus receives hippocampal fibers by way of the *fornix,* especially postcommissural fibers of this latter structure. The vegetative effects observed by *Riechert's* school on stimulation of the fornix were summarized by *Umbach* [1966]. Weak stimulation at frequencies below 3 Hz produced miosis, bradycardia, deepening of respiration, nausea, confusion, drowsiness, occasionally psychomotor attacks, anxiety, olfactory and gustatory hallucinations. At stimulus frequencies from 25 to 50 Hz there appeared arousal, desynchronization of the EEG, anxiety, tachycardia, extrasystoles, rise of blood pressure, sweating, a subjective sensation of warmth, later pallor of the face, feeling of cold, and vomiting. Weak and short stimulation tended to accelerate the respiration, strong stimulation resulted in apnea and general convulsions.

From a small area at the *lower medial quadrant of the frontal lobe, Kelly* et al. [1973] obtained autonomic changes, particularly respiratory inhibition. Stimulation of the *cingulate gyrus* or the *cingulum* elicited mainly autonomic and emotional responses. The observations of *Pool and Ranso-hoff* [1949], who noted autonomic effects on stimulation of the rostral portion of the cingulate gyrus, were extended by *Meyer* et al. [1973] who reported acute stimulation of the cingulum, and by *Escobedo* et al. [1973] who described chronic stimulation of the cingulum in patients with behavior disorders; their electrodes remained in place for a period of 2–3 weeks during which time stimulation and recording were done. *Meyer* et al. [1973] noted nausea, fear or pleasure, movements (rubbing the face, lip smacking), similar to automatisms in temporal lobe epilepsy, dysphasia or aphasia, change in the rate or volume of speech, akinetic mutism, perseveration (repetition of numbers or phrases), confusion, amnesia, generalized seizures, paresthesias or pain. In *Escobedo's* patients, the stimulation produced vegetative responses (increase of blood pressure, inhibition of respiration, swallowing, sensations of hunger, but no perceptible change in pulse rate), yawning, closing of the eyes, restlessness, confusion, auditory and taste hallucinations, abnormal feelings ('as if I were blind'), sleepiness, negativism, screaming, or psychomotor activity. He assumes that the gyrus cinguli and cingulum affect behavior through an influence over other structures of the limbic system, the temporal lobe, hypothalamus, thalamus and frontal lobe.

Afferent Mechanisms

Thalamic Inputs and Projections

The afferent and efferent relations of the thalamic nuclei will be discussed here chiefly as related to the stereotactic problems and experiences (fig. 55). For further details the reader is referred to the surveys prepared by

---

Fig. 55. Thalamic nuclei (horizontal projection) and their main connections. A = Anterior nuclei; ac = acoustic impulses; amyg = amygdala; bg = basal ganglia; CM = centrum medianum; ci = cingulate gyrus; de+ru = dentatothalamic and rubrothalamic tracts; dif = diffuse thalamic projection; DM = dorsomedial nucleus; H_1 = fasciculus thalamicus; Hy = hypothalamus; Il = intralaminar nuclei; Is = interstitial nucleus; lm = medial lemniscus; m = magnocellular, medial part of DM; mth = mammillothalamic tract; orb = orbital surface of frontal lobe; pa = pallidum; pc = parvicellular, lateral part of DM; Pf = nucleus parafascicularis; Pi = inferior part of the pulvinar; Pl = lateral part of the pulvinar; Pm = medial part of the pulvinar; PO = postcentral gyrus; POi = inferior part of PO; POs = superior part of PO; PP = posterior parietal lobe; prf = prefrontal cortex; R = nucleus

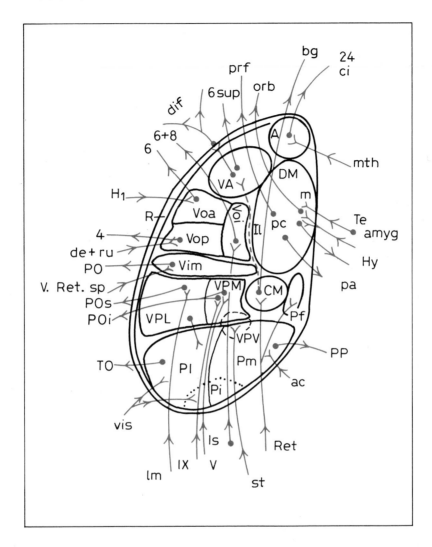

reticularis; Ret = reticular formation; sp = muscle spindle; st = spinothalamic tract; Te = temporal lobe; TO = temporooccipital region; VA = nucleus ventralis anterior; Vim = nucleus ventralis intermedius; vis = visual impulses; Voa = nucleus ventralis oralis anterior; Voi = nucleus ventralis oralis internus; Vop = nucleus ventralis oralis posterior; VPL = nucleus ventralis posterolateralis; VPM = nucleus ventralis posteromedialis; VPV = nucleus ventralis posteroventralis; 4, 6, 8, 24 = Brodmann's cortical areas; 6sup = supplementary motor area 6; V = secondary trigeminal tracts; IX = secondary glossopharyngeal tracts. Ventral thalamic nuclei partly after Hassler. Nucleus lateralis dorsalis and lateralis posterior not included.

Le Gros Clark [1932, 1936], *Walker* [1938a, b, 1966], *Kuhlenbeck* [1954], and *Hassler* et al. [1979]. The nuclei of the diffuse thalamic projection system or non- or *unspecific thalamic nuclei* [*Morison and Dempsey,* 1942, 1943; *Dempsey and Morison,* 1942], also called the thalamic reticular system, project diffusely to widespread areas of the cerebral cortex. As a rule, they are generally not subject to retrograde degeneration after cortical lesions [*Walker,* 1938b], but occasionally such degeneration was found after extensive cortical lesions [*Woolsey,* 1966]. In the development of this phenomenon, transneuronal degeneration may play a role, particularly in animals with long survival time after the cortical lesion [*Powell and Cowan,* 1956].

The axons of most of the cells of these nuclei do not enter the cortex but end partly on specific nuclei, partly in the basal ganglia, or they join chains of neurons directed cranially. They receive afferent impulses from the reticular formation of the brain stem chiefly by fibers contained in the central tegmental tract [*Nauta and Kuypers,* 1958]. These fibers are part of the ascending reticular activating system that acts upon the cortex, as shown by desynchronization of the EEG, and induces arousal and attention [*Magoun,* 1952]. These reticulothalamic fibers probably also carry pain impulses.

It would be an oversimplification to regard the neurons of the nonspecific thalamic nuclei simply as a continuation of the reticular ascending formation. It was found that cortical responses (e.g. recruiting, see later) induced by stimulation of the nonspecific thalamic nuclei can be inhibited by stimulation of the reticular formation of the medulla oblongata [*Moruzzi and Magoun,* 1949]. It also has been shown that destruction of the thalamus does not prevent the cortical activation on stimulation of the reticular formation of the medulla oblongata [*Starzl* et al., 1951]. Thus, there exists also an extrathalamic pathway for the corticopetal impulses from the reticular formation of the brain stem. The neuron chains apparently pass to the hypothalamus and subthalamus and eventually enter the internal capsule [*Nauta and Kuypers,* 1958].

The main part of the nonspecific nuclei is represented by the *intralaminar nuclei* (IL located in the lamina medullaris interna) and the centrum medianum (center médian, CM), a ventral extension of the IL nuclei (fig. 55). In the posterior part of the diencephalon, there also belong to this group the nucleus parafascicularis situated medial to the CM, the nucleus limitans, a band of cells between the habenula and the nucleus suprageniculatus; the latter caps the medial geniculate body. Not only the intralaminar nuclei, but also the CM, the nucleus limitans, and the nucleus parafascicularis receive fibers from the reticular formation of the mesencephalon.

At the cranial end of the thalamus, one finds the *nucleus ventralis anterior* (VA, nucleus lateropolaris of *Hassler)* that seems to belong partly to the nonspecific system, being partly preserved after decortication. It is supposed in part to project to the supplementary motor area on the medial aspect of the cortex, since similar reactions on its stimulation (deviation of the eyes and turning of the head to the opposite side, raising of the opposite arm and loud vocalization) were observed [*Hassler,* 1967] as on stimulation of the supplementary motor cortex. A projection to the anterior insula was also described [*Angevine* et al., 1962].

The multisynaptic chain of more posteriorly located nuclei of the nonspecific system terminates in the VA [*Jasper,* 1960]. This nucleus eventually relays the impulses to the *nucleus reticularis,* which lies between lamina medullaris externa and the capsula interna. *Ross* [1952] found that the nucleus reticularis is capable of evoking activity in at least most of the neocortex and considers it the only morphological unit within the thalamus which has been shown to possess such generalized cortical connections. This is in agreement with the view that the axons of this nucleus represent the final common path of the nonspecific nuclei to the cortex [similarly, *Hanberry and Jasper,* 1953].

There is considerable controversy among anatomists regarding whether the CM, the intralaminar nuclei and the VA project to the striatum or to the pallidum [for details see *Spiegel* et al., 1957a]. Studies of *potentials evoked in the basal ganglia* by stimulation of the nuclei of the nonspecific thalamic system, therefore, may be of interest. While *Starzl* et al. [1951] found responses in the striatum, but not in the pallidum, *Spiegel* et al. [1957a] could elicit recruitment or spindle formation in the pallidum as well as in the striatum of cats (fig. 56). On stimulation of the nuclei of the nonspecific thalamic system, the appearance of the first wave of the spindle formation was delayed up to 200 ms. Ablation of the frontal lobe or a large lesion of the head of the caudatum did not prevent the appearance of the pallidal reactions on thalamic stimulation (fig. 57, 58). In the human brain stimulation of the region of the internal medullary lamina preceding pallidotomy also elicited recruitment in the pallidum (fig. 59) [*Spiegel and Wycis,* 1961].

Stimulation in the region of the internal lamina medullaris (fig. 60) preceding thalamotomy could replace the cortical rhythm by that of the stimulation. At least in some of these records, recruitment and waxing and

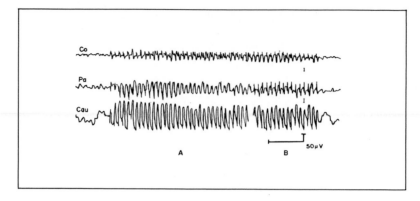

Fig. 56. Recruitment in the pallidum (Pa) and caudate nucleus (Cau) of a cat on stimulation of the lamina medullaris interna (8.5 Hz, 5 V). Between *A* and *B* continuous stimulation for 8 s. From *Spiegel* et al. [1957a]; reproduced with permission.

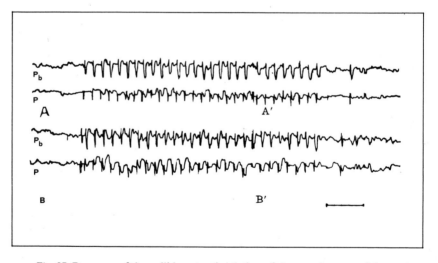

Fig. 57. Response of the pallidum to stimulation of the anterior part of the nucleus ventralis lateralis before and after the lesion of the head of the caudate nucleus shown in figure 58. The thalamic impulses may be transmitted to the pallidum by collaterals of thalamocortical fibers. *A* Record from the left pallidum (P) and from its ventral surface (Pb) before the lesion in the caudate nucleus. Stimulation of the anterior part of the left nucleus ventralis lateralis, at 10 V. Repetition of the stimulation with the same parameters after the lesion. Between *A* and *A'* and *B* and *B'*, respectively, continuous stimulation for 6 s. Same source as figure 56.

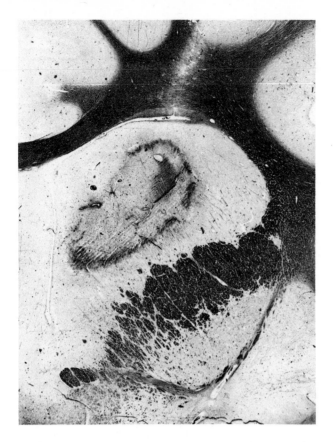

Fig. 58. Cat. Lesion of the left caudate nucleus (referred to in figure 57). Same source as figure 56.

waning of the amplitude of the cortical discharges was noted on prolonged stimulation. According to *Jasper's* [1960] experiments, the CM projects not only to the striatum but also to the nonspecific parts of the thalamus as well as to specific nuclei. It forms an intrathalamic association system. He found connections with the striatum from caudal parts of the CM, recruiting in widespread cortical areas from its rostral part.

Thalamic nuclei probably play a role in the cortical recruitment appearing on pallidal stimulation [*Spiegel and Wycis,* 1962]; the cortical recruitment induced by thalamic stimulation, however, is preserved despite elimination of both pallida [*Szekely,* 1957]. Thalamic impulses reaching the striopallidum originate not only in the nonspecific system but also in the association nuclei, e.g., the dorsomedial nucleus, and, to a certain extent, in the nucleus ventralis posterior. The influence of the nonspecific nuclei, however, is more constant and definite than that of the association nuclei.

Thus, the study of the evoked potentials indicates that the functional state of the basal ganglia is closely related to that of various parts of the thalamus. This may explain why sensory and emotional stimuli, by increasing the state of excitation of the thalamus, facilitate the involuntary movements seen in diseases of the extrapyramidal system, by enhancing the pallidofugal impulses which evoke these involuntary movements. Conversely these pallidofugal impulses are decreased if the thalamus is quiescent as in sleep or other states of decreased consciousness, and these involuntary movements stop.

Stimulation of the nonspecific system in unanesthetized animals may produce a condition described as *sleep-like* [*Hess*, 1948, 1956] or as *arrest reaction* [*Hunter and Jasper*, 1949]. The frequency and the strength of the stimulating pulses seem to be important factors in the production of these effects. When *Hess* applied frequencies of 2–4 Hz at 1–2 V lateral to the massa intermedia in cats, he obtained the sleep-like effect. With higher voltages, the animal opened its eyes and started to walk. On stimulation of the intralaminar nuclei at 5–7 Hz a sleep-like condition associated with general synchronization of the cortical electrical activity was observed by *Akimoto* et al. [1956], while higher stimulation frequencies induced awakening with desynchronization of the electrocorticogram.

The CM, the intralaminar nuclei, the nucleus parafascicularis, and the nucleus limitans have been targets in attempts to relieve chronic pain [*Hécaen* et al., 1949; *Mark* et al., 1960, 1963]. The intralaminar nuclei have been coagulated in obsessive-compulsive states [*Hassler and Dieckmann*, 1967]. Since the nonspecific system may carry epileptogenic impulses [*Mullan* et al., 1967], the VA that is supposed to receive impulses from other

Fig. 59. Recruitment in the pallidum on stimulation of the region of the lamina medullaris interna in a Parkinson patient. 1-ms pulses, 4.5 Hz, 15 V. Cap = Internal capsule; FT = frontotemporal scalp leads; Pa = pallidum. *A–C* Continuous record. From *Spiegel and Wycis* [1961]; reproduced with permission.

Fig. 60. Electrocorticographic effects in the first frontal gyrus induced by stimulation in the region of the internal medullary lamina under local anesthesia preceding thalamotomy in a patient with intractable pain. Stimulus: pulse duration 1 ms, 5.4 Hz, 10 V, 30,000 Ω resistance (stimulation between arrows); calibration: 50 µV; time: 1 s. Continuous record from *A* to *D*. Same source as figure 59.

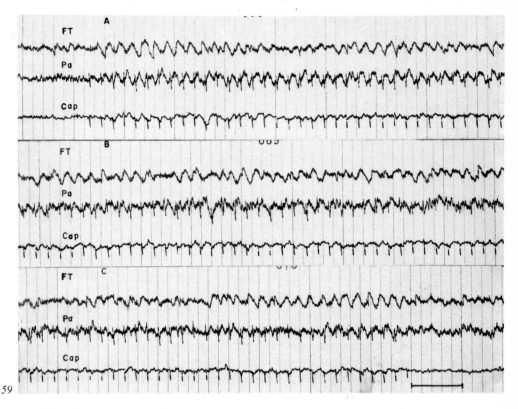

59

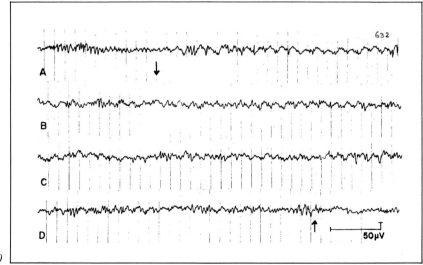

60

nuclei of the nonspecific system has been included in the areas eliminated in intractable epilepsy. *Bouchard* et al. [1975] and *Bouchard* [1976] combined lesions of the VA with fornicotomy or amygdalotomy. It may be recalled that axons of the neurons of the DM coursing to the frontal cortex pass through the VA, so that *Talairach* [1952] could succesfully treat schizophrenics by VA lesions. *Hassler* et al. [1979], however, warn that bilateral destruction of the nonspecific nuclei of the thalamus may lead to impairment of consciousness.

The *midline nuclei* (nucleus reuniens, nucleus paraventricularis, perhaps nucleus parataenialis, etc., located in the periventricular gray matter and related to the intralaminar nuclei and the hypothalamus) are rudimentary in man and, at present, hardly of interest to the stereotactic worker. The nuclei projecting to circumscribed cortical areas, the so-called *specific thalamic nuclei* include the *relay nuclei* that receive their input from the main sensory systems and the *association nuclei* that receive afferent impulses chiefly from the relay nuclei. Both groups develop retrograde degeneration after ablation of the respective cortical projection areas.

Rhythmic stimulation of the *specific nuclei* at frequencies of 6–12 Hz induces short latency (1–5 ms) *augmenting responses* in circumscribed cortical areas; there is a successive increase in the amplitude of a few initial potentials. Similar stimulation of nuclei of the *nonspecific projection* system produces, after a long latent period (15–60 ms), the so-called *recruiting responses* increasing also gradually in amplitude or developing *spindle formations* in widespread cortical areas. The long latent period probably is due to the multisynaptic structure of the nonspecific system. Measurement of the latent periods provides an important criterion for the differentiation of these two types of reactions. Such a differentiation has been attempted by *Jung and Riechert* [1955], *Alberts* et al. [1961] and *Housepian and Pool* [1962]. A projection was observed to the motor cortex, not only from the sensory relay nuclei [*Bertrand* et al., 1967], but also from the nucleus ventralis lateralis [*Yoshida* et al., 1964]. The effects upon the EEG were summarized by *Jung* [1954] as follows: diffuse bilateral responses with recruiting were obtained not only from the intralaminar nuclei but from other thalamic nuclei on unilateral stimulation. These were interpreted as activation of the nonspecific thalamic projection system. Localized homolateral responses in the postcentral cortex after stimulation of the nucleus ventralis posterior were considered to be caused by stimulation of the specific somatosensory projection system. Cortical recruitment appeared on stimulation of FH [*Spiegel* et al., 1964b] (fig. 61, 62).

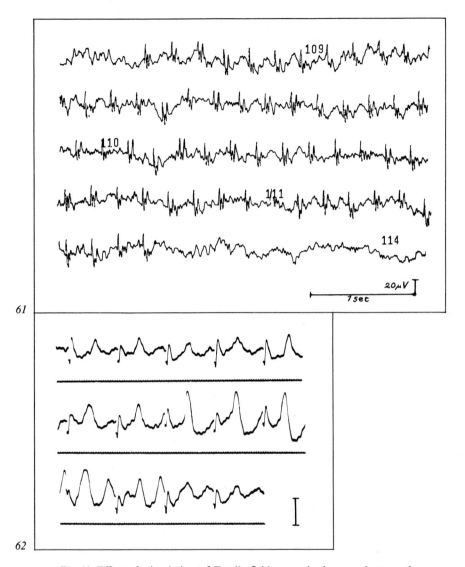

Fig. 61. Effect of stimulation of Forel's field upon the human electrocorticogram. Bipolar stimulation (1-ms pulses, 4.5 Hz, 2 mA) of left Forel's field (2 mm above inter- commissural line). Monopolar, epidural recording from left superior frontal gyrus. Contin- uous record, except for interval of 7 s preceding the last tracing. From *Spiegel* et al. [1964b]; reproduced with permission.

Fig. 62. Cat. Bipolar stimulation of left Forel's field (0.5-ms pulses, 5 Hz, 3.5 V). Monopolar record from left posterior sigmoid gyrus. Upward deflection indicates negativ- ity. Calibrations: 100 μV and 10 ms. Same source as figure 61.

The group of *relay nuclei* includes the ventral nuclei (the ventral posterior (VP), the ventral intermedius (Vim), the ventral lateral (VL), and partly the ventral anterior nucleus (VA), and the anterior nuclei (A), and in the metathalamus the medial and lateral geniculate bodies. The *ventral nuclei* serve chiefly as relays for transmission of impulses from the spinal cord, from sensory cranial nerves, from the cerebellum and from the striopallidum to the cerebral cortex. Their afferent and efferent connections are summarized in table III.

In the *nucleus ventralis posterior* (VP; nucleus ventralis caudalis, VC, *Hassler*) three subdivisions can be discerned: the nucleus ventralis posteromedialis (VPM; nucleus arcuatus or semilunaris, nucleus ventralis caudalis internus, Vci, *Hassler*); the nucleus ventralis posterolateralis (VPL; nucleus ventralis caudalis externus, Vce), and the nucleus ventralis posteroventralis (VPV; nucleus caudalis parvicellaris, Ncpc, *Hassler*). The nucleus ventralis posteromedialis receives the secondary trigeminal pathways in its lateral part and the secondary gustatory fibers in its medial part. The nucleus ventralis posterolateralis receives impulses from the arm in its medial part and from the leg in its most laterodorsal part. In this nucleus the lemniscus medialis and the spinothalamic tract end. The former carries discriminative, tactile and proprioceptive impulses (particularly from joint movements) [*Mountcastle and Powell,* 1959], the latter pain and temperature sensation. Evoked potentials induced by tactile stimulation were recorded by *Mountcastle and Henneman* [1952]. According to the studies of *Mehler* et al. [1960] in monkeys, spinothalamic fibers enter the caudal part of the VPL, spread out on the inner surface of the external medullary lamina and then reach more medial parts of the nucleus. *Bowsher's* [1957] studies of the brains of patients after cordotomy indicate that the spinothalamic fibers end in the VPL bilaterally. *Hassler* [1960] concludes from the experience that stimulation of his nucleus caudalis parvocellularis (Vcpc; corresponding to the nucleus ventralis posterior ventralis, below the VPL) in patients produced pain and its coagulation produced analgesia and thermanesthesia, that the spinothalamic tract ends in this Vcpc.

All three subdivisions of the VP project to the postcentral gyrus (areas 3, 1 and 2), with the sensory area for the face in the most ventral part and above it the representation of hand, arm, trunk, leg and foot. Orally adjacent to the VP lies the *nucleus ventralis intermedius* (Vim). Various inputs to this nucleus have been described: from the reticular formation [*Lewandowsky,* 1904], from the sensory trigeminal nucleus [*Carpenter,* 1957], from the vestibular nuclei [*Hassler* et al., 1979], and from muscle spindles [*An-*

Table III. Ventral thalamic nuclei

	Input from	Projection to
Ventroanterior nucleus (VA; W) N. lateropolaris (Lpo, H)	pallidum externum	supplementary motor cortex, insula and widespread cortical distribution
Ventrolateral nucleus (VL; W) N. ventrooralis anterior (Voa; H) N. ventrooralis posterior (Vop; H) N. ventrooralis internus (Voi; H)	pallidum internum via H_2, H_1 n. dentatus via brach. conjunct. interstitial nucl. (Cajal)	premotor cortex ($6a\alpha$) motor cortex (4γ) premotor cortex ($6a\beta$, 8) projection to mesencephalic tegmentum from VL
Ventrointermedius nucleus (Vim; W, H)	sensory 5th nucl. reticular formation; muscle spindles (vestibul. nucl. improbable)	somatic sensory-motor cortex (3a) (gyr. postcentr.)
Ventroposterior nucl. (VP; W) N. ventrocaudalis (H)	lemniscus medial.; spinothalamic, quintothalamic tracts; secondary IX fibers	gyrus postcentralis (areas 1–3)
N. ventral. posterolat. (VPL; W) N. ventral. caudal. ext. (Vce; H)	hand, arm, trunk and leg; lemniscus medialis; spinothalamic tract	
N. ventral. posteromedialis (VPM; W) N. ventral. caudal. intern. (Vci; H) (arcuate; semilunaris)	quintothalamic and taste fibers	
Basal part of VP (W) N. ventralis caudalis parvocellularis (Vcpc; H) Ventral posteroventral nucleus (VPV)	spinothalamic tract (pain and temperature sensation)	

Nomenclature: H = Hassler; W = Walker.

dersson et al., 1966]. Bilateral interruption of Forel's tegmental fasciculi in the midbrain, which are supposed to conduct labyrinthine impulses to the Vim, according to *Hassler,* does not prevent, however, the appearance of evoked potentials in the gyrus ectosylvius of cats on stimulation of the vestibular nuclei [*Spiegel* et al., 1965a]. The Vim projects to the somatic sensory-motor cortex, especially to area 3a [*Hassler* et al., 1979]. However, a cortical projection of vestibular impulses via nucleus Vim assumed by *Hassler* is improbable in view of the above-mentioned finding that interruption of Forel's tegmental fascicles does not prevent evoked potentials in the cerebral cortex on stimulation of the vestibular nuclei. Considering this finding, it seems to be rather difficult to relate to the central vestibular system the turning of the head to the same side on stimulation of the Vim.

In the *nucleus ventralis lateralis* complex (VL), three subnuclei have been distinguished, based upon their connections. The *nucleus ventralis oralis posterior* (Vop, *Hassler*) receives dentatorubrothalamic fibers. It projects to the motor cortex (area 4γ). It is the chief target in tremor at rest and in intention tremor. The *nucleus ventralis oralis anterior* (Voa, *Hassler*) receives impulses originating in the pallidum internum; these impulses are first conducted by fibers of the fasciculus lenticularis (H_2) that enter FH, course there dorsally, then laterally and continue as fasciculus thalamicus (H_1) that enters Voa. This nucleus projects to the so-called premotor cortex (area 6). It is a target for coagulation in parkinsonian rigidity. The *nucleus ventralis oralis interior* (Voi, *Hassler*) receives fibers from the nucleus interstitialis (Cajal) and is supposed to project to the premotor area (area 6aα), perhaps also to the frontal eye field (area 8). Its stimulation induces chiefly rotating movements of the body and head around the longitudinal axis to the same side [*Hassler and Hess,* 1954]. It has been the target of stereotactic coagulation in torsion dystonia of the extremities and the trunk and in spasmodic torticollis [*Hassler and Dieckmann,* 1970].

It may be inquired whether the relay of corticopetal impulses is the only function of the ventrolateral complex of the thalamus. In this respect, it has been shown by *Spuler* et al. [1962] in cats that a conduction to caudal areas exists of impulses that originate in the ventrolateral thalamic area; this conduction is independent of the frontal lobe and of the motor cortex. Degeneration of centrifugal fibers from the frontal lobe, from the motor cortex and from the pallidum did not prevent VL stimulation from producing changes in amplitude and/or frequency of a tremor induced by stimulation of the mesencephalic tegmentum (fig. 63). In agreement with this

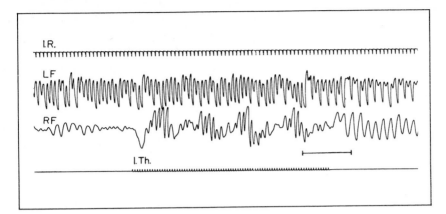

Fig. 63. Stimulation of the ventrolateral area of the left thalamus of a cat 5 weeks after left, complete frontal lobectomy combined with ablation of the left sigmoid gyri and nearly complete destruction of the left pallidum except for a small area in its most posterolateral part. Effect upon the mesencephalic tremor of the right foreleg (RF) produced by stimulation of the reticular formation (l.R.) of the left mesencephalic tegmentum. l.R. = Stimulation of the left mesencephalic reticular formation (5-ms pulses, 12 Hz, 4.5 V); l.Th. = stimulation of the ventrolateral area of the left thalamus (1-ms pulses, 20 Hz, 2 V); LF, RF = tremor of left and right foreleg; time = 1 s. From *Spuler* et al. [1962]; reproduced with permission.

finding, *Langfitt* et al. [1963] observed, on stimulation of the VL area, changes of spinal gamma motor fiber activity in chronically decorticated cats with degenerated capsula interna. The contrary negative findings of *Stern and Ward* [1960] after ablation of the motor area are probably due to the fact that they stimulated the ventrolateral area in the acute stage after ablation of the pericruciate cortex. Thus, besides its role as a relay for corticopetal impulses, the VL region is able to influence the activity of lower parts of the CNS by descending systems. In this connection, experiments conducted by *Johnson and Clemente* [1959] are of interest. These authors found degenerated fibers in the tegmentum dorsal to the nucleus ruber after lesions of the zona incerta and of the field H and they were inclined to assume the existence of fibers from the thalamus to the mesencephalic tegmentum.

Stimulation of the area of the *nucleus ventralis lateralis* changed a parkinsonian tremor (fig. 64) more easily than pallidal stimulation. *Struppler and Struppler* [1962] analyzed the factors that influenced the effect upon parkinsonian tremor on stimulation of this area. Low stimulus frequencies

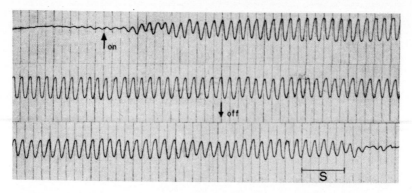

Fig. 64. In a Parkinson patient, stimulation of the area of the left nucleus ventralis lateralis markedly increases the amplitude of the tremor. The latter is recorded from the right index finger. Preceding the stimulation, the graph is flat, showing undulations of very small amplitude; on stimulation, within about 1 s, a tremor of large amplitude develops and outlasts the stimulus. Harvard Stimulator, exponential pulses, 50 ms at 0.5 A, 30 Hz, 8 V (peak); time = 1 s. From *Spuler* et al. [1962]; reproduced with permission.

(1–8 Hz) mostly inhibited the tremor, and high frequencies activated it. At frequencies of 25–50 Hz, weak stimuli activated and strong stimuli inhibited the tremor. An influence of the state of excitation of the spinal motor neurons was suggested by the observation that the effect of single supraspinal stimuli depended on the phase of the tremor at which these stimuli were applied. Passive distension of the muscles increased the effect of the supraspinal stimuli upon the tremor, so that an influence of peripheral impulses originating in the muscles was inferred.

Considering the above-mentioned experiments which showed that stimulation of the ventrolateral area of the thalamus is able to influence caudal regions, it seems that the effect of VL stimulation upon parkinsonian tremor is due to a double mechanism – impulse conduction not only to the cerebral cortex but also toward the spinal cord, probably via the reticular formation of the brain stem.

The nucleus ventralis anterior is discussed with the nonspecific nuclei [p. 149]. The *anterior nuclei* receive impulses, by way of the mammillothalamic tract (Vicq d'Azyr bundle), from the corpus mammillare, whose chief input, the fornix, carries hippocampofugal fibers. The three components of this nuclear complex project mainly to the cingulate gyrus [*Walker,* 1938b]: the largest, the nucleus anteroventralis, to its supracallosal part (posterior part of area 24 and area 23), the nucleus anteromedialis to its anterior,

precallosal part (areas 24 and 32), and the rudimentary nucleus anterodor-
salis to the retrosplenial part. A portion of the anterior thalamic radiation
carrying impulses from the anterior nuclei to the cingulate cortex also contains corticofugal fibers to these nuclei. Similarly, thalamopetal as well as
thalamofugal fibers are found in the mammillothalamic tract.

Although the mammillary body relays chiefly olfactory impulses, clinical olfactory deficits following lesions of the anterior nuclei are not known.
This has been explained by *Walker* by the diffuse connections of the olfactory system. Functionally it is more important that these nuclei are *part of
the Papez circuit* (fig. 67) and thus participate in mechanisms related to
emotions. In agreement with this concept, *Spiegel* et al. [1951a] reported a
favorable influence of bilateral lesions of the anterior nuclei upon emotional
disturbances in some schizophrenic patients.

Stimulation of the anterior nuclei in anesthetized cats [*Baird* et al.,
1952] and man [*Spiegel and Wycis,* 1961] induces slowing or arrest of respiration (fig. 65, 66). The effect upon the blood pressure in cats is variable; a
depressor effect is frequently observed. Stimulation of these nuclei in unanesthetized cats produces an alertness reaction. The head is raised, the eyes
are opened, the animal looks around and starts to walk. These effects are
probably caused by an activation of hypothalamic mechanisms. These reactions persist after ablation of the cingulate gyrus and of the fornix. These
observations suggest the existence of centrifugal systems from the anterior
nucleus that transmit these stimulation effects: fibers descending from the
anterior nucleus to the mammillary body in Vicq d'Azyr's bundle, then the
mammillotegmental tract to the nucleus dorsalis tegmenti. The inhibition
of respiration induced by stimulation of the cingulate gyrus is not prevented
by elimination of the anterior nucleus. Apparently impulses from the cingulate gyrus may reach the lower centers partly by a pathway coursing outside the anterior nucleus, perhaps by fibers descending in the internal capsule. *Bilateral lesions of the anterior nuclei* in cats produce a brief state of
catalepsy followed by a transient period of reduced reactivity to threatening
or painful stimuli.

In the metathalamus, the *medial and the lateral geniculate bodies* are
relay nuclei. The dorsal parvicellular part of the former transmits cochlear
impulses to Heschl's transverse gyri (areas 41 and 42), the latter optic
impulses to the calcarine cortex (area 17). They are, of course, off limits for
the stereotactic surgeon in view of their functional importance. The magnocellular part of the medial geniculate body probably receives collaterals of
pain tracts.

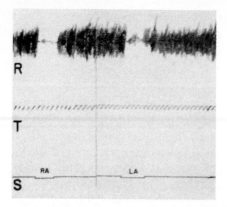

Fig. 65. Marked respiratory depression induced by stimulation of the right (RA) and left (LA) anterior nuclei of a cat. The left cingulate gyrus has been completely removed. R = Respiration; T = time intervals (5 s); S = stimulus marker. From *Baird* et al. [1952].

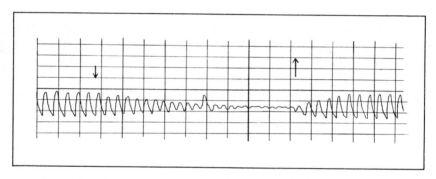

Fig. 66. Inhibition of respiration induced by stimulation of the anterior nucleus of the thalamus in a schizophrenic patient, preceding production of a lesion in this nucleus. Stimulus: pulse duration 10 ms, 10 Hz, 15 V, 30,000 Ω resistance (stimulation between arrows). Time interval between vertical lines: 5 s. From *Spiegel and Wycis* [1961]; reproduced with permission.

The *association nuclei* include the dorsomedial nucleus, the pulvinar, and the lateral nuclei (nucleus lateralis dorsalis and nucleus lateralis posterior). The *dorsomedial nucleus* (DM, medial nucleus) consists of a medial, smaller, phylogenetically older magnocellular and a lateral, larger, phylogenetically younger parvocellular part. There is no sharp limit between these nuclei [*Kuhlenbeck,* 1954]. The magnocellular part receives impulses from and sends fibers to the hypothalamus, chiefly by way of the periventricular fibers. The magnocellular part projects chiefly to the orbital surface of the frontal lobe (areas 11, 12 and 47 of Brodmann). The parvocellular part, which is developed particularly in primates and in man, receives impulses from adjacent thalamic nuclei (n. ventralis posterior, n. lateralis, intralaminar nuclei, centrum medianum). It projects to the phylogenetically young frontal granular cortex (prefrontal cortex), chiefly areas 9 and 10 at the frontal pole, areas 45 and 46 behind it in the inferior part of the frontal lobe. *Walker* [1938b] emphasizes the precise organization of this projection. Afferent impulses enter the DM also from the temporal lobe (it is uncertain whether the medial or lateral part predominantly receives them), probably particularly from the amygdala. They are carried by part of the inferior thalamic radiation. The DM is peculiar in that it may be considered an association nucleus, since it develops retrograde degeneration of the parvocellular part after ablation of the frontal cortex, but it can also be included in the nonspecific projection system, since stimulation of its lower part may induce recruiting [*Starzl and Whitlock*, 1952] in the cortex.

In the dorsomedial nucleus, an integration of the somesthetic impulses mediated chiefly by the ventroposterior nuclei and of the visceral impulses relayed by the hypothalamus takes place. It is probable that this integration and the projection of the resulting impulses to the prefrontal cortex play an important role in the elaboration of the affective component of mental activities. The importance of the reciprocal thalamofrontal connections in the mechanism of emotions was recognized in the era of prefrontal lobotomies. *Freeman and Watts* [1950, p. 541] noted, in the course of their prefrontal lobotomies, the importance of emotional changes in the treatment of mental disorders, and that a striking change occurs almost at the moment of sectioning of the (frontothalamic) fibers. This change consists of a reduction in affect connected with ideas and acts, while, despite interruption of large numbers of association fibers of the cerebrum, the pathologic phenomena persist.

The relief of emotional disturbances obtained, at least in some instances, by frontal lobotomy that interrupts the thalamofrontal circuits and the experience that this procedure produces degeneration of the parvocellular part of the DM, induced *Spiegel* et al. [1947] to coagulate the DM, particularly in cases of pathologic anxiety, depression and agitation.

Fibers from frontal areas descending to the DM seem to be less numerous than ascending thalamofrontal fibers [*Kuhlenbeck*, 1954]. Impulses carried by frontofugal fibers may be relayed by the DM to the hypothalamus [*Mettler*, 1935] and may serve emotional expression [*Crosby* et al., 1962].

Stimulation of the DM in the macaque [*Showers,* 1958] produced a pattern of movements similar to those obtained from the supplementary motor areas. These responses could still be elicited after extensive cortical ablation, but were eliminated by added large basal ganglia lesions.

The circuit between the magnocellular part of the DM and hypothalamus may also participate in the genesis of emotions, since *Spiegel and Wycis* [1962] observed that emotional disturbances recurring after prefrontal lobotomy could be relieved, in some cases, by lesions of the DM nuclei, apparently of the undegenerated magnocellular part. Dorsomedial thalamotomy was performed not only to relieve pathologic anxiety, depression and aggression related to emotional disturbances, but also to mitigate the emotional component of pain [*Spiegel and Wycis,* 1948, 1953], and to interrupt epileptogenic impulses originating in the temporal lobe [*Ganglberger,* 1976]. After extensive destruction of the dorsomedial nuclei, a *slowing of the cortical rhythm* was found in about 75% of the patients during the first postoperative week; the preoperative rhythm returned within a few months [*Spiegel and Wycis,* 1962].

In the *pulvinar,* three nuclei can be distinguished – a lateral, a medial and an inferior. It is said to receive impulses from both geniculate bodies and from the nucleus ventralis posterior of the thalamus. In the macaque, *Walker* [1938b] described an input into the posterior and medial parts of the pulvinar from the medial geniculate body, into the lateral part from the lateral geniculate, and into the anterior and medial parts from the nucleus ventralis posterior. In his report dealing mainly with the human brain, *Walker* [1966] outlined that afferent visual impulses pass mainly into the inferior nucleus, while the input from the medial geniculate body and from the ventral posterior nucleus of the thalamus is less well defined. In this ganglion, visual, auditory and somatic sensory impulses are integrated, and the resulting impulses are projected into occipital, parietal and temporal areas. For the chimpanzee, *Walker* [1938b] found a projection from the lateral part of the pulvinar to the superior parietal lobe, from the medial part to the supramarginal gyrus, and from the inferior nucleus to the temporooccipital region. According to his later report [*Walker,* 1966], the fibers from the medial portion end in the posterior parietal lobe, those from the lateral part in the temporooccipital region, and those from the inferior nucleus in the vicinity of the striate cortex.

Stereotactic experiences in recent years suggest a relation of the pulvinar to the mechanisms of pain [see p. 50] and of dyskinesias and spasticity [p. 69]. The *effect of pulvinar lesion upon chronic pain* may be due to interruption of the input from the ventral posterior thalamic nuclei. It is more difficult to explain the *reduction of muscular hypertonus* in spasticity and of *dyskinesias* observed after pulvinotomy. Tentatively, I should like to point to the close vicinity of the pulvinar to the centrum medianum (fig. 55). If one considers that the CM sends fibers to the basal ganglia, and that it was coagulated in order to reduce spasticity and dyskinesias, it may be worthwhile to ascertain whether fibers originating in the pulvinar can be traced to the CM.

The *nucleus lateralis (lateralis posterior)* is located between pulvinar and nucleus ventrolateralis, lateral to the dorsomedial nucleus, and between lamina medullaris interna and externa. It receives fibers from the ventral nuclei, being regarded by *Walker* [1938b] as a functionally higher thalamic center than the latter. It relays impulses to the posterior part of the postcentral gyrus and the superior and inferior parietal lobules [*Walker*, 1938b]. The *nucleus lateralis dorsalis* is found dorsomedial to the nucleus lateralis. It receives impulses from the stria medullaris and from the pallidum [*Glees*, 1945] and projects to the parietal lobe and the cingulate gyrus.

Somatotopic Localization in the Thalamus

The projections of various somatic areas to *sensory thalamic nuclei* proved to be similar in man to those found in animal experiments: the arcuate nucleus (n. ventralis posteromedialis) receiving impulses from head, face and intraoral areas, laterally adjacent cell groups of the nucleus ventralis posterolateralis receiving chiefly impulses from the arm, the most lateral and dorsal part of the nucleus ventralis posterolateralis receiving impulses from the leg [*Hassler and Riechert*, 1961]. Cutaneous impulses from the arm may extend into the arcuate nucleus [*Gaze and Gordon*, 1954, in cat and monkey; *Spiegel and Wycis*, 1962, in man]. A more precise localization in the human somesthetic thalamus was developed by *Tasker and Emmers* [1969] and *Emmers and Tasker* [1975]: (1) a discrete somatotopic, contralateral representation (tongue and inside of mouth, 8–9 mm lateral, leg, 19 mm lateral); (2) a less discrete bilateral representation between 12 and 17 mm lateral, with the body hanging down; (3) a representation of large portions of the contralateral side, possibly via medial lemniscus impulses. In further studies by *Tasker* et al. [1978], threshold stimulation of lemniscal fibers in the upper human brain stem elicited a sensation of tingling or vibration; stimulation of spinothalamic fibers a sensation of warm or cold, tingling, or rarely burning; stimulation of vestibular fibers caused a sense of movement; stimulation of visual fibers produced visual obscuration or white phosphenes.

The somatotopic array within the *nucleus ventralis oralis* of the thalamus (*Walker's* nucleus ventralis lateralis) was studied by *Rümler* et al. [1972] using the effects of bipolar electric stimulation (tonic changes of position, activation or suppression of tremor and of speech). The representation of the leg was found in the most dorsal part of the nucleus, then in a dorsoventral direction the proximal part of the arm, the hand and the head. Speech and hand representation were more diffuse than that of leg, arm and head. Speech was influenced with few exceptions from the left nucleus. Suppression was mostly obtained from dorsal parts, activation from ventral parts of the nucleus; these effects were plotted without respect to the body segments.

Further studies seem to be desirable in order to reconcile these observations with those of *Hassler and Riechert* [1961], according to which head and neck are represented in medial parts of the ventral oral nuclei and the legs in the most lateral area.

Disturbances of the Body Scheme and Evoked Potential Studies

Disturbances of the body scheme, finger agnosia and right-left disorientation were observed by *Bechterewa* [1969] when the ventrolateral nucleus of the thalamus of the left or right hemisphere and the adjacent white matter were eliminated. In *evoked potentials studies,* pain-conducting fibers could be located in the mesencephalon [*Spiegel and Wycis,* 1962; *Liberson* et al., 1970] and their thalamic endings in the thalamus determined [*Umbach,* 1966]. Evoked potentials were recorded from FH [*Spiegel* et al., 1964b], probably from reticulothalamic fibers passing through the prerubral field.

Especially important for an understanding of the functional organization of the ventral thalamic nuclei were studies of the spontaneous discharges and of the evoked potentials of single neurons [*Albe-Fessard* et al., 1962; *Jasper and Bertrand,* 1964, 1966]. A tactile area was located in the ventral posterior nuclei responding to light touch and bending of hairs; more anteriorly relay cells reacted to deep pressure, then in a posteroanterior direction, 'joint cells' responded to active or passive joint movements, then cells discharged on stretching or isometric contraction of muscles; eventually rhythmically firing cells were located in the most anterior part of the ventral posterior nuclei. A small area behind the nucleus ventralis lateralis (probably corresponding to *Hassler's* nucleus ventralis intermedius) reacted to stimulation of fibers probably originating in muscle spindles [*Goto* et al., 1968]. *Bertrand and Hardy* [1977] found cell units responding to tactile stimuli in the anterior portion of the nucleus ventralis caudalis of *Hassler;* units discharging on pressure and limb movement were encountered more anteriorly in an area overlapping the nucleus ventralis intermedius.

The three-dimensional distribution of somatosensory-evoked responses in the nuclei ventrales posteriores was determined with the use of microelectrodes by *Giorgi* et al. [1980]. The positions of the evoked responses were plotted within the subdivisions of a three-dimensional computer-generated atlas. Thus, the relative volume and three-dimensional projection of each body part was determined within the ventral posterior nuclei. This aided the placement of chronic stimulating electrodes for treatment of pain.

Subjective Sensations

Pain Conduction and Levels of Pain Perception

The biologic importance of reactions to noxious stimuli explains the multiplicity of *pain conducting systems* and of levels of pain perception [*Spiegel and Wycis,* 1968]. Section of the phylogenetically young lateral spinothalamic system that seems to serve the transmission of discrete, localized pain usually results in pain relief for a limited time only. The same applies to interruption of the phylogenetically old spinoreticulothalamic system [*Spiegel and Wycis,* 1966] which conducts diffuse, poorly localized pain. After elimination of the lateral spinothalamic, the spinoreticulothalamic tract may compensate for its loss and vice versa; the remaining system even may become hypersensitive, and a hyperpathia develops, particularly after elimination of the fast-conducting spinothalamic system. Recurrence of the pain was observed even after apparent elimination of both systems [*Spiegel and Wycis,* 1966]. It probably was incomplete or lower centers compensated for the loss of perception by higher ones.

Several *levels of pain perception* have been recognized: (1) cortical areas [*Schilder and Stengel,* 1932; *Biemond,* 1956]; (2) thalamic nuclei (nuclei ventrales posteriores, intralaminar nuclei, centrum medianum, nucleus parafascicularis, thalamic reticular nucleus, nucleus limitans, posterior nuclear thalamic group, pulvinar) [*Kudo* et al., 1966; *Richardson* and Zorub, 1970]; (3) hypothalamic cell groups [*Karplus and Kreidl,* 1928; *Spiegel* et al.,

1954b]; (4) reticular formation of the caudal mesencephalon [*Spiegel* et al., 1954a] and rhombencephalon, and (5) the periaqueductal gray [*Spiegel* et al., 1954a]. In a case of chronic facial pain, *Nashold and Wilson* [1966] recorded paroxysmal discharges of the mesencephalic tegmentum accompanying the attacks of pain.

Other Subjective Sensations on Electrical Stimulation

Electrical stimulation of the systems ascending from the spinal cord and entering the diencephalon, of their thalamic endings or of the thalamo-cortical fibers in the internal capsule produced rather unspecific subjective responses, at least at frequencies below 25 Hz – sensations of vibration, tingling, electric shock, or of 'pins and needles'. While *Hassler* et al. [1960] stated that pain could be elicited from the nucleus ventralis caudalis parvo-cellularis, *Tasker and Emmers'* [1969] patients apparently experienced only paresthesias, no matter which part of the somatosensory thalamic nuclei was stimulated, perhaps due to the relatively low voltage and frequency applied. In our experience the subjective effect was greatly influenced by the patient's condition. Only in patients suffering from a painful disorder could pain be easily elicited by stimulation of the afferent systems [similarly *Obrador and Dierssen*, 1966]. We found, for instance, that in patients suffering from thalamic pain, this pain was greatly increased by stimulation of the afferent fibers in the mesencephalic tegmentum [*Spiegel and Wycis*, 1962].

It has been mentioned already that the *stimulus frequency* proved to be an important factor. *Hassler and Riechert* [1961] obtained pain responses only on application of stimulus frequencies above 25 Hz (25–50 Hz) to the nucleus ventralis caudalis parvocellularis. The sensation of warmth could be elicited in some instances by stimulation of the medial lemniscus [*Johansson*, 1968] or of the centrum medianum [*Sugita and Doi*, 1967]. On stimulation of the dorsomedial nucleus [*Spiegel and Wycis*, 1962], of the prerubral field [*Spiegel* et al., 1964b] or of the subthalamus [*Obrador*, 1962], indefinite dizziness was occasionally reported. On stimulation of the dorsomedial nucleus with high frequencies an alerting effect was observed [*Hassler and Riechert*, 1967]. It could not be decided whether this was due to excitation of this nucleus or of the adjacent intralaminar nuclei. On stimulation of the basilar thalamic region adjacent to FH and of medial thalamic areas, olfactory hallucinations sometimes were elicited [*Nashold and Wilson*, 1966]. When the Vim was stimulated at 60 Hz, weak stimulation produced paresthesias, stronger stimulation complex contralateral arm movements [*Ohye* et al., 1975].

Elementary visual responses could be elicited not only from the primary visual cortex (area 17) and the secondary visual cortex (areas 18 and 19) [*Penfield and Rasmussen,* 1950], but sometimes also from the hippocampus [*Adams and Rutkins,* 1970] and from deeper areas. Photopsia and noise perception were occasionally experienced on stimulation of Forel's field [*Obrador,* 1962], white phosphenes on stimulation of the superior colliculus [*Nashold,* 1970] or between it and the pulvinar, visual obscurations from the same area, the tegmentum or the subthalamus [*Tasker* et al., 1980]. Colored phosphenes were noted on stimulation of the optic tract and of the lateral geniculate body [*Marg and Dierssen,* 1965; *Boëthius* et al., 1976].

Emotions

Effects of Stereotactic Psychosurgery Related to the Neural Mechanisms of Emotions

It may be of interest to examine whether and to what extent the effects of stereotactic lesions upon psychic disturbances confirm the prevailing concepts of neural circuits (fig. 67) subserving the central mechanisms of emotions, and whether they suggest some additions to this theory.

(1) Interruption of the *thalamofrontothalamic circuit* in the dorsomedial nuclei [*Spiegel* et al., 1947, 1951b; *Spiegel and Wycis,* 1962] relieved anxiety, depression, and tension at least in some patients. Thalamic projections to the orbital frontal cortex could be interrupted by incision below the orbital cortex [*Scoville,* 1949] or by implantation of radioactive ^{90}Y seeds in the subcaudate region (the so-called substantia innominata, *Knight's* [1964] subcaudate tractotomy. Severance of the frontothalamic fibers in the anterior limb of the internal capsule (anterior capsulotomy) benefitted particularly patients suffering from obsessional neurosis [from *Leksell's* clinic; *Herner,* 1961].

(2) *Papez circuit* [*Papez,* 1937] (also called medial limbic circuit) involves the cingulate gyrus (with the cingulum), gyrus hippocampi, hippocampus-fornix (with its endings in the septal region, in the preoptic region, in the hypothalamus, in the mammillary bodies, and in the central gray of the midbrain) [*Nauta,* 1960]; the mammillothalamic tract to the anterior nuclear complex of the thalamus, and the thalamic radiation to the cingu-

late gyrus. This system was successfully interrupted in the cingulate gyrus, chiefly area 24 [*Ward,* 1948; *Cairns* et al., 1952; *Le Beau,* 1952; *Livingston,* 1953], in the cingulum in 'neuropsychiatric illness' [*Ballantine* et al., 1967; *Brown and Lighthill,* 1968] and in so-called intractable pain [*Foltz and White,* 1962][18] [see also *Mac Lean's* studies of the limbic system, 1955].

Lesions of the anterior nuclei of the thalamus [*Spiegel and Wycis,* 1951, 1962] were beneficial in severe anxiety neurosis relapsed after dorsomedial thalamotomy, and in schizophrenia with paranoid and catatonic manifestations, after lesions of the dorsomedial nuclei and of the hypothalamus had been only transitorily effective.

(3) The *amygdaloid system* (also called basolateral limbic circuit) [*Livingston and Escobar,* 1971]. One efferent system of the amygdala is represented by the *Stria terminalis* which ends chiefly in the septum, the preoptic area and the hypothalamus; its discharges reach caudally as far as the mesencephalic tegmentum. There is also a *ventral amygdalofugal* pathway transmitting impulses caudalward similarly as the stria terminalis [*Gloor,* 1960]. Corticopetal impulses from the amygdala reach the piriform cortex, possibly also the rostral part of the temporal lobe, the insula and the frontal orbital cortex. Both the stria terminalis and the ventral system also carry afferent fibers. Besides olfactory impulses, the amygdala, particularly the basolateral part, receives impulses from various receptors.

Regarding *amygdaloid stimulation in animals,* the most significant effects are behavioral responses: arousal, alerting, attention (orienting reaction) progressing to fear, flight, defense reaction (crouching of cat, raising of

---

[18] Stereotactic cingulotomy was also performed in drug-resistant epilepsy [*Diemath* et al., 1966], and section of the fornix in temporal lobe epilepsy [*Hassler and Riechert,* 1957; *Umbach and Riechert,* 1959, 1964].

Fig. 67. Circuits related to the mechanism of emotions. I = Between medial thalamic nuclei (Me) and frontal lobe (Fro). II = Papez circuit: cingulate gyr (C) with cingulum (Ci), hippocampus (Hi), fornix (Fo), corpus mammillare (M), mammillothalamic tract (from M to A), anterior nuclei (A), cingulate gyrus. C sends fibers into the internal capsule. III = Amygdaloid system, chiefly connections between the amygdala (Amy) and hypothalamus (Hy) by way of the stria terminalis (St) and by a ventral system. IV = Possibly the unspecific thalamocortical projection system (usp). V = Intradiencephalic circuits: between medial nucleus and hypothalamus, and between anterior nuclei and mammillary body. VI = Between frontal lobe and hypothalamus; the path from Fro to Hy is interrupted in the septum (Sp) and in the zona incerta. Amygdala and fornix send fibers to the mesencephalic

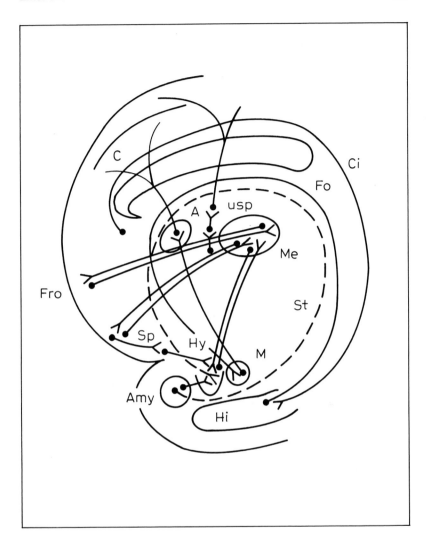

tegmentum. Afferent impulses to Me: from the centrum medianum and from the ventral thalamic nuclei. Afferent impulses to the hypothalamus: from ventral thalamic nuclei, the mesencephalic tegmentum, the vagus, the amygdala (system III). Afferent impulses to the mammillary bodies: from the fornix, from the hypothalamus, and perhaps from the medial lemniscus according to Papez. In the hippocampal gyrus and hippocampus, olfactory impulses received by way of the lateral olfactory striae seem to be integrated with auditory, visual and tactile impulses received via fornix and septum [see *Crosby* et al., 1962]. The stria terminalis ascends from the amygdala, surrounds the thalamus and ends in the hypothalamus (Hy).

forepaw with protruded claws) or attack (biting, fighting with claws) and rage reactions [see reviews by *Gloor,* 1960; *Kaada,* 1972]. In contrast, on stimulation of the ventral part of the cortical and medial amygdaloid nuclei and of the periamygdaloid cortex sleep and synchronization of the electro-corticogram were observed. Self-stimulation experiments on rats indicate that stimulation, particularly of medial parts of the amygdala, may induce a pleasurable or rewarding sensation.

Closely related to the alerting, fear and rage reactions are the *desynchronization* of the electrocorticogram and the *vegetative changes:* dilatation of the pupils, piloerection, salivation, micturition, defecation, alterations of respiration, of blood pressure, pulse rate, gastrointestinal motility and secretion. In the last systems excitatory as well as inhibitory responses were observed depending partly on stimulus frequency and depth of anesthesia.

Some *somatomotor effects* are part of the behavioral responses, e.g., arrest of spontaneous movements such as walking, searching movements, contraversive turning of the head, sniffing accompanying orienting reactions. Some postural responses such as raising a forepaw are part of the defense reaction. Other responses are due to the convulsive reactivity, e.g., ipsilateral facial cloni. There are, however, some motor responses that can hardly be part of other activities, such as the rhythmic movements related to eating (licking, mastication, swallowing, gagging, retching).

The amydgala as well as the hippocampus have an extremely *low convulsive threshold.* Microinjection of ACh (1 μg) and particularly of carbachol into the basolateral portion of the amygdala in cats [*Grossman,* 1963] induced local spike discharges spreading rapidly from the amygdala to other parts of the temporal lobe, psychomotor seizures and behavioral changes. Viciousness was observed in the cats for periods of 5 months. Subthreshold stimulations of the amygdala repeated once every day led to convulsions. This progressive development of seizure responses to repeated stimuli has been called a kindling effect [*Goddard,* 1972].

Endocrine effects, release of gonadotropic hormones inducing ovulation, of luteinizing hormone, of ACTH, of epinephrine leading to hyperglycemia are caused by an influence of the amygdala upon the pituitary gland by way of the hypothalamus.

In *man* confusion, unresponsiveness, in some instances fear [*Chapman,* 1958] or rage reactions [*Heath,* 1971; *Stevens* et al., 1969] were observed on amygdaloid *stimulation. Feindel* [1961] and *Chapman* [1958] emphasize the interference with memory-recording mechanisms inducing amnesia regarding occurrences taking place at the time of stimulation. Hallucinations were evoked in temporal lobe epilepsy.

Similarly as in animal experiments, *Narabayashi* [1972] observed on high frequency stimulation of the amygdala pupillary dilatation and arrest of respiration in the inspiratory phase. The close relationship between emotional and behavioral mechanisms and the central apparatus mediating autonomic responses is indicated by *Narabayashi's* observation that destruction of the area from where the most prominent autonomic responses could be elicited induced a particular calming effect.

Using chronic electrodes, *Stevens* et al. [1969] and *Mark* et al. [1972] observed on stimulation (2–3 ma, for 10–30 s) long latency, long-lasting psychological effects of periamygdaloid and hippocampal stimulation. They suggested that these effects may be due to secretion of biologically active transmitters.

There are conflicting reports in the literature regarding the behavioral and emotional effects of *ablation* of the amygdala. *Kaada* [1972] pointed out that emotional responses are obtained from dorsal areas of the amygdaloid complex at the level of its middle and posterior parts in addition to the anterior amygdala and the prepiriform cortex. Ventral portions of the amygdaloid complex and the overlying piriform cortex seem to exert an inhibitory influence on flight and defense reactions, adrenocortical and cardiovascular responses, feeding and mating behavior, and release of luteinizing hormones. He explained the apparent discrepancy between the taming effect of bilateral, extensive or complete amygdalectomy and the aggressiveness and savage behavior following some partial amygdaloid lesions [*Bard and Rioch*, 1937; *Spiegel* et al., 1940; *Bard and Mountcastle*, 1947] by elimination of the inhibitory regions induced by such partial lesions.

Aggressiveness, violence became the chief indication for *amygdalotomy* in adults [*Narabayashi* et al., 1963] besides the elimination of a focus in temporal lobe epilepsy.

Lesions were placed in the *hypothalamus* by *Spiegel and Wycis* [1951, 1962] chiefly in aggressive schizophrenia, also by *Sano* [1962], *Sano* et al. [1970a, posteromedial hypothalamotomy] in the treatment of aggressive behavior.

Since both the medial and the basolateral limbic system are continued caudally, partly by the medial forebrain bundle, into the midbrain tegmentum, they may influence the reticular activating system in the midbrain [*Nauta*, 1960]. This author pointed out that parts of the Papez circuit (the hippocampus) and of the basolateral circuit (the amygdala) project to the same septal, preoptic, hypothalamic and mesencephalic areas and suggested that there may be, at least partly, a mutual antagonism between these two systems. The experiences in patients in whom one or the other circuit was interrupted do not offer support for this idea, since hyperactivity of the uninjured system, after severing the other supposedly antagonistic pathway, was not observed. There are, however, functional differences between these circuits, indicated by the fact that amygdalotomy benefits chiefly patients suffering from aggressiveness, while interruption of the Papez circuit relieves anxiety and depression.

(4) If it should be proven that lesions of the *intralaminar nuclei* reduce obsessive-compulsive symptoms [*Hassler and Dieckmann,* 1967] also if limited to these nuclei and not encroaching upon adjacent systems (particularly the mammillothalamic tract, a part of the Papez circuit), the beneficial effect of such a procedure would suggest that the *unspecific thalamocortical projection system* participates in mechanisms responsible for pathologic deviations of emotions and behavior.

(5) *Intradiencephalic circuits,* particularly connections between the dorsomedial nuclei and the hypothalamus. Their participation in the mechanism of emotions became manifest in patients who had relapsed after extensive frontal leukotomies, and in whom cell groups of the dorsomedial nuclei projecting to the frontal lobes were degenerated. Yet in about 40% of such patients lesions of the dorsomedial nuclei reduced the emotional reactions [*Spiegel and Wycis,* 1962], apparently by interrupting connections between the dorsomedial nuclei and the hypothalamus. Fibers between the anterior nuclei and the mammillary bodies may also be a part of intradiencephalic mechanisms.

(6) *Frontoseptalhypothalamic connections.* Septal lesions [*Heath,* 1963, 1968] produced emotional flattening, apparently by elimination of septal influences upon the hypothalamus.

Affective Responses on Cerebral Stimulation

Stimulation of various cerebral areas could elicit pleasurable (so-called positive) reactions, relaxation, euphoria, sexual satisfaction, as well as anxiety, depression (negative reactions) [*Heath,* 1954, 1963; *Sem-Jacobsen,* 1960; 1968; *Obrador and Dierssen,* 1967]. On septal stimulation, the patient felt more comfortable, became more alert *[Heath];* these effects, however, were not quite consistent. The points from which positive effects were elicited were sometimes rather close to those producing negative effects in the ventromedial part of the frontal lobe [*Sem-Jacobsen,* 1960,

1968]. In animal experiments, self-stimulation of pleasure-producing areas sometimes became automatic and was repeated so vigorously that convulsive seizures appeared. Psychological effects of excitation in the limbic system were summarized by *King* [1961].

Regarding the *mechanism of pleasure* induced by central gray stimulation and related self-stimulation, experiments on rats are of interest. *Stein and Belluzzi* [1978] administered the opioid antagonist naloxone before the self-stimulation test. In further experiments, they injected diethyldithiocarbamate, an inhibitor of noradrenaline synthesis, 1 h preceding the self-stimulation experiment. They obtained a dose-related decrease in self-stimulation rates after administration of either agent. These observations suggested that central gray self-stimulation depends on the activation of enkephalin-containing neurons as well as of noradrenaline-containing neurons.

Caudate stimulation in *man* [*Heath* et al., 1952] induced drowsiness, perhaps a precursor of the catatonia-like condition produced in cats by chemical stimulation of this area [*Spiegel and Szekely,* 1961]. These observations may be related to the high enkephalin content of the striatum [*Bloom* et al., 1978]. Rage reactions sometimes appeared on stimulation of the *posterior hypothalamus;* anxiety and discomfort, besides flushing and pounding of the head, developed on stimulation of the *anterior hypothalamus* [*Heath* 1971]. *Kelly* et al. [1973] also reported anxiety on hypothalamic stimulation. From points *close to the third ventricle,* particularly in the vicinity of the midbrain, euphoria and laughing, as well as depression and horror, could be elicited [*Sem-Jacobsen,* 1968]. Positive reactions were also observed on activation of the *nucleus ventralis oralis internus* [*Hassler,* 1967]. Anxiety states elicited by high frequency stimulation of the *nucleus ventralis oralis anterior* or of the *pallidum* may be explained, at least partly, by impairment of the cardiac blood supply. Furthermore some depressed Parkinson patients become euphoric when relieved of tremor and rigidity. This may be a factor in the euphoria appearing in such patients after coagulation of the pallidum.

The important role of the *amygdala* and *hippocampus* in emotional mechanisms is well illustrated by observations reported by *Stevens* et al. [1969]. Episodes of anger and aggressive behavior were accompanied by bilateral discharges of sharp waves and spikes and high-voltage slow and sharp waves in the amygdala and hippocampus. Relaxation and euphoria were obtained by stimulation of the most medial part of the amygdala after a latent period of 15–30 s and lasted for minutes or hours following the stimulation. Lesions at the area of the maximum spike activity prevented the rage attacks. In two further cases deep temporal stimulation also induced long-lasting psychic changes, perhaps by secretion of biologically active substances.

On stimulation of the *amygdala* [*Kim and Umbach*, 1973], autonomic responses and subjective sensations were elicited at 25–50 Hz, and seizures at 4–8 Hz. As to the sensations obtained by stimulation of the amygdala, these authors noted anxiety and occasionally paranoid ideas in patients with psychomotor epilepsy and phobia, in 50% on stimulation of the medial, in 14% on stimulation of the lateral part. Reduced vigilance, dreamy states or vertigo were elicited chiefly from the lateral part. Aggressiveness on stimulation was observed only in violent cases [regarding the cingulate gyrus, see p. 146].

In view of the dependence of *behavior* on the individual's emotional state, it is understandable that abnormal behavior, e.g., restlessness, violence, aggression, or obsessive-compulsive states, could be improved by acting upon some of the above-mentioned circuits. It may be sufficient to mention briefly the beneficial effect of lesions of the dorsomedial nuclei and/or of the anterior nuclei, of hypothalamotomy, anterior cingulumectomy, or cingulotomy in restlessness or violence due to anxiety, of anterior capsulotomy in obsessive-compulsive states, and of amygdalotomy in aggressiveness.

Higher Cerebral Functions

Memory and Cognitive Functions
Neural mechanisms involved in the mechanism of *memory* could be influenced not only by stimulation of the surface of the temporal lobe [*Penfield and Perot*, 1963] but also by activating subcortical structures. *Arrest of memory recording*, automatic behavior and poststimulation amnesia were noted on stimulation of the *amygdaloid complex* [*Feindel and Penfield*, 1954; *Feindel*, 1961]. Bilateral *hippocampal lesions* [*Penfield and Milner*, 1958] produced pronounced memory defects. Similarly, transection of the efferent fibers of the hippocampus on both sides *(fornicotomy)* [*Umbach and Riechert*, 1964; *Umbach*, 1966; *Hassler*, 1967] induced loss of memory for recent events, failure of retention, and disturbances of temporal, spatial and situational orientation. Recollections were evoked by stimulation of medial parts of the temporal lobe close to the hippocampus, and hallucina-

tions by stimulation of posterior temporal areas [*Sem-Jacobsen and Tor-kildsen*, 1960].

In confirmation of *Hess'* [1948, 1956] experiments on cats, weak low-frequency stimuli applied to the *intralaminar nuclei* and to medial areas of the thalamus in man produced a dampening of consciousness and occasionally *sleep* [*Umbach*, 1966]. *Arousal effects* on high frequency stimulation could be elicited from various thalamic target points, but more rarely than on stimulation of the *limbic system.*

Amnesic states, acoustic hallucinations and blocking of recent memory were induced by hippocampal stimulation [*Brazier*, 1964], and paralysis of recall occurred on stimulation of the white matter in the middle of the temporal lobe [*Bickford* et al., 1958]. Stimulation of the mediobasal part of the amygdaloid complex or of the adjacent hippocampal area revived old memories [*Velasco-Suarez and Escobedo*, 1970]; deeper stimulation sometimes elicited pleasant childhood experiences, and periamygdaloid stimulation produced recall of terrifying memories. The body scheme may be affected following stimulation. These memories could temporarily be suppressed by instillation of 0.01 mg of atropine sulfate. One must conclude that the amygdaloid complex and hippocampus participate in memory mechanisms, besides the surface of the temporal lobe.

After unilateral *ventrolateral thalamotomy* in nonparkinsonian dyskinesic patients, *Blumetti and Modesti* [1980] observed deterioration of both receptive and expressive *verbal performance* immediately after operation in all 10 patients. More loss was noted after left than after right VL thalamotomy. There was significant improvement over time. Nonverbal memory impairment was noted after right VL thalamotomy; there was also improvement after some time. Only in patients with familial tremor was there no residual loss of processing, memory, attention and emotion on long-term observation. In all other cases minimal to moderate impairment was found in at least two of the above categories [see also *Modesti and Blumetti*, 1980].

Spatial Orientation

In healthy individuals, the subjective vertical or horizontal orientation deviates to the opposite or same side on inclination of the head. In parkinsonian patients, the deviation from the objective vertical or horizontal is significantly larger than in normal subjects. This disturbance of orientation in space is increased after lesions of the pallidum or of the nucleus ventralis oralis anterior or posterior [*Metzel* et al., 1966].

Temporal Orientation

Following small, circumscribed thalamic lesions, confusion regarding the time of day and the date as well as an under- or overestimation of time, was observed transitorily, with and without anosognosia *(chronotaraxis)* [*Spiegel* et al., 1956e]. Regarding localization of lesions disrupting temporal orientation, the disturbance was observed after bilateral lesions of the dorsomedial and/or the anterior nuclei. A participation of the intralaminar nuclei is possible, whereas lesion of the nuclei ventrales posteriores or of the pallidum did not induce temporal disorientation. Since lesions of the parietal lobe [*Pötzl*, 1928; *Critchley*, 1953], the projection areas of the nucleus lateralis dorsalis and of the nucleus lateralis posterior, also produce temporal disturbances, it may be suspected that impairment of these latter nuclei may have a similar effect, but observations in this respect are lacking.

It seems tempting to relate the disturbances of temporal orientation to memory defects in view of their frequent association with amnesic states [*Williams and Zangwill*, 1950]. Such an explanation, however, could not be applied to all our observations. One of our patients, for instance, was disturbed by the feeling that the day finished within a few hours, although she was aware that only a few hours had elapsed since the morning. She complained that this feeling was repeated several times during the day. In view of such observations, it would seem that isolated disturbances of the perception of time exist and may be caused by circumscribed thalamic lesions. This would support the assumption of an elementary time sense and suggest its relationship to thalamic function.

Possible Participation of the Striatum in Higher Cerebral Functions

Relatively little is known regarding the possible importance of the striatum for higher integrative functions in man. After unilateral caudate lesions, *Meyers* [1957] failed to find consistent psychological defects in his patients. Our experiences on patients subjected to unilateral caudate lesions for relief of bradykinesia are in agreement with *Meyers'* observations. In patients with bilateral involvement of the caudatum, e.g., in Huntington's chorea, mental deficiency is frequent; one finds in these patients, however, impairment of other areas, particularly of the frontal lobe, so that the question remains unanswered whether the caudate lesions participate in the genesis of the mental symptoms. A study of this problem in patients who suffered isolated bilateral caudate injury would be desirable in view of animal experiments that can only briefly be mentioned here.

Caudate lesions in monkeys induced *memory defects* leading to difficulties in performing tasks where forced time delay was involved [*Dean and Davis,* 1959]. On stimulation as well as after coagulation of the head of the caudate nucleus, impairment of delayed alternation performance was observed [*Rosvold and Delgado,* 1956]. The striatum may also play a part in avoidance behavior [*Brady* et al., 1954; *Pribram and Kruger,* 1954]. In *Thompson's* [1959] decorticated cats, avoidance behavior was acquired and then caudectomy was performed; resistance to extinction, number of trials required for retraining, and latency of escape-responding in retraining seemed to depend on the size of the caudate lesions. *Mettler* [1957] ablated more than 50% of the head of the caudate nuclei in cats; the animals became unable to relate themselves to the environment. Severe lesions caused a loss of unlearned adaptive behavior. Monkeys had a stupid, uncomprehending appearance after extensive lesions of the nucleus caudatus and of the putamen. Further studies will have to decide whether and to what extent inferences from these experiments are permissible regarding the possible role of the striatum in higher cerebral mechanisms.

Psychiatric Symptoms in Parkinsonian Patients

It has been controversial whether the psychiatric symptoms of parkinsonian patients are caused by the basic disease process or whether they are a reaction to the motor disturbances. For a clarification of this problem, stereotactic operations followed by complications, e.g., by hallucinations after bilateral lesions of the internal part of the pallidum [*Hartmann-von Monakow,* 1959] are hardly suitable. *Fünfgeld* [1967], therefore, subjected 129 parkinsonian patients to psychiatric examinations preoperatively and several months after pallidotomy or ventrolateral thalamotomy performed by *Riechert* and his associates without complications. All his patients had psychiatric anomalies before operation, in the milder forms, reactive depression, emotional lability or rigidity; in the more severely diseased patients decreased spontaneity up to severe personality changes, with decreased initiative, interest and volition, and eventually decreased attention, perception and concentration, with impaired registration, loss of memory, particularly for recent events, and of judgment. Before operation 25.6% of his patients showed severe psychic alterations. 6–10 months after the first stereotactic procedure he found marked neurological disturbances reduced in 94% and an improvement in the psychic state in 83% of the patients. In 77.5%, their psychic states had become inconspicuous. In 67 patients a second operation on the opposite side was performed. In 32.4% of these, the psychic status became worse after this second operation, and their akinesia became pronounced. The author concluded that the psychiatric changes are to a large extent reversible and he is inclined to regard, in most cases, these changes as reactions to the motor disturbances. This view is plausible as far as the emotional reactions are concerned; for the memory defects, the lack of initiative, bradykinesia and akinesia, it is rather debatable, particularly since the important part played by dopamine deficiency has become recognized. Thus, it seems that a uniform explanation of the psychiatric disturbances in paralysis agitans and parkinsonism is hardly justified. While the emotional disturbances may be regarded as reactions to the patients' motor impairment, the memory defects, lack of initiative, and changes related to akinesia seem to depend on alterations associated with biochemical defects.

An *organic syndrome*, confusion, impairment of orientation, memory, apperception, knowledge, judgment, and an amnesic confabulatory (Korsakoff) syndrome [*Noyes*, 1954] appear not infrequently in aged persons under stress, e.g., after air encephalography [*Fünfgeld*, 1967]. Such disturbances have been found not only following pallidotomy and ventrolateral thalamotomy [*Mundinger and Riechert*, 1961, 1962; *Müller and Yasargil*, 1959], but also after campotomy [*Spiegel* et al., 1963b]. In the latter group a depression of consciousness, ranging from drowsiness to deep sleep, also appeared transiently in 21.2% (mostly unilateral lesions). Besides the unspecific effect of stress, partial interruption of fibers of the reticular activating system passing through Forel's field may play a part, particularly in the genesis of the temporary depression of consciousness. *Fünfgeld* [1967] and also *Riechert* [1980] emphasized that a severe form of psychoorganic syndrome is a contraindication for a stereotactic operation, although in some patients a transient syndrome appeared only after air encephalography, but not after the stereotactic procedures.

Concluding Survey of Stereotactic Procedures

Reviewing this report, the following seem to be most promising and/or the most frequently used chiefly stereotactic procedures:

(1) Anterior cingulotomy in drug-resistant anxiety and depression and emotionally charged pain.

(2) Subcaudate tractotomy (stereotactic lesion in and/or anterior to the substantia innominata) in drug-resistant depression and anxiety with a depressive element. Combined (1) and (2) in obsession and compulsion.

(3) Anterior capsulotomy in obsessive-compulsive states.

(4) Amygdalotomy in aggressiveness, violence of adults, hyperactivity, destructive behavior of feebleminded children, if necessary, combined with posterior hypothalamotomy.

(5) Hypothalamotomy for sedation of aggressive patients, either following inefficient lesions of the dorsomedial and anterior thalamic nuclei or after amygdalotomy or without lesions of these nuclei. Hypothalamotomy involving chiefly the ventromedial nucleus served as a last resort in sexual perversions, occasionally in severe alcoholism and drug addiction.

(6) Experiences with stereotactic subcortical lesions in emotional and behavioral disorders indicate a multiple representation of the mechanisms upon which emotions depend. Besides connections between the frontal, particularly orbital, cortex and the dorsomedial nuclei, the importance of the Papez circuit, of amygdalohypothalamic, fronto-septal-hypothalamic, and intradiencephalic circuits became evident. The unspecific thalamocortical projection system may also participate in the genesis of pathologic deviations of emotions and behavior.

(7) Percutaneous chordotomy in chronic, drug-resistant pain.

(8) Combination of lesions of pain conducting and perceiving systems with dorsomedial thalamotomy for relief of chronic, apparently intractable pain with an emotional component.

(9) Deep temporal electroencephalography and combined amygdalofornicotomy and anterior commissurotomy in temporal lobe epilepsy.

(10) The experiences with ventralis anterior thalamotomy in convulsive disorders are not sufficient as yet to permit a definite statement.

(11) Pallidoamygdalotomy or CM lesions in salaam convulsions.

(12) Pallidotomy (chiefly lesion of the pallidum internum) and pallidoansotomy were initially applied in paralysis agitans and parkinsonism, mainly for relief of tremor and rigor, also in some instances of choreatic and athetotic hyperkinesia, hemiballism and torsion spasm. It became replaced by ventrolateral thalamotomy in Parkinson's disease, parkinsonism, hyperkineses (athetosis, hemiballism, myoclonia, torsion spasm). The effect of ventrolateral thalamotomy is longer lasting than that of pallidotomy.

In Parkinson's disease and in parkinsonism the indication for operative treatment became restricted to cases resistant to L-dopa plus a decarboxylase inhibitor or ineffectiveness of such medication on prolonged application. Parkinson tremor as well as intention tremor could be relieved by lesions of parts of the ventrolateral nuclear complex, particularly the nucleus ventralis oralis posterior. For treatment of the parkinsonian rigidity, the target of choice, besides the pallidum internum, is the ending of the pallidothalamic fibers, the nucleus ventralis oralis anterior.

Two rather similar types of subthalamic lesions were successfully performed: (1) lesion of Forel's field H (campotomy) in Parkinson's disease and parkinsonism, athetosis and myoclonia, and (2) lesions of the zona incerta, including the fields H, H_1, and H_2, in Parkinson's disease (particularly in oculogyric crises), in action myoclonus, intention tremor and spasmodic torticollis.

(13) The initial enthusiasm for dentatotomy in spasticity has been replaced by the experience that the reduction of the muscular hypertonus becomes less marked after several years. Thus, the necessity of sequential, multiple lesions in spasticity of cerebral palsy became recognized, e.g., the combination of lesions of the contralateral zona incerta, of the ventrooral, the ventral intermedius and ventral posterior nuclei, of the pulvinar and eventually of the homolateral dentate nucleus.

(14) In spasmodic torticollis central lesions were performed contralateral to the hyperactivity of deep neck muscles, recognizable by electromyography, mostly, but not always, homolateral to the hypertrophic sternocleidomastoideus muscle. The lesions involved, e.g., the nucleus ventralis oralis internus and Forel's field H or the nucleus ventralis oralis internus and the pallidum. Such procedures may prove insufficient, so that peripheral lesions have to be added, e.g., interruption of spinal accessory fibers to the hypertrophied sternocleidomastoideus muscle and eventually bilateral

section of the anterior rami of C_1–C_3, and possibly C_4 unilaterally, innervating the hyperactive deep neck muscles.

(15) In chronic pain, favorable results were experienced on intermittent transdermal stimulation of peripheral nerves, on application of stimuli at relatively high frequencies (30–200 Hz) to the posterior columns, to the area of the mesencephalic medial lemniscus, to the ventral posterior and some other thalamic nuclei, to the periaqueductal or periventricular gray, and to the posterior limb of the internal capsule.

(16) Therapeutic success was reported also on stimulation of the posterior columns in spasticity, of the ventral posterior thalamic nuclei in dyskinesias, and of the posterior columns or of the ventrooral thalamic nuclei and of the zona incerta in spasmodic torticollis. These observations justify further studies. Chronic cerebellar stimulation hardly can be recommended in view of the undesirable side effects.

(17) Obliteration of the lumen of intracranial aneurysms, angiomas, arteriovenous malformations, chiefly by production of a local thrombosis.

(18) Evacuation of intracerebral hematomas, aspiration of intracerebral abscesses.

(19) Removal of foreign bodies.

(20) Implantation of radioactive isotopes in deep-seated cerebral tumors, or their elimination by laser beams.

(21) Hypophysectomy in pituitary tumors; for inhibition of tumor growth and pain relief in metastasizing, sex-linked tumors; in diabetic retinopathy.

(22) There is now a close cooperation in many institutions between the stereotactic neurosurgeon, the roentgenologist and the computer specialist. This promises further to refine the technique of guided brain operations and to minimize unnecessary damage to the patient's brain.

References

References marked with an asterisk* are not cited in the text but have been included for the purpose of completeness.

*Adams, J.E.: Technique and technical problems associated with implantation of neuroaugmentive devices. Appl. Neurophysiol. *40:* 111–123 (1977).

Adams, J.E.; Hosobuchi, Y.; Fields, H.L.: Stimulation of internal capsule for relief of chronic pain. J. Neurosurg. *41:* 740–744 (1974).

Adams, J.E.; Hosobuchi, Y.; Rutkins, B.B.: Central stimulation in the treatment of pain. Confinia neurol. *37:* 279 (1975).

Adams, J.E.; Rutkins, B.B.: Lesions of the centrum medianum in movement disorders. Confinia neurol. *26:* 231–236 (1965).

Adams, J.E.; Rutkins, B.B.: Visual responses to subcortical stimulation in the visual and limbic system. Confinia neurol. *32:* 158–164 (1970).

*Adey, W.R.; Rand, R.W.; Walter, R.D.: Depth stimulation and recording in thalamus and globus pallidus of patients with paralysis agitans. J. nerv. ment. Dis. *129:* 417–428 (1959).

Afshar, F.; Watkins, E.S.; Yap, J.C.: Stereotaxic atlas of the human brainstem and cerebellar nuclei (Raven Press, New York 1978).

Akert, K.; Andersson, B.: Experimenteller Beitrag zur Physiologie des Nucleus caudatus. Acta physiol. scand. *22:* 281–298 (1951).

Akil, H.; Mayer, D.J.: Antagonism of stimulation-produced analgesia by *p*-CPA, a serotonin synthesis inhibitor. Brain Res. *44:* 692–697 (1972).

Akil, H.; Watson, S.J.; Berger, P.A.; Barchas, J.D.: Endorphins, β-LPH and ACTH; in Costa, Trabucchi, The endorphins, pp. 125–129 (Raven Press, New York 1978).

Akimoto, H.; Yamaguchi, N.; Okabe, K.; Nakagawa, T.; Nakamura, I.; Abe, K.; Torii, H.; Masahashi, K.: On the sleep induced by electrical stimulation on dog thalamus. Folia psychiat. neurol. jap. *10:* 117 (1956).

Albe-Fessard, D.; Arfel, G.; Guiot, G.: Activités électriques caractéristiques de quelques structures cérébrales chez l'homme. Annls Chir. *17:* 1185–1214 (1963).

Albe-Fessard, D.; Arfel, G.; Guiot, G.; Hardy, J.; Vourc'h, G.; Hertzog, E.; Aleonard, P.; Derome, P.: Dérivations d'activités spontanées et évoquées dans les structures cérébrales profondes de l'homme. Revue neurol. *106:* 89–105 (1962).

Albe-Fessard, D.; Gillett, L.: Convergence vers le centre médian. Electroenceph. clin. Neurophysiol. *13:* 257–269 (1961).

Albe-Fessard, D.; Guiot, G.; Lamarre, Y.; Arfel, G.: Activation of thalamocortical projections related to tremorogenesis; in Purpura, Yahr, The thalamus, pp. 237–253 (Columbia University Press, New York 1966).

Albe-Fessard, D.; Oswaldo-Cruz, E.; Rocha-Miranda, C.E.: Activités évoquées dans le noyau caudé du chat en réponse à des types divers d'afférences, I. Etude macrophysiol. II. Etude microphysiol. Electrenceph. clin. Neurophysiol. *12:* 405–420, 649–661 (1960).

Alberts, W.W.; Wright, E.W.; Levin, G.; Feinstein, B.; Mueller, M.: Threshold stimulation of the lateral thalamus and globus pallidus. Electroenceph. clin. Neurophysiol. *13:* 68–74 (1961).

Alexander, G.L.; Szekely, E.G.; Spiegel, E.A.: Influence of cerebellar stimulation upon tremor of tegmental origin. Confinia neurol. *19:* 454–461 (1959).

Alexander, G.L.; Szekely, E.G.; Spiegel, E.A.: Effect of stimulation of the pallidum on experimental tegmental tremor in the cat. J. Neuropath. exp. Neurol. *19:* 116–124 (1960).

Alksne, J.F.; Fingerhut, A.G.; Rand, R.W.: Magnetic probe for the stereotactic thrombosis of intracranial aneurysm. J. Neurol. Neurosurg. Psychiat. *30:* 159–162 (1967).

Amano, K.; Iseki, H.; Notani, M.; Kawabatake, H.; Tanikawa, T.; Kawamura, H.; Kitamura, K.: Rostral mesencephalic reticulotomy for pain relief. Report of 15 cases. Acta neurochir. *30:* suppl., pp. 391–394 (1980a).

Amano, K.; Kitamura, K.; Kawamura, H.; Tanikawa, T.; Kawabatake, H.; Notani, M.; Iseki, H.; Shiwaku, T.; Suda, T.; Demura, H.: Alterations of immunoreactive beta-endorphin in the third ventricular fluid in response to electrical stimulation of the human periaqueductal grey matter. Appl. Neurophysiol. *43:* 150–158 (1980b).

Andersson, S.A.; Landgren, S.; Wolsk, D.: The thalamic relay and cortical projection of group I muscle afferents from the forelimb of the cat. J. Physiol., Lond. *183:* 576–591 (1966).

Andrew, J.; Rice Edwards, J.M.; Rudolf, N. de: The placement of stereotaxic lesions for involuntary movements other than in Parkinson's disease. Acta neurochir. *21:* suppl., pp. 39–47 (1974).

Andrew, J.; Watkins, E.S.: A stereotaxic atlas of the human thalamus (Williams & Wilkins, Baltimore 1969).

Andy, O.J.: Diencephalic coagulation in the treatment of hemiballism. Confinia neurol. *22:* 346–350 (1962).

Andy, O.J.: Thalamotomy in hyperactive and aggressive behavior. Confinia neurol. *32:* 322–325 (1970).

Andy, O.J.: Parafascicular-center median nuclei stimulation for intractable pain and dyskinesia (painful dyskinesia). Appl. Neurophysiol. *43:* 133–144 (1980).

Andy, O.J.; Turko, M.F.; Sias, F.R.; Jr.: Subthalamotomy in treatment of Parkinsonian tremor. J. Neurosurg. *20:* 860–870 (1963).

Angeleri, F.; Ferro-Milone, F.; Parigi, S.: Electrical activity and reactivity of the rhinencephalic, pararhinencephalic and thalamic structures. Electroenceph. clin. Neurophysiol. *16:* 100–129 (1964).

Angevine, J.B., Jr.; Locke, S.; Yakovlev, P.I.: Thalamocortical projection of the ventral anterior nucleus in man. Archs Neurol. *7:* 518–528 (1962).

Arjona, V.E.: Stereotactic hypothalamotomy in erethic children. Acta neurochir. *21:* suppl., pp. 185–191 (1974).

Arnold, A.; Bailey, P.; Laughlin, J.S.: Effects of betatron radiation on the brain of primates. Neurology *4:* 165–178 (1954).

Aronow, S.: The use of radiofrequency power in making lesions in the brain. J. Neurosurg. *17:* 431–438 (1960).

Aronson, E.; Sachs, J.: Die Beziehungen des Gehirns zur Körperwärme und zum Fieber. Experimentelle Untersuchungen. Pflügers Arch. ges. Physiol. *37:* 232–301 (1885).

Aronson, N.I.; Becker, B.E.; McGovern, W.A.: A study in experimental tremor. Confinia neurol. *22:* 397–429 (1962).

Aronson, N.I.; Walker, A.E.; McGovern, W.A.: A simplified approach to pallidotomy. Sth. med. J., Nashville *52:* 136–142 (1959).

Asenjo, A.; Imbernón, A.; Rocamora, R.; Chiorino, R.; Aranda, L.: Tecnica estereotáxica con el aparato Asenjo-Imbernón. Neurocirugia *22:* 86–91 (1964).

Austin, B.; Hayward, W.; Tsai, C.; Hill, C.: Stereotaxic localization with midline bony landmarks and electrical stimulation. Confinia neurol. *29:* 230–237 (1967).

Austin, B.; Lee, A.: A plastic ball and socket type of stereotaxic detector. J. Neurosurg. *15:* 264–268 (1958).

Austrogesilo, A.; Borges-Fortes, A.: Sur un cas d'hémichorée avec lésion du noyau caudé. Revue neurol. *67:* 477–488 (1937).

Austrogesilo, A.; Gallotti, O.: Sur un cas d'hémiparésie et d'hémichorée avec lésion du corps caudé. Revue neurol. *40:* 41–43 (1924).

Babb. I.L.; Ottino, C.A.; Crandall, P.H.: Chronic cerebellar stimulation in experimental limbic seizures. Meeting of the European Society for Stereotactic and Functional Neurosurgery, Paris 1979. Abstr., p. J20.

*Backlund, E.O.: Stereotaxic treatment of craniopharyngiomas. Acta neurochir. *21:* suppl., pp. 177–183 (1974).

Backlund, E.O.: Solid craniopharyngiomas treated by stereotactic radiosurgery. Meeting of the European Society for Stereotactic and Functional Neurosurgery, Paris 1979. Abstr., p. V28.

Backlund, E.O.; Bergstrand, G.; Laurell, U.; Rosenborg, M.; Wajngot, A.: Single dose effects after stereotactic radiosurgery in non-active pituitary adenomas. Meeting of the European Society for Stereotactic and Functional Neurosurgery, Paris 1979. Abstr., p. V22.

Backlund, E.O.; Holst, H. von: Controlled subtotal evacuation of intracerebral hematomas by stereotactic technique. Surg. Neurol. *9:* 99–101 (1978).

Backlund, E.; Leksell, L.: A new instrument for stereotaxic brain tumor biopsy. Acta chir. scand. *137:* 825 (1971).

Bagg, H.J.: The effect of radium emanation. Am. J. Roentg. *8:* 547 (1921).

Bailey, P.; Stein, S.N.: Stereotaxic apparatus. Exhibit AMA, Atlantic City. June 1951.

Baird, H.W.; Guidetti, B.; Reyes, V.; Wycis, H.T.; Spiegel, E.A.: Stimulation and elimination of the anterior nuclei. Pflügers Arch. ges. Physiol. *255:* 58–67 (1952).

Baird, H.W.; Wycis, H.T.; Spiegel, E.A.: Convulsions in tuberous sclerosis controlled by elimination of impulses in the basal ganglia. J. Pediat. *49:* 165–172 (1956a).

Baird, H.W.; Wycis, H.T.; Spiegel, E.A.: Treatment of convulsions in tuberous sclerosis by pallidoansotomy. Archs Neurol. Psychiat. *75:* 446–447 (1956b).

Bakay, L.; Hueter, T.F.; Ballantine, H.T., Jr.; Sosa, D.: Ultrasonically produced changes in the blood-brain barrier. Archs Neurol. Psychiat. *76:* 457–467 (1956).

*Balasubramaniam, V.; Kanaka, T.S.: Amygdalotomy and hypothalamotomy. Confinia neurol. *37:* 195–201 (1975).

Balasubramaniam, V.; Kanaka, T.S.: Why hemispherectomy? Appl. Neurophysiol. *38:* 196–205 (1975a).

Balasubramaniam, V.; Kanaka, T.S.; Ramanujam, P.B.: Stereotaxic cingulumotomy for drug addiction. Indian Neurology, Madras *21:* 63–66 (1973).

Balasubramaniam, V.; Ramamurthi, B.: Stereotaxic amygdalotomy in behavior disorders. Confinia neurol. *32:* 367–373 (1970).

Ballantine, H.T., Jr.; Cassidy, W.L.; Brodeur, J.; Giriunas, I.: Frontal cingulotomy for mood disturbances; in Hitchcock, Laitinen, Vaernet, Psychosurgery, p. 221 (Thomas, Springfield 1972).

Ballantine, H.T., Jr.; Cassidy, W.L.; Flanagan, N.B.; Marino, R.: Stereotaxic anterior cingulotomy for neuropsychiatric illness and intractable pain. J. Neurosurg. *26:* 488–495 (1967).

Bancaud, J.; Talairach, J.; Bonis, A.; Schaub, C.; Szikla, G.; Morel, P.; Bordas-Ferer, M.: La stéréo-électroencéphalographie dans l'épilepsie (Masson, Paris 1965).

Bancaud, J.; Talairach, J.; Morel, P.; Brisson, M.: La corne d'Ammon et le noyau amygdalien; effects cliniques et électriques de leur stimulation chez l'homme. Revue neurol. *115:* 329–352 (1966).

Bantli, H.; Bloedel, J.R.; Long, D.M.; Thienprasit, P.: Distribution of activity in spinal pathways evoked by dorsal column stimulation. J. Neurosurg. *42:* 290–294 (1975).

Bantli, H.; Bloedel, J.R.; Tolbert, D.: Activation of neurons in the cerebellar nuclei and ascending reticular formation by stimulation of the cerebellar surface. J. Neurosurg. *45:* 539–554 (1976).

Bárány, R.: Lokalisation in der Rinde der Kleinhirnhemisphären. Dt. med. Wschr. *39:* 637–642 (1913).

Barbeau, A.; Chase, T.; Paulson, G.W.: Advances in neurology, I. Huntington's chorea (Raven Press, New York 1980).

Barcia-Salorio, J.L.; Barberá, J.; Broseta, J.; Soler, F.: Tomography in stereotaxis. Acta neurochir. *24:* suppl., pp. 77–83 (1977).

Barcia-Salorio, J.L.; Broseta, J.; Hernandez, G.; Roldan, P.; Bordes, V.: A new approach for directed CT localization in stereotaxis. Appl. Neurophysiol. *45:* 383–386 (1982).

Barcia-Salorio, J.L.; Hernandez, G.; Broseta, J., et al.: Radiosurgical treatment of a carotic cavernous fistula. Meeting of the European Society for Stereotactic and Functional Neurosurgery, Paris 1979. Abstr., p. V41.

Barcia-Salorio, J.L.; Martinez Carrillo, J.A.: Calculation of the target point by means of an analogue field plotter; in Gillingham, Donaldson, 3rd Symp. on Parkinson's Disease, pp. 223–232 (Livingstone, London 1969).

Bard, P.; Mountcastle, V.B.: Some forebrain mechanisms involved in the expression of rage. Res. Publs Ass. nerv. ment. Dis. *27:* 362–404 (1947).

Bard, P.; Rioch, D.Mc.: A study of four cats deprived of neocortex and additional portions of the forebrain. Johns Hopkins Hosp. Bull. *60:* 73–148 (1937).

Bates, J.: Computer techniques in the analysis of electrophysiological data from the human thalamus. Confinia neurol. *36:* 310–311 (1974).

*Battig, K.; Rosvold, H.E.; Mishkin, M.: Comparison of the effects of frontal and caudate lesions on delayed response and alternation in monkeys. J. comp. physiol. Psychol. *53:* 400–404 (1960).

Baudoin, A.; Puech, P.: Premiers essais d'intervention directe sur le thalamus. Revue neurol. *81:* 78–81 (1949).

Bechterew, W.: Die Funktionen der Nervenzentren, Bd. 1–3 (Fischer, Jena 1908–1911).

Bechterewa, N.P.: Physiologie und Pathophysiologie der tiefen Hirnstrukturen des Menschen (Volk und Gesundheit, Berlin 1969).

Bechterewa, N.P.; Bondortchuk, A.N.; Smirnov, V.M.; Meliutcheva, L.A.: Pain therapy by electric stimulation of deep encephalic structures. Vop. Neurokhir. *36:* 1–7 (1972).

*Bechterewa, N.P.; Bondartchuk, A.N.; Smirnov, V.M.; Meliutcheva, L.A.; Shandurina, A.N.: Method of electrostimulation of the deep brain structures in treatment of some chronic diseases. Confinia neurol. *37:* 136–140 (1975).

Benabid, A.L.; Persat, J.C.; Cirossel, J.P.; de Rougemont, J.; Barge, M.; Salmon, G.; Farnarier, P.: Correlative study between computerized transverse scanning and stereoimpedoencephalography in space-occupying lesions of the brain. Acta neurochir. *46:* 219–232 (1979).

Bergstrom, M.; Boëthius, J.; Collins, V.P.; Edner, G.; Lewander, R.; Willems, J.: A combined study of computed tomography and stereotactic biopsy in gliomas; in Carrea, Neurological surgery with emphasis on non-invasive methods of diagnosis and treatment, pp. 45–50 (Excerpta Medica, Amsterdam 1978).

Bergstrom, M.; Boëthius, J.; Eriksson, L.; Greitz, T.; Ribbe, T.; Widen, L.: Head fixation device for reproducible position alignment in transmission CT and positron emission tomography. J. Comput. assist. Tomogr. *5:* 136–141 (1981).

Bergstrom, M.; Greitz, T.: Stereotaxic computed tomography. Am. J. Roentg. *127:* 167–170 (1976).

Bernis, W.J.; Spiegel, E.A.: Die Zentren der statischen Innervation und ihre Beeinflussung durch Klein- und Grosshirn. Arb. neurol. Inst. Wien. Univ. *27:* 197–224 (1925).

Bertler, A.; Rosengren, E.: Occurrence and distribution of catecholamines in brain. Acta Physiol. Scand. *47:* 350–361 (1959).

Bertrand, C.: A pneumotaxic technique producing localized cerebral lesions and its use in the treatment of Parkinson's disease. J. Neurosurg. *15:* 251–264 (1958).

Bertrand, C.: Long-term results of stereotactic surgery for uncontrollable seizures originating outside of the temporal lobes. Meeting of the European Society for Stereotactic and Functional Neurosurgery, Paris 1979. Abstr., p. J16.

Bertrand, C.; Martinez, N.; Hardy, J.: Fronto-thalamic section for intractable pain; in Knighton, Dumke, Pain Symp., Detroit 1964, pp. 531–535 (Churchill, London 1966).

Bertrand, C.; Molina-Negro, P.; Martinez, S.N.: Combined stereotactic and peripheral surgical approach in spasmodic torticollis. Appl. Neurophysiol. *41:* 122–133 (1978).

Bertrand, G.; Hardy, T.: Computerized graphic study of the distribution, in the human thalamus, of neurones responding to tactile stimuli. Meeting of the World Society for Stereotactic and Functional Neurosurgery, São Paulo 1977, p. 40.

Bertrand, G.; Jasper, H.: Microelectrode recording of unit activity in the human thalamus. Confinia neurol. *26:* 205–208 (1965).

Bertrand, G.; Jasper, H.; Wong, A.: Microelectrode study of the human thalamus: functional organization in the ventrobasal complex. Confinia Neurol. *29:* 81–86 (1967).

Bertrand, G.; Olivier, A.; Thompson, C.J.: Computer display of stereotaxic brain maps and probe tracts. Acta neurochir. *21:* suppl., pp. 235–243 (1974).

Besson, J.M.; Oliveras, J.L.: Analgesia induced by electrical stimulation of the brain stem in animals: involvement of serotoninergic mechanisms. Acta. neurochir. *30:* suppl., pp 201–207 (1980).

Bickford, R.G.: Discussion of Brazier (1964).

Bickford, R.G.; Keith, H.M.; MacCarthy, C.S.: Some observations on the mechanism of petit mal. 80th Meet. Trans. Am. neurol. Ass., 1955, p. 13–15.

Bickford, R.G.; MacDonald, H.N.A.; Dodge, H.W., Jr.; Svien, H.J.: Distant evoked responses to single pulse stimulation; in Sheer, Electrical stimulation of the brain, pp. 91–98 (University of Texas Press, Austin 1961).

Bickford, R.G.; Mulder, D.W.; Dodge, H.W., Jr.; Swien, H.J.; Rome, H.P.: Changes in memory function produced by electrical stimulation of the temporal lobe in man. Res. Publs Ass. Res. nerv. ment. Dis. 36: 227–243 (1958).

Biemond, A.: The conduction of pain above the level of the thalamus opticus. Archs Neurol. Psychiat., Chicago 75: 231–244 (1956).

Bingley, T.; Leksell, L.; Meyerson, B.A.; Rylander, G.: Stereotactic anterior capsulotomy and obsessive-compulsive states; in Laitinen, Livingston, Surgical approaches in psychiatry, pp. 159–164 (Medical and Technical Publishing, Lancaster 1973).

Birg, W.; Mundinger, F.: Computer calculation of target parameters for a stereotactic apparatus. Acta neurochir. 29: 123–129 (1973).

Birg, W.; Mundinger, F.: Direct target point determination for stereotactic brain operations from CT data and the calculation of setting parameters for polar-coordinate stereotactic devices. Appl. Neurophysiol. 45: 387–391 (1982).

Birg, W.; Mundinger, F.; Klar, M.: A computer programme system for stereotactic neurosurgery. Acta neurochir. 24: suppl., pp. 99–108 (1977).

Birkmayer, W.; Hornykiewicz, O.: Der L-dioxyphenylalanin (L-Dopa) Effekt beim Parkinson-Syndrome des Menschen. Zur Pathogenese und Behandlung der Parkinson-Akinese. Arch. Psychiat. NervKrankh. 203: 560–574 (1962).

Bischof, W.: Die longitudinale Myelotomie. Zentbl. Neurochir. 11: 79–88 (1951).

Bishop, G.H.: The relationship between nerve fiber size and sensory modality: phylogenetic implication of the afferent innervation of cortex. J. nerv. ment. Dis. 128: 89–114 (1959).

Bjorndal, N.; Casey, D.E.; Gerlach, J.: Enkephalin, morphina and naloxone in tardive dyskinesia. Psychopharmacology 69: 133–136 (1980).

Black, P.; Nematsu, S.; Walker, A.E.: Stereotaxic hypothalamotomy for control of violent, aggressive behavior. Confinia neurol. 37: 187–188 (1975).

Bloom, F.E.; Costa, E.; Salmoirachi, G.C.: Anesthesia and the responsiveness of individual neurons of the caudate nucleus of the cat to acetylcholine, norepinephrine and dopamine administered by microelectrophoresis. J. Pharmac. exp. Ther. 150: 244 (1965).

Bloom, F.E.; Rossier, J.; Battenberg, E.L.F.; Bayon, A.; French, E.; Henrikson, S.J.; Siggins, G.R.; Browne, R.; Ling, N.; Guillemin, R.: Beta-endorphin: cellular localization, electrophysiological and behavioral effects; in Costa, Trabucchi, The endorphins. Advances in biochemical psychopharmacology, vol. 18, pp. 89–109 (Raven Press, New York 1978).

Bloom, F.E.; Segal, D.; Ling, N.; Guillemin, R.: Endorphins: profound behavioral effects in rats suggest new etiological factors in mental illness. Science 94: 630–632 (1976).

Blumetti, A.; Modesti, L.M.: Long-term cognitive effects of stereotactic thalamotomy on non-parkinsonian dyskinetic patients. Appl. Neurophysiol. 43: 259–262 (1980).

Boëthius, J.; Bergstrom, G.; Collins, V.P.; Edner, G.; Tribukait, B.: DNA distribution various parts of malignant gliomas assayed on stereotactic biopsies. Appl. Neurophysiol. *43:* 216–221 (1980b).

Boëthius, J.; Bergstrom, M.; Greitz, T.: Stereotaxic computerized tomography with a GE 8800 scanner. J. Neurosurg. *52:* 794–800 (1980a).

Boëthius, J.; Bergstrom, M.; Greitz, T.; Ribbe, T.: CT localization in stereotactic surgery. Appl. Neurophysiol. *43:* 164–169 (1980c).

Boëthius, J.; Collins, V.P.; Edner, G.; Lewander, R.; Zajicek, J.: Stereotactic biopsies and computer tomography in gliomas. Acta neurochir. *40:* 223–232 (1978).

Boëthius, J.; Levander, B.; Lindquist, C.: Intraventricular pressure monitoring – a stereotactic approach for compressed ventricular systems. Acta neurochir. *28:* suppl., pp. 582–584 (1979).

Boëthius, J.; Lindblom, U.; Meyerson, B.A.; Widen, L.: Effect of multifocal brain stimulation on pain and somatosensory functions; in Zotterman, Sensory functions of the skin, pp. 531–546 (Pergamon Press, Oxford 1976).

Boëthius, J.; Meyerson, B.A.: Chronic, percutaneous deep brain stimulation in cancer pain. Meeting of the World Society for Stereotactic and Functional Neurosurgery, São Paulo 1977, p. 21.

Borison, R.L.; Davis, J.M.: Amantadine and Gilles de la Tourette syndrome; in Duvoisin, Trans. Am. neurol. Ass., vol. 105, pp. 471–473 (Springer, New York 1980).

*Borison, H.L.; Wang, S.C.: Quantitative effects of radon implanted in the medulla oblongata. J. comp. Neurol. *94:* 33–53 (1951).

Bosch, D.A.: Indications for stereotactic biopsy in brain tumors. Acta neurochir. *54:* 167–179 (1980a).

Bosch, D.A.: Indications for stereotactic biopsy in brain tumors. Acta neurochir. *54:* 167–179 (1980b).

*Bosch, D.A.; Hindmarsch, T.; Larsson, S.; Backlund, E.O.: Intraneoplastic administration of bleomycin in intracerebral gliomas: a pilot study. Acta. neurochir. *30:* suppl., pp. 441–444 (1980).

Bosch, D.A.; Rahn, T.; Backlund, E.O.: Treatment of colloid cysts of the third ventricle by stereotactic aspiration. Surg. Neurol. *9:* 15–18 (1978).

Bouchard, G.: Stereotactic operations in generalized forms of epilepsy. Acta neurochir. *21:* suppl., pp. 15–24 (1974).

Bouchard, G.: Basic targets of the different epilepsies. Acta neurochir. *23:* suppl., pp. 193–199 (1976).

Bouchard, G.; Kim, Y.K.; Umbach, W.: Stereotaxic methods in different forms of epilepsy. Confinia neurol. *37:* 232–238 (1975).

Bowsher, D.: Termination of the central pain pathway; the conscious appreciation of pain. Brain *80:* 606–622 (1957).

Boyesen, S.; Campbell, J.B.: Stereotaxic implantation of palladium-109 and yttrium-90 spheres. Yale J. Biol. Med. *28:* 216–224 (1955).

Brady, J.V.; Schreiner, L.; Geller, I.; Kling, A.: Subcortical mechanisms in emotional behavior: the effect of rhinencephalic injury upon the acquisition and retention of a conditioned avoidance response in cats. J. comp. physiol. Psychol. *47:* 179–186 (1954).

Brazier, M.A.B.: Stimulation of the hippocampus in man using implanted electrodes; in Brazier, Brain function. II. RNA and brain function, memory and learning, pp. 299–310 (University of California Press, Berkeley 1964).

Brazier, M.A.B.: Interactions of deep structures during seizures in man; in Petsche, Brazier, Synchronization of EEG activity in epilepsies, pp. 409–424 (Springer, Wien 1972).

Brazier, M.A.B.; Barlow, J.S.: Some applications of correlation analysis to clinical problems in electroencephalography. Electroenceph. clin. Neurophysiol. 8: 325 (1956).

*Brazier, M.A.B.; Kjellberg, R.N.; Sweet, W.N.; Barlow, J.S.: Electrographic recording and correlation analysis from deep structures within the brain; in Ramey, O'Doherty, Electrical studies on the unanesthetized brain, pp. 311–333 (Hoeber, New York 1960).

Brierley, J.B.; Beck, E.: The significance in human stereotactic brain surgery of individual variation. J. Neurol. Neurosurg. Psychiat. 22: 287–298 (1959).

Broager, B.: Experiences with chemopallidectomy and chemothalamectomy (Nord. Neurokirurgisk Forenings, Copenhagen 1958).

Broggi, G.; Franzini, A.: Value of serial stereotactic biopsies and impedance monitoring in the treatment of deep brain tumors. J. Neurol. Neurosurg. Psychiat. 44: 397–401 (1981).

Broseta, J.; Barcia-Salorio, J.L.; Barberá, J.: Septal stimulation in painful and symbolic stress. Experimental study. Acta neurochir. 30: suppl., pp. 275–278 (1980).

Broseta, J.; Gonzalez-Darder, J.; Barcia-Salorio, J.L.: Stereotactic evacuation of intracerebral hematomas. Appl. Neurophysiol. 45: 443–448 (1982).

Brown, M.H.: Further experience with multiple limbic targets for schizophrenia and aggression; in Laitinen, Livingstone, Surgical approaches in psychiatry, pp. 189–195 (Medical and Technical Publishing, Lancaster 1973).

Brown, M.H.: Limbic target surgery in the treatment of intractable pain with drug addiction. Acta neurochir. 24: suppl., p. 233 (1977).

Brown, M.H.; Lighthill, J.A.: Selective anterior cingulotomy. J. Neurosurg. 29: 513–519 (1968).

Brown, R.A.: A computerized tomography-computer graphics approach to stereotaxic localization. J. Neurosurg. 50: 715–720 (1979a).

Brown, R.A.: A stereotactic head frame for use with CT body scanners. Investve Radiol. 14: 30–304 (1979b).

Brown, R.A.: Computer graphic approach to stereotactic procedures; in Newton, Potts, Radiology of the skull and brain: technical aspects of computed tomography, pp. 4296–4300 (Mosby, St. Louis, 1981).

Brown, R.A.; Roberts, T.S.; Osborn, A.G.: Stereotaxic frame and computer software for CT-directed neurosurgical localization. Investve Radiol. 15: 308–312 (1980).

Brown, R.A.; Roberts, T.S.; Osborn, A.G.: Simplified CT-guided stereotaxic biopsy. Am. J. Neuroradiol. 2: 181–184 (1981).

Bruyn, G.W.: Huntington's chorea; in Vinken, Bruyn, Handbook of clinical neurology, vol. 6: Diseases of the basal ganglia, pp. 298–378 (North-Holland, Amsterdam 1968).

Buchwald, N.A.; Wieck, H.H.; Wyers, E.J.: Effects of stimulation of caudate nucleus on outflow of globus pallidus. Anat. Rec. 133: 256 (1950).

Buño, W.J.; Martin-Rodriguez, J.G.; Garcia-Austt, E.; Obrador, S.: Electrophysiological set-up for data acquisition and processing during stereotaxic surgery. Acta neurochir. 24: suppl., pp. 109–119 (1977).

Burchiel, K.J.; Ojemann, G.A.; Bolender, N.: Localization of stereotaxic centers by computerized tomographic scanning. Technical note. J. Neurosurg. 53: 861–863 (1980).

Burton, C.V.; Mozley, J.M.; Walker, A.E.; Braitmann, H.E.: Inductive heating. IEEE Trans. biomed. Engng *13:* 114 (1966).

Burzaco, J.A.: Fundus striae terminalis, an optional target in sedative stereotactic surgery; in Laitinen, Livingston, Surgical approaches in psychiatry, pp. 135–137 (Medical and Technical Publishing, Lancaster 1973).

Cail, W.S.; Morris, J.L.: Localization of intracranial lesions from CT scans. Surg. Neurol. *11:* 35–37 (1979).

Cairns, H.; Duffield, J.E.; Tow, P.M.; Whittey, C.W.: Anterior cingulectomy in the treatment of mental disease. Lancet *i:* 75 (1952).

Callan, J.P.: Electroconvulsive therapy. Editorial. J. Am. med. Ass. *242:* 545–546 (1979).

Calne, D.B.: Bromocriptine in Parkinson's disease. Symp. Am. Acad. of Neurology, 1981.

*Calne, D.B.; Kebabian J.W.; Silbergeld, E., et al.: Advances in the neuropharmacology of parkinsonism. Ann. intern. Med. *90:* 219–229 (1979).

Campbell, R.L.; Campbell, J.A.; Heimburger, R.F.; Klasbeck, J.E.; Mealey, J.: Ventriculography and myelography with absorbable radiopaque medium. Radiology *82:* 286–289 (1964).

Campbell, J.B.; Rossi, H.H.; Biavati, M.H.; Biavati, B.J.: Production of subcortical lesions by implantation of radioactive substances. Confinia neurol. *22:* 178–182 (1962).

Cannon, W.B.; Rosenblueth, A.: The supersensitivity of denervated structures (Macmillan, New York 1949).

Carlsson, A.; Lindquist, M.: Effects of chlorpromazine and haloperidol on the formation of 3-methoxytyramine and normetanephrine in mouse brain. Acta pharmac. tox. *20:* 140–144 (1963).

Carmel, P.W.: Sympathetic deficits following thalamotomy. Archs Neurol., Chicago *18:* 378–387 (1968).

Carpenter, M.B.: Dorsal trigeminal tract in rhesus monkey. J. Anat., Lond. *91:* 82–90 (1957).

Carpenter, M.B.; McMasters, R.E.: Lesions of the substantia nigra in the rhesus monkey. Efferent fiber degeneration and behavioral observations. Am. J. Anat. *114:* 293–312 (1964).

Carpenter, M.B.; Whittier, J.R.; Mettler, F.A.: Analysis of choreoid hyperkinesia in the rhesus monkey. J. comp. Neurol. *92:* 293–331 (1950).

Carrea, R.M.E.; Mettler, F.A.: Physiologic consequences following extensive removals of the cerebellar cortex and deep cerebellar nuclei and effect of secondary cerebral ablations in the primate. J. comp. Neurol. *87:* 169–288 (1947).

Carrea, R.M.E.; Mettler, F.A.: Function of the primate brachium conjunctivum and related structures. J. comp. Neurol. *102:* 151–327 (1955).

Casey, D.E.; Korsgaard, S.; Gerlach, J.; Jorgensen, A.; Simmelsgaard, H.: Effect of des-tyrosine-γ-endorphin in tardive dyskinesia. Archs gen. Psychiat. *38:* 158–160 (1981).

Castellanos, F.X.: Naloxone effects. Neurology *29:* 1318–1319 (1979).

Cerroni, M.; DeMichele, D.; Hamilton, B.; Norman, W.; Sinks, L.; McCullough, D.; Manz, H.; Schellinger, D.; O'Doherty, D.: Some methods for extracting quantitative data from CT scans. J. Comput. assist. Tomogr. *3:* 571 (1979).

Chapman, W.R.: Studies of the periamygdaloid area in relation to human behavior. Res.
    Publs Ass. Res. nerv. ment. Dis. 36: 258–277 (1958).

Chapman, W.P.: Depth electrode studies in patients with temporal lobe epilepsy; in
    Ramey, O'Doherty, Electrical studies on the unanesthetized brain, pp. 334–350
    (Hoeber, New York 1960).

Chatrian, G.E.; Chapman, W.P.: Electrographic study of the amygdaloid region with
    implanted electrodes in patients with temporal lobe epilepsy; in Ramey, O'Doherty,
    Electrical studies on the unanesthetized brain, pp. 351–368 (Hoeber, New York
    1960).

Check, W.A.: Alcohol injections relieving intractable pain. Editorial. J. Am. med. Ass. 242:
    2164–2169 (1979).

Chescotta, R.; Stella, O.; Chinela, A.; Gotusso, C.: Experience with stereotaxic surgery in
    treating extrapyramidal disorders. Meeting of the World Society for Stereotactic and
    Functional Neurosurgery, São Paulo 1977, p. 70.

Chitanondh, H.: Stereotaxic amygdalotomy in the treatment of olfactory seizures and psy-
    chiatric disorders with olfactory hallucinations. Confinia neurol. 27: 181–196 (1966).

Choppy, M.; Zimbacca, N.; LeBeau, J.: Psychological changes after selective frontal sur-
    gery (especially cingulumotomy) and after stereotactic surgery of the basal ganglia; in
    Laitinen, Livingston, Surgical approaches in psychiatry, pp. 174–181 (Medical and
    Technical Publishing, Lancaster 1973).

Clark, W.E. Le Gros: The structure and connections of the thalamus. Brain 55: 406–470
    (1932).

Clark, W.E. Le Gros: Functional localization in the thalamus and hypothalamus. J. ment.
    Sci. 82: 99–118 (1936).

Cohen, D.J.; Detlor, J.; Young, J.G.; Shaywitz, B.A.: Clonidine ameliorates Gilles de la
    Tourette syndrome. Archs. gen. Psychiat. 37: 1350–1357 (1980).

Colombo, F.; Angrilli, F.; Zanardo, A.; Pinna, A.; Benedetti, A.: A new method for utiliz-
    ing CT data in stereotactic surgery: measurement and transformation technique. Acta
    neurochir. 57: 195–203 (1981).

Colombo, F.; Angrilli, F.; Zanardo, A.; Pinna, V.; Alexandre, A.; Benedetti, A.: A universal
    method to employ CT scanner spatial information in stereotactic surgery. Appl. Neu-
    rophysiol. 45: 352–365 (1982).

Colombo, F.; Benedetti, A.; Alexandre, A.: Stereotactic exploration of deep-seated or sur-
    gically unamenable intracranial space-occupying lesions. J. neurol. Sci. 24: 173–177
    (1980).

Conger, K.B.: Quoted by Spiegel and Wycis (1962).

Cook, A.W.; Weinstein, S.P.: Chronic dorsal column stimulation in multiple sclerosis.
    N.Y. St. J. Med. 73: 2868–2872 (1973).

Cooper, I.W.: Chemopallidectomy. Science 121: 217 (1955).

Cooper, I.S.: Neurosurgical alleviation of intention tremor of multiple sclerosis and cere-
    bellar disease. New Engl. J. Med. 263: 441–444 (1960).

Cooper, I.S.: Parkinsonism (Thomas, Springfield 1961).

Cooper, I.S.; Amin, I.; Chandra, R.; Waltz, I.: A surgical investigation of the clinical
    physiology of the pulvinar complex in man. J. neurol. Sci. 18: 89–110 (1973a).

Cooper, I.S.; Amin, I.; Gilman, S.: The effect of chronic cerebellar stimulation upon epi-
    lepsy in man. Trans. Am. neurol. Ass. 1973, pp. 192–196 (Springer, New York
    1973b).

Cooper, I.S.; Bravo, G.J.: Chemopallidectomy and chemothalamectomy. J. Neurosurg. *15:* 244–250 (1958a).

Cooper, I.S.; Bravo, G.J.: Implications of a five year study of 700 basal ganglia operations. Neurology *8:* 701–717 (1958b).

Cooper, I.S.; Gioino, G.; Terry, R.: The cryogenic lesion. Confinia neurol. *26:* 161–177 (1965).

Cooper, I.S.; Lee, A. St. J.: Cryostatic congelation. J. nerv. ment. Dis. *133:* 259–263 (1961).

Cooper, I.S.; Poloukhine, N.: Chemopallidectomy. J. Am. Geriat. Soc. *3:* 838–859 (1955).

Cooper, I.S.; Riklan, M.; Snider, R.S.: Cerebellum, epilepsy and behavior (Plenum Press, New York 1974).

*Cooper, I.S.; Upton, A.R.M.; Rappaport, Z.H.: Correlation of clinical and physiological effects of cerebellar stimulation. Acta neurochir. *55:* suppl. 30, pp. 339–344 (1980).

Cooper, I.S.; Waltz, J.M.; Amin, I.; Fuita, S.: Pulvinectomy: a preliminary report. J. Am. Geriat. Soc. *19:* 553–554 (1971).

Cordeau, J.P.: Microelectrode studies in monkeys with a postural tremor. Revue Can. Biol. *20:* 147–157 (1961).

Cordeau, J.P.; Gybels, J.M.; Jasper, H.; Poirier, L.J.: Microelectrode studies of unit discharges in the sensorimotor cortex: investigations in monkeys with experimental tremor. Neurology *10:* 691–600 (1960).

Corkin, S.; Twitchell, T.E.; Sullivan, E.V.: Safety and efficacy of cingulotomy for pain and psychiatric disorder; in Hitchcock, Alterations of brain function (Elsevier, Amsterdam 1979).

Corssen, G.: Alcohol induced adenolysis of the pituitary gland. A new approach to control intractable cancer pain. Anesth. Analg. *56:* 414–421 (1977).

*Costa, E.; Fratta, W.; Hong, J.S.; Moroni, F.; Yang, H.-Y.T.: Interactions between enkephalin and other neuronal systems; in Costa, Trabucchi, The endorphins. Advances in biochemical psychopharmacology, pp. 217–226 (Raven Press, New York 1978).

Cox, A.W.; Brown, M.H.: Results of multitarget limbic surgery in the treatment of schizophrenia and aggressive states; in Sweet, Obrador, Martin-Rodriguez, Neurosurgical treatment of psychiatry, pain and epilepsy, pp. 369–479 (University Park Press, Baltimore 1977).

Critchley, M.: The parietal lobes (Arnold, London 1953).

Crosby, E.C.; Humphrey, T.; Lauer, E.W.: Correlative anatomy of the nervous system (Macmillan, New York 1962).

Crow, T.J.; Longden, A.; Johnstone, E.C.; Owen, F.: Dopamine and schizophrenia; in Roberts, Woodruff, Iversen, Advances of biochemical pharmacology, vol. 19, pp. 301–309 (Raven Press, New York 1978).

Crue, B.L.; Todd, E.M.; Carregal, E.J.A.; Kilham, O.: Percutaneous trigeminal tractotomy. Bull. Los Ang. neurol. Soc. *32:* 86–92 (1967).

Dahlstrom, A.; Fuxe, K.: Evidence for the existence of monoamine containing neurons in the central nervous system. I. Demonstration of monoamines in the cell bodies of brain stem neurons. Acta physiol. scand. *62:* 1–55 (1964).

Davis, K.L.; Hollister, L.E.; Stahl, S.M.; Berger, P.A.: Choline chloride in Huntington's disease; in Duvoisin, Trans. Am. neurol. Ass., vol. 105, pp. 464–467 (Springer, New York 1980).

Davis, R.; Barolat-Romana, G.; Engle, H.: Chronic cerebellar stimulation for cerebral palsy. Five-year study. Acta neurochir. *30:* suppl., pp. 317–332 (1980).

Davison, C.: The role of the globus pallidus and substantia nigra in the production of rigidity and tremor. Diseases of the basal ganglia. Res. Publs Ass. nerv. ment. Dis. *21:* 267–333 (1942).

Davison, C.; Goodhart, S.P.: Monochorea and somatotopic localization. Archs Neurol. Psychiat. *43:* 792–803 (1940).

*Dawson, B.H.; Dervin, E.; Heywood, O.B.: The development of a mechanical analogy for directing and tracking of the electrode during stereotaxic operations. J. Neurosurg. *31:* 361–366 (1969).

Dean, W.H.; Davis, G.D.: Behavior changes following caudate lesions in rhesus monkey. J. Neurophysiol. *22:* 524–537 (1959).

Delgado, J.M.R.; Mark, V.H.; Sweet, W.H., et al.: Intracerebral radiostimulation and recording in completely free patients. J. nerv. ment. Dis. *147:* 329–340 (1968).

Delgado, J.M.R.; Obrador, S.; Martin-Rodriguez, J.G.: Two-way radio communication with the brain in psychosurgical patients; in Laitinen, Livingston, Surgical approaches in psychiatry, pp. 215–223 (Medical and Technical Publishing, Lancaster 1973).

Delmas-Marsalet, V.A.P.: Contribution expérimentale à l'étude des fonctions du noyau caudé; thèse Bordeaux (1925).

Delmas-Marsalet, V.A.P.: Essais de chirurgie physiologique dans le traitement du parkinsonisme. Revue neurol. *63:* 550–553 (1935).

Dempsey, E.W.; Morison, R.S.: The production of rhythmically recurrent cortical potentials after localized thalamic stimulation. Am. J. Physiol. *135:* 293–300 (1942).

Denny-Brown, D.: The basal ganglia (Oxford University Press, London 1962).

Diamond, B.I.; Borison, R.L.: Enkephalins and nigrostriatal functions. Neurology *28:* 1085–1088 (1978).

Diamond, B.I.; Borison, R.L.: Enkephalins and experimental extrapyramidal movement disorders; in Duvoisin, Trans. Am. neurol. Ass., vol. 105, pp. 467–468 (Springer, New York 1980).

Diamond, B.I.; Rajan, K.S.; Borison, R.L.: Therapeutic forms of *L*-dopa; in Duvoisin, Trans. Am. neurol. Ass., vol. 105, pp. 469–471 (Springer, New York 1980).

Dieckmann, G.; Gabriel, E.; Hassler, R.: Size, form and structural peculiarities of experimental lesions obtained by thermocontrolled radiofrequency. Confinia neurol. *26:* 134–142 (1966).

Dieckmann, G.; Hassler, R.: Stereotaxic treatment of extrapyramidal myoclonus. Confinia neurol. *34:* 57–63 (1972).

Dieckmann, G.; Hassler, R.: Unilateral hypothalamotomy in sexual delinquents. Confinia neurol. *37:* 177–186 (1975).

Dieckmann, G.; Schneider, H.: Influence of stereotactic hypothalamotomy on alcohol and drug addiction. Appl. Neurophysiol. *41:* 93–98 (1978).

Diemath, H.E.; Heppner, F.; Enge, S.; Lechner, H.: Die stereotaktische vordere Cingulotomie bei therapieresistenter generalisierter Epilepsie. Confinia neurol. *27:* 124–128 (1966).

Diemath, H.E.; Nievoll, A.: Stereotaktische Ausschaltungen im Nucleus amygdalae und im gegenseitigen Dorsomedial-Kern bei erethischen Kindern. Confinia neurol. *27:* 172–180 (1966).

Dierssen, G.: Treatment of dystonic and athetoid symptoms by lesions in the sensory portion of the internal capsule. Confinia neurol. *26:* 404–406 (1966).

Dierssen, G.; Bergmann, L.L.; Gioino, G.; Cooper, I.S.: Hemiballism following surgery for Parkinson's disease. Archs Neurol., Chicago *5:* 627–637 (1961).

Dierssen, G.; Bergmann, L.L.; Giono, G.; Cooper, I.S.: Surgical lesions affecting Parkinsonian symptomatology. Acta neurochir. *10:* 125–133 (1962).

Dittmar, C.: Über die Lage des sogenannten Gefässzentrums in der Medulla oblongata. Ber. sächs. Ges. Wiss., Leipzig (Math. phys.) *25:* 449–469 (1973).

Divitii, E. de; D'Errico, A.; Cerillo, A.: Stereotactic surgery in Gilles de la Tourette syndrome. Acta neurosurg. *24:* suppl., p. 73 (1977).

Doerner, G.; Doecke, F.; Hinz, G.: Homo- and hypersexuality in rats with hypothalamic lesions. Neuroendocrinology *4:* 20–24 (1969).

Doerner, G.; Doecke, F.; Moustafa, S.: Differential localization of a male and a female hypothalamic mating center. J. Reprod. Fertil. *17:* 583–586 (1968).

Dumas-Duport, C.; Monsaingeon, V.; Szenthe, L.; Szikla, G.: Serial stereotactic biopsies: a double histological code of gliomas according to malignancy and 3-D configuration, as an aid to therapeutic decision and assessment of results. Appl. Neurophysiol. *45:* 431–437 (1982).

Edner, G.: Stereotactic biopsy in tumours of the sellar region other than adenomas. Acta neurochir. *28:* suppl., pp. 326–328 (1979).

Edner, G.: Stereotactic biopsy of intracranial space occupying lesions. Acta neurochir. *57:* 213–234 (1981).

Ehringer, H.; Hornykiewicz, O.: Verteilung von Noradrenalin und Dopamin im Gehirn des Menschen und ihr Verhalten bei Erkrankungen des extrapyramidalen Systems. Klin. Wschr. *38:* 1236–1239 (1960).

Emmers, R.: Pain: a spike-interval coded message in the brain (Raven Press, New York 1981).

Emmers, R.; Tasker, R.R.: The human somesthetic thalamus (Raven Press, New York 1975).

Engel, J., Jr.: Crandall, P.; Brown, W.: Significance of focal, regional and bilaterally independent ictal EEG onsets recorded from mesial temporal depth electrodes. Abstr. Meet. Am. EEG Soc., Boston 1980, p. 11.

Ervin, F.R.; Brown, C.E.; Mark, V.H.: Striatal influence on facial pain. Confinia neurol. *27:* 75–86 (1966).

Escobedo, F.; Fernández-Guardiola, A.; Solls, G.: Chronic stimulation of the cingulum in humans with behavior disorders; in Laitinen, Livingston, Surgical approaches in psychiatry, pp. 65–68 (Medical and Technical Publishing, Lancaster 1973).

Essen, C. von; Augustinsson, L.; Lindqvist, G.: VOI thalamotomy in spasmodic torticollis. Appl. Neurophysiol. *43:* 159–163 (1980).

Evans, R.D.: Isotopes; in Glasser, Medical physics, pp. 643–658 (Yearbook, Chicago 1944).

Fairman, D.: Roentgenologic principles of a new stereotactic apparatus. Am. J. Roentg. *81:* 1001–1003 (1959).

Fairman, D.: Hypothalamotomy as a new perspective for alleviation of intractable pain and regression of metastatic malignant tumors; in Fusek, Kunc, Present limits of neurosurgery, pp. 525–528 (Avicenum, Prague 1971).

Fairman, D.: Neurophysiological basis for the hypothalamic lesions and stimulation by chronic implanted electrodes for the relief of intractable pain in cancer. Adv. Pain Res. Ther. *1:* 842–847 (1976).

*Fairman, D.; Lavallol, M.A.: New method of stereotactic hypophysectomy. Confinia neurol. *37:* 172–176 (1975).

Fasano, V.A.; Morgando, E.; Baggiore, P.; Monticone, G.F.: Risultati del trattamento chirurgico di 35 casi di sindromi parkinsoniane. Boll. Soc. Piemont. Chir. *31:* 1–7 (1961).

Feindel, W.: Response patterns elicited from the amygdala and deep temporo-insular cortex; in Sheer Electrical stimulation of the brain, pp. 519–532 (Hogg Foundation, Austin 1961).

Feindel, W.; Penfield, W.: Localization of discharges in temporal lobe automatism. Archs Neurol. Psychiat. *72:* 605–630 (1954).

Fernandez-Molina, A.; Hunsperger, R.W.: Organization of the subcortical system governing defense and flight reactions in the cat. J. Physiol., Lond. *160:* 200 (1962).

Foerster, O.: Zur Analyse und Pathophysiologie der striären Bewegungsstörungen. Z. ges. Neurol. Psychiat. *72:* 1–164 (1921).

Folkerts, J.F.; Spiegel, E.A.: Tremor on stimulation of the midbrain tegmentum. Confinia neurol. *13:* 193–202 (1953).

Foltz, E.L.; White, L.E., Jr.: Pain relief by frontal cingulumotomy. J. Neurosurg. *19:* 89–100 (1962).

Forrest, A.P.M.; Blair, D.W.; Valentine, J.S.: Screw implantation of the pituitary with yttrium-90. Lancet *ii:* 192–193 (1958).

*Forrest, A.P.M.; Roberts, M.M.; Stewart, H.J.: Pituitary ablation by yttrium-90. Acta neurochir. *21:* suppl., pp. 137–143 (1974).

Fraioli, B.; Guidetti, B.: Effects of stereotactic lesions of the pulvinar and lateralis posterior nucleus on intractable pain and dyskinetic syndromes in man. Appl. Neurophysiol. *38:* 23–30 (1975).

Fraioli, B.; Guidetti, B.; LaTorre, E.: The stereotaxic dentatotomy in the treatment of spasticity and dyskinetic disorders. J. neurolog. Sci. *17:* 49–52 (1973).

*Frazier, R.; Joplin, G.F.; Laws, J.W.; Morrison, R.; Steiner, R.E.: Needle implantation of yttrium seeds for pituitary ablation in cases of secondary carcinoma. Lancet *i:* 382–384 (1959).

Freeman, G.L.; Krasno, L.: Inhibitory functions of the corpus striatum. Archs Neurol. Psychiat. *44:* 323–327 (1940).

Freeman, W.; Watts, J.W.: Psychosurgery; 2nd ed. (Thomas, Springfield 1950).

French, L.A.; Story, J.L.; Galicich, J.H.; Schultz, E.A.: Some aspects of stimulation and recording from the basal ganglia in patients with abnormal movements. Confinia neurol. *22:* 265–273 (1962).

Friedman, H.; Nashold, B.S.; Senjen, G.: Physiological effects of dorsal column stimulation; in Bonica, Advances of neurology, pp. 769–773 (Raven Press, New York 1974).

Fukamachi, A.; Ohye, C.; Saito, Y.; Narabayashi, H.: Estimation of the neural noise within the human thalamus. Acta neurochir. *24:* suppl., pp. 121–136 (1977).

Fünfgeld, E.W.: Psychopathologie und Klinik des Parkinsonismus vor und nach stereotaktischen Operationen (Springer, Berlin 1967).

Galanda, M.; Nádvornik, P.; Fodor, S.: Stereotactic approach to therapeutic stimulation of cerebellum for spasticity. Acta neurochir. *30:* suppl., pp. 345–350 (1980).

Ganglberger, J.A.: The effect of stereotaxic lesions in pallidum or thalamus upon the EEG. Excerpta Med. Int. Congr. Ser., No. 37, pp. 71–72 (1961).

Ganglberger, J.A.: New possibilities of stereotactic treatment of temporal lobe epilepsy. Acta neurochir. *23:* suppl., pp. 211–214 (1976).

Gaze, R.M.; Gillingham, F.J.; Kalyanaram, S.; Porter, R.W.; Donaldson, A.A.; Donaldson, I.M.L.: Microelectrode recordings from the human thalamus. Brain *87:* 691–706 (1964).

Gaze, R.M.; Gordon, G.: The representation of cutaneous sense in the thalamus of the cat and monkey. Q. Jl exp. Physiol. *39:* 279–304 (1954).

Gildenberg, P.L.: Variability of subcortical lesions produced by a heating electrode and Cooper's balloon cannula. Confinia neurol. *20:* 53–65 (1960).

Gildenberg, P.L.: Survey of stereotactic and functional neurosurgery in the United States and Canada. Appl. Neurophysiol. *38:* 31–37 (1975).

Gildenberg, P.L.: Radiofrequency lesion making procedures. Symposium. Appl. Neurophysiol. *39:* 69–132 (1976/77).

Gildenberg, P.L.: Treatment of spasmodic torticollis with dorsal column stimulation. Acta neurochir. *24:* suppl., pp. 65–66 (1977).

Gildenberg, P.L.; Hirshberg, R.: Limited myelotomy for the treatment of intractable pain. Meeting of the European Society for Stereotactic and Functional Neurosurgery, Paris 1979, p. S30.

Gildenberg, P.L.; Kaufman, H.H.: Direct calculation of stereotactic coordinates from CT scans. Appl. Neurophysiol. *45:* 347–351 (1982).

Gildenberg, P.L.; Kaufman, H.H.; Murthy, K.S.K.: Calculation of stereotactic coordinates from computed tomographic scan. Neurosurgery *10:* 580–586 (1982).

Gillingham, F.J.: Small localized lesions of the internal capsule in the treatment of dyskinesias. Confinia neurol. *22:* 385–392 (1962).

Gillingham, F.J.; Campbell, D.: Surgical interruption of the conduction pathways for the control of intractable epilepsy. Acta neurochir. *30:* suppl., pp. 67–74 (1980).

Gillingham, F.J.; Kalyanaraman, S.: The surgical treatment of oculogyric crises. Confinia neurol. *19:* 237–245 (1965).

Gillingham, F.J.; Kalyanaraman, S.; Donaldson, A.A.: Bilateral stereotaxic lesions in the management of parkinsonism and the dyskinesias. Br. med. J. *ii:* 656–659 (1964).

Gillingham, F.J.; Walsh, E.G.; Zogada, L.F.: Stereotactic lesions of the pulvinar for hypertonus and dyskinesias. Acta neurochir. *24:* suppl., pp. 15–20 (1977).

Gillingham, F.J.; Watson, W.S.; Donaldson, A.A.; Cairns, V.M.: Stereotactic lesions for the control of epilepsy. Acta neurochir. *23:* 263–269 (1976).

Gilman, S.; Dauth, G.W.; Tennyson, V.M.; Kremzner, L.T.; Defendini, R.: Morphological and biochemical effects of chronic cerebellar stimulation in monkey. Trans. Am. neurol. Ass., pp. 9–11 (Springer, New York 1975).

Giorgi, C.; Kelly, P.J.; Eaton, D.C.; Guiot, G.; Derome, P.: A study on the tridimensional distribution of somatosensory, evoked responses in human thalamus to aid the placement of stimulating electrodes for treatment of pain. Acta neurochir., suppl. 30, pp. 279–288 (1980).

Gleason, C.A.; Wise, B.L.; Feinstein, B.: Stereotactic localization with computerized tomographic scanning, biopsy and radiofrequency treatment of deep brain lesions. Neurosurgery *2:* 217–222 (1978).

Glees, P.: The interrelation of the striopallidum and the thalamus in the macaque monkey. Brain *68:* 331–346 (1945).

Gloor, F.: Amygdala; in Field, Magoun, Hall, Handbook of physiology; section I, Neurophysiology, vol. 2, pp. 1395–1420 (American Physiological Society, Washington 1960).

Goddard, G.V.: Long-term alteration following amygdaloid stimulation; in Eleftheriou, Neurobiology of the amygdala, pp. 581–596 (Plenum Press, New York 1972).

Gol, A.: Relief of pain by electrical stimulation of the septal area. J. neurol. Sci. *5:* 115–120 (1967).

Goldring, S.; Anthony, L.U.; Stohr, P.E.; O'Leary, J.L.: Caudate induced cortical potentials; comparison between monkey and cat. Science *139:* 772 (1963).

Goldstein, K.: Das Kleinhirn; in Bethe, Bergmann, Emden, Ellinger, Handbuch der normalen und pathologischen Physiologie, Bd. 10, pp. 222–317 (Springer, Berlin 1927).

Goto, A.; Kosaka, K.; Nakamura, R.; Narabayashi, H.: Thalamic potentials from muscle afferents in the human. Archs Neurol., Chicago *19:* 302–309 (1968).

Granit, R.: Systems for control of movements. 1st Int. Congr. Neurol. Sci. Acta med. belg. *1:* 63–80 (1957).

Granit, R.; Kaada, B.: Influence of stimulation of central nervous structures on muscle spindles in cat. Acta physiol. scand. *27:* 130–160 (1952).

Greitz, T.; Bergstrom, M.: Stereotactic computed tomography of the head; in Newton, Potts, Radiology of the skull and brain: technical aspects of computed tomography, pp. 4286–4295 (Mosby, St. Louis 1981).

Greitz, T.; Bergstrom, M.; Boëthius, J.; Kingsley, D.; Ribbe, T.: Head fixation system for integration of radiodiagnostic and therapeutic procedures. Neuroradiology *19:* 1–6 (1980).

Grossman, S.P.: Chemically induced epileptiform seizures in the cat. Science *142:* 409–411 (1963).

Guidetti, B.; Fraioli, B.: Neurosurgical treatment of spasticity and dyskinesias. Acta neurochir. *24:* suppl., pp. 27–39 (1977).

Guillemin, R.; Vargo, T.; Rossier, J.; Minick, S.; Lint, N.; Rivier, C.; Vale, W.; Bloom, B.: β-endorphin and adrenocorticotropin are secreted concomitantly by the pituitary. Science *197:* 1367–1369 (1977).

Guiot, G.; Brion, S.: Traitement des mouvements anormaux par la coagulation pallidale. Revue neurol. *89:* 578–580 (1953).

Guiot, G.; Brion, S.; Fardeau, M.; Bettaier, A.; Molina, P.: Dyskinésie volitionelle d'attitude supprimée par la coagulation thalamo-capsulaire. Revue neurol. *102:* 220–229 (1960).

Guiot, G.; Hardy, J.; Albe-Fessard, D.: Délimitation précise des structures sous-corticales et identification des noyaux thalamiques chez l'homme par l'électrophysiologie stéréotaxique. Neurochirurgia *5:* 1–18 (1962).

Guiot, G.; Hertzog, E.; Rondot, P.; Molina, P.: Arrest or acceleration of speech evoked by thalamic stimulation in the course of stereotaxic procedures for parkinsonism. Brain *84:* 368–379 (1961).

Guiot, G.; Sachs, M.; Hertzog, E.; Brion, S.; Rougerie, J.; Dalloz, J.C.; Napoleone, F.: Stimulation électrique et lésions chirurgicales de la capsule interne: déductions anatomiques et physiologiques. Neuro-Chirurgie *5:* 17–42 (1959).

Gybels, J.M.: The neural mechanism of parkinsonian tremor (Editions Arscia, Brussels 1963).

Gybels, J.M.; Dom, R.; Cosyns, P.: Electrical stimulation of the central gray for pain relief in human: autopsy data. Acta neurochir. *30:* suppl., pp. 259–268 (1980).

Gye, R.S.; Adams, C.B.T.; Stanworth, P.A.; Stewart, G.A.: Cryohypophysectomy for bone pain of metastatic breast cancer. Pain *6:* 201–206 (1979).

Hahn, J.F.; Levy, W.J.; Weinstein, M.J.: Needle biopsy of intracranial lesions guided by computerized tomography. Neurosurgery *5:* 11–15 (1979).

Hanberry, J.; Jasper, H.: Independence of the diffuse thalamic cortical projection system shown by specific nuclear destruction. J. Neurophysiol. *16:* 252–271 (1953).

Harman, P.J.; Carpenter, M.B.: Volumetric comparison of the basal ganglia of various primates including man. J. comp. Neurol. *23:* 125–137 (1950).

Hartmann-von Monakow, K.: Halluzinosen nach doppelseitiger stereotaktischer Operation bei Parkinson-Kranken. Arch. Psychiat. NervKrankh. *199:* 477–486 (1959).

Hassler, R.: Über Kleinhirnprojection zum Mittelhirn und Thalamus beim Menschen. Dt. Z. NervHeilk. *163:* 629–671 (1950).

Hassler, R.: Gezielte Operationen gegen extrapyramidale Bewegungsstörungen; in Schaltenbrand, Bailey, Einführung in die stereotaktischen Operationen, Bd. 1, pp. 472–488 (Thieme, Stuttgart 1959).

Hassler, R.: Die zentralen Systeme des Schmerzes. Acta neurochir. *8:* 353 (1960).

Hassler, R.: Discussion of pain symposium. Confinia neurol. *27:* 89 (1966).

Hassler, R.: Funktionelle Neuroanatomie und Psychiatrie; in Gruhle, Psychiatrie der Gegenwart I. Part A, pp. 152–285 (Springer, Berlin 1967).

Hassler, R.: Physiopathology of rigidity; in Siegfried, Parkinson's disease, vol. 1, pp. 20–45 (Huber, Bern 1972).

Hassler, R.: Fiber connections within the extrapyramidal system. Confinia neurol. *36:* 237–255 (1974).

Hassler, R.: Central interactions of the systems of the rapidly and slowly conducted pain. Adv. Neurosurg. *3:* 143–156 (1975).

Hassler, R.; Dieckmann, G.: Stereotaxic treatment of compulsive and obsessive symptoms. Confinia neurol. *29:* 153–158 (1967).

Hassler, R.; Dieckmann, G.: Stereotaxic treatment of different kinds of spasmodic torticollis. Confinia neurol. *32:* 135–143 (1970).

Hassler, R.; Hess, W.R.: Experimentelle und anatomische Befunde über die Drehbewegungen und ihre nervösen Apparate. Arch. Psychiat. Nervkrankh. *192:* 488–526 (1954).

Hassler, R.; Mundinger, F.; Riechert, T.: Correlation between clinical and autoptic findings in stereotaxic operations of parkinsonism. Confinia neurol. *26:* 282–290 (1965).

Hassler, R.; Mundinger, F.; Riechert, T.: Stereotaxis in Parkinson syndrome (Springer, Berlin 1979).

Hassler, R.; Mundinger, F.; Riechert, T.; Umbach, W.; Ganglberger, J.A.: Physiologic observations in stereotaxic operations in extrapyramidal motor disturbances. Brain *83:* 337–350 (1960).

Hassler, R.; Riechert, T.: Indikationen und Lokalisationsmethode der gezielten Hirnoperationen. Nervenarzt *25:* 441–447 (1954).

Hassler, R.; Riechert, T.: Über einen Fall von doppelseitiger Fornicotomie bei sogenannter temporaler Epilepsie. Acta neurochir. *5:* 330–340 (1957).

Hassler, R.; Riechert, T.: Wirkungen der Reizungen und Koagulationen in den Stammganglien bei stereotaktischen Hirnoperationen. Nervenarzt *32:* 97–109 (1961).

Hayne, R.A.; Belinson, L.; Gibbs, F.A.: Electrical activity of subcortical areas in epilepsy. Electroenceph. clin. Neurophysiol. *1:* 437–445 (1949).

Heath, R.G.: Studies in schizophrenia (Harvard University Press, Cambridge 1954).

Heath, R.G.: Electrical self-stimulation of the brain in man. Am. J. Psychiat. *120:* 571–577 (1963).

Heath, R.G.: The pleasure response; in Kline, Laska, Computers and electronic devices in psychiatry (Grune & Stratton, New York 1968).

Heath, R.G.: Depth recording and stimulation studies in patients; in Winter, Surgical control of behavior (Thomas, Springfield 1971).

Heath, R.G.; Hodes, R.: Induction of sleep by stimulation of the caudate nucleus in Macaccus rhesus and in man. Trans. Am. neurol. Ass. *77:* 204–210 (1952).

Heath, R.G.; Weber, G.G.; Hogan, C.; Price, T.D.: Metabolic changes following destructive lesions in the forebrain in cats; in Heath, Studies in schizophrenia, p. 61 (Harvard University Press, Cambridge 1954).

Hécaen, H.; Talairach, J.; David, M.; Dell, M.D.: Coagulations limitées du thalamus dans les algies du syndrome thalamique. Revue neurol. *81:* 917–931 (1949).

Heggs, N.M.; Kelly, D.; Richardson, A.E.: Stereotactic limbic leucotomy; in Sweet, Obrador, Martin-Rodriguez, Neurosurgical treatment in psychiatry, pain and epilepsy, pp. 367–379 (University Park Press, Baltimore 1977).

Heimburger, R.F.: Dentatectomy in the treatment of dyskinetic disorders. Confinia neurol. *29:* 101–106 (1967).

Heimburger, R.F.: Putamenotomy as an aide to upper extremity control. Confinia neurol. *37:* 16–23 (1975a).

Heimburger, R.F.: Multiple sequential stereotaxic surgery for cerebral palsy. Confinia neurol. *37:* 270 (1975b).

Heimburger, R.F.; Whitlock, C.C.: Stereotaxic destruction of the human dentate nucleus. Confinia neurol. *26:* 346–358 (1965).

Heimburger, R.F.; Whitlock, C.C.; Kalsbeck, J.E.: Stereotaxic amygdalotomy for epilepsy with aggressive behavior. J. Am. med. Ass. *198:* 741–745 (1966).

Henny, G.C.; Wycis, H.T.; Spiegel, E.A.: Studies in stereoencephalotomy. XIII. Refinements in roentgen technique during stereotaxic operations. Confinia neurol. *21:* 501–504 (1961).

Hermann, K.; Turner, J.W.; Gillingham, F.J.; Gaze, R.M.: The effect of destructive lesions and stimulation of the basal ganglia on speech mechanisms. Confinia neurol. *27:* 197–207 (1966).

Herner, T.: Treatment of mental disorders with frontal stereotaxic thermolesions. Acta psychiat. neurol. scand. *36:* suppl. 158 (1961).

Herz, A.; Zieglgänsberger, W.: Synaptic excitation of the corpus striatum inhibited by microelectrophoretically administered dopamine. Experientia *22:* 839 (1966).

Hess, W.R.: Die funktionelle Organisation des vegetativen Nervensystems (Schwabe, Basel 1948).

Hess, W.R.: Hypothalamus und Thalamus. Experimentelle Dokumente (Thieme, Stuttgart 1956).

Hickey, R.C.; Fry, W.J.; Meyers, R.; Fry, F.J.; Bradbury, J.: Human pituitary irradiation with focal ultrasound in advanced breast cancer. Archs Surg., Chicago *83:* 620–630 (1961).

Higgins, A.C.; Nashold, B.S., Jr.: Stereotactic evacuation of large, intracerebral hematoma. Appl. Neurophysiol. *43:* 96–103 (1980).

Higgins, A.C.; Nashold, B.S., Jr.: Modification of instrument for stereotactic evacuation of intracerebral hematoma. Technical note. Neurosurgery *7:* 604–604 (1980a).

Higgins, A.C.; Nashold, B.S., Jr.: Stereotactic evacuation of large intracerebral hematoma. Appl. Neurophysiol. *43:* 96–103 (1980b).

Higgins, A.C.; Nashold, B.S., Jr.; Cosman, E.: Stereotactic evacuation of primary intracerebral hematomas. New instrument. Appl. Neurophysiol. *45:* 438–442 (1982).

Hill, R.C.; Roemer, D.; Buescher, H.H.: Some pharmacological qualities of FK-33-824; in Costa, Trabucchi, The endorphins, pp. 211–216 (Raven Press, New York 1978).

Hillman, P.; Wall, P.D.: Inhibitory and excitatory factors influencing the receptive fields of lamina 5 spinal cord cells. Exp. Brain Res. *9:* 284–306 (1969).

Hilton, S.M.; Zbrozyna, A.W.: Amygdaloid region for defense reactions and its efferent pathway to the brain stem. J. Physiol., Lond. *165:* 160–173 (1963).

Hirsch, C.; Müller, O.: Beiträge zur Wärmetopographie des Warmblütlers im normalen Zustande, bei Abkühlung und Überhitzung, im Fieber und nach Wärmestich. Dt. Arch. klin. Med. *75:* 278–307 (1903).

Hitchcock, E.R.: Stereotaxic spinal surgery. J. Neurosurg. *31:* 386–396 (1969a).

Hitchcock, E.R.: An apparatus for spinal stereotactic surgery. Lancet *i:* 703–706 (1969b).

Hitchcock, E.R.: Stereotactic trigeminal tractotomy. Ann. clin. Res. *2:* 131–135 (1970).

Hitchcock, E.R.; Ashcroft, G.W.; Cairns, V.M.; Murray, L.G.: Observations on the development of an assessment scheme for amygdalotomy; in Laitinen, Livingston, Surgical approaches in psychiatry, pp. 142–155 (Medical and Technical Publishing, Lancaster 1973).

Hoefer, P.F.A.; Putnam, T.J.: Action potentials of muscle rigidity and tremor. Archs Neurol. Psychiat., Chicago *43:* 704–725 (1940).

Hongo, T.; Kubota, K.; Shimazu, H.: EEG spindle and depression of gamma motor activity. J. Neurophysiol. *27:* 568–580 (1963).

Hornykiewicz, O.: Metabolism of brain dopamine in human Parkinsonism. Neurochemical and clinical aspects; in Costa, Côté, Yahr, Biochemistry and pharmacology of the basal ganglia, pp. 171–185 (Raven Press, New York 1966).

Horowitz, M.D.; Adams, J.E.: Hallucinations on brain stimulation: evidence for revision of the Penfield hypothesis; in Kemp, Origin and mechanism of hallucination, pp. 13–22 (Plenum Press, New York 1970).

Horsley, V.; Clarke, R.H.: The structure and function of the cerebellum examined by a new method. Brain *31:* 45–124 (1908).

Hosobuchi, Y.: The current status of analgesic brain stimulation. Acta neurochir. *30:* suppl., pp. 219–228 (1980).

*Housepian, E.M.; Pool, J.L.: An evaluation of pallidoansal surgery; in Fields, Pathogenesis and treatment of parkinsonism, pp. 317–324 (Thomas, Springfield 1958).

Housepian, E.M.; Pool, J.L.: The accuracy of human stereoencephalotomy. J. nerv. ment. Dis. *130:* 520–525 (1960).

Housepian, E.M.; Pool, J.L.: Application of stereotaxic methods to histochemical, electronmicroscopic and electrophysiological studies of human, subcortical structures. Confinia neurol. *22:* 171–177 (1962).

Housepian, E.M.; Purpura, D.P.: Electrophysiological studies of subcortical-cortical relations in man. Electroenceph. clin. Neurophysiol. *15:* 20–28 (1963).

Hughes, B.: A new, versatile stereotactic instrument. J. Neurol. Neurosurg. Psychiat. *23:* 351 (1960).

Huk, W.; Baer, U.: A new targeting device for stereotaxic procedures within the CT scanner. Neuroradiology *19:* 13–17 (1980).

Hunsperger, R.W.; Wyss, O.A.M.: Ausschaltung von Nervengewebe durch Hochfrequenz-Koagulation. Helv. physiol. Acta *11:* 283–304 (1953).

Hunter, J.; Jasper, H.H.: Effects of thalamic stimulation in unanesthetized animals. Electroenceph. clin. Neurophysiol. *1:* 305–324 (1949).

Hurt, R.W.; Ballantine, H.T.: Stereotactic anterior cingulate lesions for persistent pain. A report of 68 cases. Clin. Neurosurg. *21:* 334–351 (1974).

*Iisuka, J.: Development of a stereotaxic endoscopy of the ventricular system. Confinia neurol. *37:* 141–149 (1975).

Ito, Z.; Kato, H.; Matsuoka, S.; Sakurai, Y.: Effects on the speech function after stereotaxic amygdalotomy for behavior disordered children. Neurol. Med. Chir., Tokyo *12:* 368–369 (1972).

Ivan, L.P.; Ventureyra, E.C.G.; Wiley, J.; Pressman, E.; Knights, R.; Guzman, C.; Uttley, D.: Chronic cerebellar stimulation in cerebral palsy. Surg. Neurol. *15:* 81–84 (1981).

Jacques, S.; Shelden, H.; McCann, G.D.: A computerized microstereotactic method to approach 3-dimensionally, reconstruct, remove and adjuvantly treat small CNS lesions. Appl. Neurophysiol. *43:* 176–182 (1980b).

Jacques, S.; Shelden, C.H.; McCann, G.D.; Freshwater, D.B.; Rand, R.: Computerized three-dimensional stereotaxic removal of small central nervous system lesions in patients. J. Neurosurg. *53:* 816–820 (1980b).

Jasper, H.H.: Unspecific thalamocortical relations; in Field, Magoun, Hall, Handbook of physiology: Section I. Neurophysiology, vol. 2, pp. 1307–1321 (American Physiological Society, Washington 1960).

*Jasper, H.H.; Andrews, H.L.: Brain potentials and voluntary muscle activity in man. J. Neurophysiol. *1:* 87–100 (1938).

Jasper, H.H.; Bertrand, G.: Stereotaxic microelectrode studies of single thalamic cells and fibers in patients with dyskinesia. Trans. Am. neurol. Ass. *89:* 79–82 (1964).

Jasper, H.H.; Bertrand, G.: Thalamic units involved in somatic sensation and voluntary and involuntary movements in man; in Purpura, Yahr, The thalamus, pp. 365–390 (Columbia University Press, New York 1966).

Jasper, H.H.; Hunter, J.: A stereotaxic instrument for man. Electroenceph. clin. Neurophysiol. *1:* 523–526 (1949).

Jelasic, F.: Relation of the lateral part of the amygdala to pain. Confinia neurol. *27:* 53–55 (1966).

Jelsma, R.; Bertrand, C.; Martinez, S.; Molina-Negro, P.: Stereotaxic treatment of frontal lobe and centrencephalic epilepsy. J. Neurosurg. *39:* 42–51 (1973).

Jenkner, F.L.; Ward, A.A., Jr.: Bulbar reticular formation and tremor. Archs Neurol. Psychiat., Chicago *70:* 489–502 (1953).

Jinnai, D.; Nishimoto, A.: Stereotaxic destruction of Forel H for treatment of epilepsy. Neurochirurgia *6:* 164–176 (1963).

Johansson, G.G.: Sensory responses evoked by electric stimulation of human diencephalic brain structures. Scand. J. clin. Lab. Invest. *21:* suppl. 101, p. 63 (1968).

Johansson, G.G.: Electric stimulation of a human ventrolateral, subventrolateral thalamic target area. Acta physiol. scand., preprints I–IV (1969).

Johansson, G.G.; Laitinen, L.: Electric stimulation of the thalamic and subthalamic area in Parkinson's disease. Confinia neurol. *26:* 445–450 (1965).

Johnson, T.N.; Clemente, C.D.: An experimental study of the fiber connections between the putamen, glob. pallidus, ventral thalamus and midbrain tegmentum in cat. J. comp. Neurol. *113:* 83–102 (1959).

Jung, R.: Physiologische Untersuchungen über den Parkinson Tremor und andere Zitterformen beim Menschen. Z. ges. Neurol. Psychiat. *173:* 263–322 (1941).

Jung, R.: Correlation of bioelectrical and autonomic phenomena with alteration of consciousness and arousal in man; in Delafresnaye, Brain mechanisms and consciousness, pp. 310–339 (Blackwell, Oxford 1954).

Jung, R.; Riechert, T.: EEG Befunde bei Thalamusreizung am Menschen. Nervenarzt *26:* 35 (1955).

Jung, R.; Toennies, J.F.: Hirnelektrische Untersuchungen über Entstehung und Erhaltung von Krampfentladungen. Arch. Psychiat. NervKrankh. *185:* 701–735 (1950).

Kaada, B.R.: Somato-motor, autonomic and electrocorticographic responses to electric stimulation of rhinencephalic and other structures in primates, cat and dog. Acta physiol. scand. *24:* suppl. 83, pp. 1–285 (1951).

Kaada, B.R.: Stimulation and regional ablation of the amygdaloid complex with reference to functional representation; in Eleftheriou, The neurobiology of the amygdala, pp. 205–281 (Plenum Press, New York 1972).

Kalyanaraman, S.; Ramamurthi, B.: Stereotaxic surgery for generalized epilepsy. Neurology, Madras *18:* suppl., pp. 34–41 (1970).

Kanaka, T.S.; Balasubramaniam, V.: Dentato-thalamotomy in infantile hemiplegia. Confinia neurol. *37:* 271–276 (1975).

Kanaka, T.S.; Balasubramaniam, V.: Experiences with pulvinar lesions. Appl. Neurophysiol. *41:* 86–93 (1978).

Kandel, E.I.: The Parkinson syndrome and its surgical treatment (Russian) (Moscow 1965).

Kandel, E.I.; Chebotaryova, N.M.: Conray ventriculography in stereotaxic surgery. Confinia neurol. *34:* 34–40 (1972).

Kandel, E.I.; Peresedov, V.V.: Stereotaxic clipping of arterial and arteriovenous aneurysms of the brain. Acta neurochir., *30:* suppl., pp. 405–412 (1980).

Karplus, J.P.; Kreidl, A.: Gehirn und Sympathicus VIII. Pflügers Arch. ges. Physiol. *219:* 613 (1928).

Kato, M.: Studies on effects of pyramid stimulation upon flexor and extensor motoneurons and gamma motoneurons. Jap. J. Physiol. *14:* 34–44 (1964).

Katz, J.; Levin, A.B.: Treatment of diffuse metastatic cancer pain by instillation of alcohol into the sella turcica. Anesthesia *46:* 115–121 (1977).

Kaufman, H.H.; Catalano, L.W., Jr.: Diagnostic brain biopsy: a series of 50 cases and a review. Neurosurgery *4:* 129–136 (1979).

Kaufman, H.H.; Gildenberg, P.L.: New head-positioning system for use with computed tomographic scanning. Neurosurgery *7:* 147–149 (1980).

Kebabian, J.W.; Calne, D.B.: Multiple receptors for dopamine. Nature, Lond. *277:* 93–96 (1979).

Kelly, D.; Richardson, A.; Mitchell-Hess, N.: Technique and assessment of limbic leu-cotomy; in Laitinen, Livingston, Surgical approaches in psychiatry, pp. 165–173 (Medical and Technical Publishing, Lancaster 1973).

Kelly, P.J.: Microelectrode recording for the somatotopic placement of stereotactic tha-lamic lesions in the treatment of parkinsonian and cerebellar intention tremor. Appl. Neurophysiol. *43:* 263–267 (1980).

Kelly, P.J.; Alker, G.J.: A method for stereotactic laser microsurgery in the treatment of deep-seated CNS neoplasms. Appl. Neurophysiol. *43:* 210–215 (1980).

Kelly, P.J.; Olson, M.H.; Wright, A.E.: Stereotactic implantation of iridium 192 into CNS neoplasms. Surg. Neurol. *10:* 349–354 (1978).

*Kim, Y.K.: Effects of basolateral amygdalotomy; in Umbach, Special topics in stereotaxis (Hippocrates, Stuttgart 1972).

Kim, Y.K.; Goettsching, G.: Topometric relationship of the amygdala to the surrounding structures. Confinia neurol. *37:* 207–214 (1975).

Kim, Y.K.; Umbach, W.: Combined stereotactic lesions for treatment of behavior disor-ders and severe pain; in Laitinen, Livingston, Surgical approaches in psychiatry, pp. 183–188 (Medical and Technical Publishing, Lancaster 1973).

King, H.E.: Psychological effects of excitation in the limbic system; in Sheer, Electrical stimulation of the brain, pp. 477–486 (University of Texas Press, Austin 1961).

Kingsley, D.P.; Bergstrom, M.; Berggren, B.M.: A critical evaluation of two methods of head fixation. Neuroradiology *19:* 7–12 (1980).

Kirschner, M.: Die Punktionstechnik und Elektrokoagulation des Ganglion Gasseri. Arch. klin. Chir. *176:* 581–620 (1933).

Kjellberg, R.N.; Kliman, B.; Adams, R.D.: Bragg peak proton radiosurgery of pituitary adenomas, arteriovenous malformations and other benign and malignant tumors. Meeting of the European Society for Stereotactic and Functional Neurosurgery, Paris 1979. Abstr., p. V42.

Kjellberg, R.N.; Koehler, A.M.; Preston, W.M.; Sweet, W.H.: Stereotaxic instrument for use with the Bragg peak of a proton beam. Confinia neurol. *22:* 183–189 (1962).

Klawans, H.L.; Goetz, C.G.; Perlik, S.: Tardive dyskinesia: review and update. Am. J. Psychiat. *137:* 900–908 (1980).

Klein, M.R.: Essai de traitement de l'athétose par destruction de l'anse lenticulaire. Sem. Hôp. Paris *31:* 1059 (1955).

Klüver, H.; Bucy, P.C.: Preliminary analysis of functions of the temporal lobes in mon-keys. Archs Neurol. Psychiat., Chicago *42:* 978–1000 (1939).

Knight, G.C.: The orbital cortex as an objective in the surgical treatment of mental illness. The results of 450 cases of open operation and the development of the stereotactic approach. Br. J. Surg. *51:* 114–124 (1964).

Knight, G.C.: Additional stereotactic lesions in the cingulum following failed tractotomy in the subcaudate region; in Laitinen, Livingston, Surgical approaches in psychiatry, pp. 101–106 (Medical and Technical Publishing, Lancaster 1973).

Kodama, S.: Über die sogenannten Basalganglien; morphogenetische und pathologisch-anatomische Untersuchungen. Schweizer Arch. Neurol. Psychiat. *23:* 179–265 (1929).

Koslow, M.; Abele, M.G.: A fully interfaced computerized tomographic-stereotactic surgi-cal system. Appl. Neurophysiol. *43:* 174–175 (1980).

Koslow, M.; Abele, M.D.; Griffith, R.C.; Mair, G.A.; Chase, N.E.: Stereotactic surgical system controlled by computed tomography. Neurosurgery *8:* 72–82 (1981).

Koslow, M.; Abele, M.; Ng, J.: Considerations for a CT-directed stereotactic surgical system. Appl. Neurophysiol. (in press, 1982).

Krainick, J.U.; Thoden, U.; Strassburg, H.M.; Wenzel, D.: The effect of electrical spinal cord stimulation on spastic movement disorders. Adv. Neurosurg. *4:* 257–260 (1977).

Krauthamer, G.; Albe-Fessard, D.: Inhibition of nonspecific sensory activities following striopallidal and capsular stimulation. J. Neurophysiol. *28:* 100–124 (1965).

Krayenbühl, H.: Prof. Ernest A. Spiegel's 80th birthday. Confinia neurol. *37:* 357–363 (1975).

Krayenbühl, H.; Siegfried, J.: La chirurgie stéréotaxique du noyau dentelé dans le traitement des hyperkinesies et des états spastiques. Neuro-Chirurgie *15:* 51–58 (1969).

Krayenbühl, H.; Siegfried, J.; Kohenof, M.; Yasargil, M.G.: Is there a dominant thalamus? Confinia neurol. *26:* 246–249 (1965).

Krayenbühl, H.; Siegfried, J.; Yasargil, M.G.: Résultats tardifs des opérations stéréotaxiques dans le traitement de la maladie de Parkinson. Revue neurol. *108:* 485–494 (1963).

Krayenbühl, H.; Wyss, O.A.M.; Yasargil, M.G.: Bilateral thalamotomy and pallidotomy as treatment for bilateral parkinsonism. J. Neurosurg. *18:* 429–444 (1961).

Krayenbühl, H.; Yasargil, M.G.: Bilateral thalamotomy in parkinsonism. J. nerv. ment. Dis. *130:* 538–541 (1960).

Krayenbühl, H.; Yasargil, M.G.: Ergebnisse der stereotaktischen Operationen beim Parkinsonismus, insbesonders der doppelseitigen Eingriffe. Dt. Z. NervHeilk. *182:* 530–541 (1961).

Krayenbühl, H.; Yasargil, M.G.: Relief of intention tremor due to multiple sclerosis by stereotaxic thalamotomy. Confinia neurol. *22:* 368–374 (1962).

Kudo, T.; Yoshii, N.; Shimizu, S.; Aikawa, S.; Nakahama, H.: Effects of stereotaxic thalamotomy to intractable pain and numbness. Kejo J. Med. *15:* 151–194 (1966).

Kudo, T.; Yoshii, N.; Shimizu, S.; Aikawa, S., et al.: Stereotactic thalamotomy for pain relief. Tohoku J. exp. Med. *96:* 219–230 (1968).

Kuhlenbeck, H.: The human diencephalon. Confinia neurol. *14:* suppl., pp. 1–230 (1954).

Kullberg, G.: Differences in effect of capsulotomy and cingulotomy; in Sweet, Obrador, Martin-Rodriguez, Neurosurgical treatment in psychiatry, pain and epilepsy, pp. 301–308 (University Park Press, Baltimore 1977).

Kullberg, G.; Cronquist, S.; Brismar, J.: Stereotactic lesions studied by computer tomography. Acta neurochir. *30:* suppl., pp. 395–400 (1980).

Kwak, R.; Okudaira, Y.; Sakamoto, T.; Otabe, K.; Ohi, T.; Niizuma, H.; Suzuki, J.; Saso, S.: Arrest reaction in man. Motor arrest response by electrical stimulation of the deep structures of the cerebrum. Appl. Neurophysiol. *41:* 209–216 (1978).

Laitinen, L.V.: Stereotaxic treatment of spasmodic torticollis. Acta neurol. Scand. *39:* suppl. 4, pp. 231–236 (1963).

Laitinen, L.V.: Stereotactic lesions in the knee of the corpus callosum in the treatment of emotional disorders. Lancet *i:* 472 (1972).

Laitinen, L.V.: Anterior pulvinotomy in the treatment of intractable pain. Acta neurochir. *24:* suppl., pp. 223–235 (1977).

Laitinen, L.V.; Arsalo, A.; Hanninen, A.: Combination of thalamotomy and longitudinal myelotomy in the treatment of multiple sclerosis. Acta neurochir. *21:* suppl., pp. 89–91 (1974).

Laitinen, L.V.; Livingston, K.E.: Surgical approaches in psychiatry (Medical and Technical Publishing, Lancaster 1973).

Laitinen, L.V.; Singounas, E.: Longitudinal myelotomy in the treatment of spasticity of the legs. J. Neurosurg. *35:* 536–540 (1971).

Laitinen, L.V.; Toivakka, E.: Locating brain tumors through depth EEG probes. Confinia neurol. *34:* 101–105 (1972).

Laitinen, L.V.; Toivakka, E.: Depth EEG and electrical stimulation of the human amygdala. Acta neurochir. *30:* suppl., pp. 177–182 (1980).

Laitinen, L.V.; Vílkki, J.: Observation on the transcallosal emotional connections; in Laitinen, Livingston, Surgical approaches in psychiatry, pp. 74–80 (Medical and Technical Publishing, Lancaster 1973).

Lamarre, Y.; Cordeau, J.P.: Central unit activity in monkeys with postural tremor. Fed. Proc. *22:* 1993 (1962).

Lamarre, Y.; Cordeau, J.P.: Activité des neurones centraux chez le singe porteur d'un tremblement expérimental. J. Physiol., Paris *56:* 589–591 (1964).

Langfitt, T.W.; Kamel, K.; Koff, G.Y.; Peacock, S.M., Jr.: Gamma neuron control by thalamus and globus pallidus. Archs Neurol., Chicago *9:* 593–606 (1963).

Lapras, C.: Chirurgie stéréotaxique des dyskinésies; thèse Lyon (1960).

Laursen, A.M.: Electrical signs of the relation between caudate nucleus and cerebral cortex in cats. Acta physiol. scand. *53:* 218–232 (1961a).

Laursen, A.M.: Caudate nucleus and electrocortical activity. Acta physiol. scand. *53:* 233–238 (1961b).

Laursen, A.M.: Movements evoked from the region of the caudate nucleus in cats. Acta physiol. scand. *54:* 175–184 (1962a).

Laursen, A.M.: Inhibition evoked from the region of the caudate nucleus in cats. Acta physiol. scand. *54:* 185–190 (1962b).

Law, J.D.; Cacak, R.E.: Progress in developing a CT-compatible adapter for the Leksell stereotach. Appl. Neurophysiol. *45:* 381–382 (1982).

Le Beau, J.: La résection bilatérale de certaines aires corticales préfrontales. Sem. Hôp. Paris *24:* 1937–1942 (1948).

Le Beau, J.: The cingular and precingular areas in psychosurgery (agitated behavior, obsessive compulsive states, epilepsy). Acta psychiat. neurol. scand. *27:* 305–306 (1952).

Le Beau, J.: Anterior cingulectomy in man. J. Neurosurg. *11:* 268–277 (1954).

Lee, S.H.; Villafana, T.; Lapayowker, M.S.: CT intracranial localization with a new marker system. Neuroradiology *16:* 570–571 (1978).

Leksell, L.: The action potential and excitatory effects of the small ventral root fibers to skeletal muscle. Acta physiol. scand. *10:* suppl. 31, pp. 1–84 (1945).

Leksell, L.: A stereotaxic apparatus for intracerebral surgery. Acta chir. scand. *99:* 229–233 (1949).

Leksell, L.: The stereotaxic method and radiosurgery of the brain. Acta chir. scand. *102:* 316–319 (1951).

Leksell, L.: Stereotaxis and radiosurgery. An operative system (Thomas, Springfield 1971).

Leksell, L.; Herner, T.; Lidén, K.: Stereotaxic radiosurgery of the brain. K. fysiogr. Sällsk. Lund. Förh. *25:* 1–10 (1955).

Leksell, L.; Jernberg, B.: Stereotaxis and tomography. A technical note with 6 figures. Acta neurochir. *52:* 1–7 (1980).

Leksell, L.; Larsson, B.; Andersson, P.; Rexed, B.; Sourander, P.; Mair, W.: Lesions in the depth of the brain produced by a beam of high energy protons. Acta radiol. *54:* 251–264 (1960).

Leksell, L.; Lidén, K.: A therapeutic trial with radioactive isotopes in cystic brain tumor; in Radioisotope techniques. Proc. Isotope Technique Conf., Oxford, vol. 1, pp. 76–78 (HMSO, London 1953).

*Leksell, L.; Lidén, K.; Hertz, C.H.: Gezielte Hirnoperationen; in Handbuch der Neurochirurgie, vol. 6, pp. 178–218 (Springer, Berlin 1957).

*Lesser, R.P.; Fahns, S.; Snider, S.R., et al.: Analysis of the clinical problems in parkinsonism and the complications of long-term levodopa therapy. Neurology *29:* 1253–1260 (1979).

Lévy, A.; Monnier, M.; Krupp, P.: Elektrophysiologische Analyse funktioneller Verbindungen zwischen den Hauptstrukturen des extrapyramidalen Systems. Confinia neurol. *19:* 334–348 (1954).

Lewander, R.; Bergstrom, M.; Boëthius, J.; Collins, V.P.; Edner, G.; Greitz, T.; Willems, J.: Stereotactic computer tomography for biopsy of gliomas. Acta radiol. (Diag.) *19:* 867–888 (1978).

Lewandowsky, M.: Untersuchungen über die Leitungsbahnen des Truncus cerebri; in Vogt, Neurobiologische Arbeiten, Serie 2, vol. 1/2, pp. 63–150 (Fischer, Jena 1904).

Lewin, W.: Selective leucotomy. A review; in Laitinen, Livingston, Surgical approaches in psychiatry, pp. 69–73 (Medical and Technical Publishing, Lancaster 1973).

Liberson, W.; Voris, H.; Uematsu, S.: Recording of somatosensory evoked potentials during mesencephalotomies for intractable pain. Confinia neurol. *32:* 185–194 (1970).

Lin, P.M.; Gildenberg, P.L.; Polakoff, P.P.: An anterior approach to percutaneous lower cervical cordotomy. J. Neurosurg. *25:* 553–560 (1966).

Lipton, S.; Dervin, E.; Heywood, O.B.: A stereotactic approach to the anterior percutaneous electrical chordotomy.Acta neurochir. *21:* suppl., pp. 125–133 (1974).

Lipton, S.; Miles, J.; Williams, N.; Bark-Jones, N.: Pituitary injection of alcohol for widespread cancer pain. Pain *5:* 73–82 (1978).

Lister, W.C.; Sherwood, S.L.: A lightweight stereotaxic instrument. Electroenceph. clin. Neurophysiol. *7:* 311–314 (1955).

Livingston, K.E.: Cingulate cortex isolation for the treatment of psychoses and psychoneuroses. Res. Publs Ass. Res. nerv. ment. Dis. *31:* 374–378 (1953).

Livingston, K.E.; Escobar, A.: The anatomical bias of the limbic system concept: a proposed reorientation. Archs Neurol., Chicago *24:* 17–21 (1971).

Llamas, A.; Reinoso-Suarez, F.: Projection of the substantia nigra and ventral tegmentalmesencephalic area; in Gillingham, Donaldson, 3rd Symp. Parkinson's Disease, pp. 81–87 (Livingstone, Edinburgh 1969).

Lobato, R.D.; Riva, J.J.; Cabello, A.; Roger, R.: Stereotactic biopsy of brain lesions visualized with computed tomography. Appl. Neurophysiol. *45:* 426–430 (1982).

Loewenthal, M.; Horsley, V.: On the relation between the cerebellar and other centers (namely cerebral and spinal) with special reference to the action of antagonistic muscles. Proc. R. Soc. Lond. *61:* 20–25 (1897).

Long, D.M.: External electrical stimulation as a treatment of chronic pain. Minn. Med. *57:* 195 (1974).

Lunsford, L.D.: A dedicated CT system for the stereotactic operating room. Appl. Neurophysiol. *45:* 374–378 (1982).

Maccagnani, F.; Vizioli, R.: Considerazioni sulla patogenesi degli spasmi infantili alla luce di un caso operato di asportazione di un nodulo di sclerosi tuberosa ad evoluzione neoplastica situato nella testa del nucleo caudato. Soc. ital. Electroencefalog. *22:* XI (1958).

MacLean, P.D.: The limbic system ('visceral brain') and emotional behavior. AMA Archs Neurol. Psychiat. *73:* 130–134 (1955).

Magoun, H.H.: An ascending reticular activating system in the brain stem. Archs Neurol. Psychiat. *67:* 145–154 (1952).

Magoun, H.W.; Rhines, R.: Spasticity. The stretch reflex and extrapyramidal systems (Thomas, Springfield 1948).

Manrique, M.; Vaquero, J.; Oya, S.; Lozano, A.P.; Bravo, G.: Side effects and long-term results of chronic cerebellar stimulation in man. Acta neurochir. *30:* suppl., pp. 333–338 (1980).

Marg, E.; Dierssen, G.: Reported visual perceptions from stimulation of the human brain with microelectrodes during therapeutic surgery. Confinia neurol. *26:* 57–75 (1965).

Mark, V.H.: The destruction of both anterior thalamic nuclei in a patient with intractable depression. J. nerv. ment. Dis. *150:* 266–272 (1970).

Mark, V.H.; Chato, J.C.; Eastman, F.G.; Aronow, S.; Ervin, F.R.: Localized cooling in the brain. Science *134:* 1520–1521 (1961).

Mark, V.H.; Chiba, T.; Ervin, F.R.; Hamlin, H.: The comparison of heat and cold for the production of localized lesions in the central nervous system. Confinia neurol. *26:* 178–184 (1965).

Mark, V.H.; Ervin, F.R.: Violence and the brain (Harper & Row, New York 1970).

*Mark, V.H.; Ervin, F.R.: The effect of amygdalotomy on violent behavior in patients with temporal lobe epilepsy; in Hitchcock, Psychosurgery (Thomas, Springfield 1972).

Mark, V.H.; Ervin, F.R.; Hackett, T.P.: Clinical aspects of stereotactic thalamotomy in the human. Part I. Archs Neurol., Chicago *3:* 351–367 (1960).

Mark, V.H.; Ervin, F.R.; Sweet, W.H.: Deep temporal lobe stimulation in man; in Eleftheriou, Neurobiology of the amygdala, pp. 485–507 (Plenum Press, New York 1972).

Mark, V.H.; Ervin, F.R.; Sweet, W.H.; Delgado, J.: Remote telemeter stimulation and recording from implanted temporal lobe electrodes. Confinia neurol. *31:* 86–93 (1969a).

Mark, V.H.; Ervin, F.R.; Yakovlev, P.I.: Stereotactic thalamotomy. Part III. Archs Neurol., Chicago *8:* 528–538 (1963).

Mark, V.H.; Folkman, J.; Ervin, F.R.; Sweet, W.: Focal brain suppression by means of a silicone rubber chemode. J. Neurosurg. *30:* 195–199 (1969b).

*Mark, V.H.; McPherson, P.M.; Sweet, W.H.: A new method for correcting distortion in cranial roentgenogram. With special reference to a new human stereotaxic instrument. Am. J. Roentg. *71:* 435–444 (1954).

Maroon, J.C.; Brank, W.O.; Drayer, B.P.; Rosenbaum, A.E.: Intracranial biopsy assisted by computerized tomography. J. Neurosurg. *46:* 740–744 (1977).

Marshall, J.: Tremor; in Vinken, Bruyn, Handbook of clinical neurology, vol. 6, pp. 809–825 (North-Holland, Amsterdam 1968).

Martin, J.P.: Remarks on the functions of the basal ganglia. Lancet *i:* 999–1005 (1959).

Martin, J.P.: Further remarks on the functions of the basal ganglia. Lancet *i:* 1362–1365 (1960).

Martin, J.P.; Hurwitz, L.J.: Locomotion and the basal ganglia. Brain *85:* 261–267 (1962).

Martin-Rodriguez, J.G.; Obrador, S.: Evaluation of stereotaxic pulvinar lesions. Confinia neurol. *37:* 56–62 (1975).

Martinez, S.N.; Bertrand, C.; Botana-Lopez, C.: Motor fiber distribution within the cerebral peduncle. Confinia neurol. *29:* 117–122 (1967).

Martinez, S.N.; Bertrand, C.; Molina Negro, P.: Alteration of pain perception by stereotactic lesions of the frontothalamic pathways. Confinia neurol. *37:* 113–118 (1975).

Martins, L.F.; Umbach, W.: Size and position of stereotaxic lesions in comparison with clinical pain relief. Confinia neurol. *37:* 80–85 (1975).

Maspes, P.E.; Beduschi, A.; Cassinari, V.: Implantation d'électrodes de profondeur chroniques. Neuro-Chirurgie *9:* 118–125 (1961).

Matthews, P.B.C.; Rushworth, G.: The relative sensitivity of muscle nerve fibers to procaine. J. Physiol., Lond. *135:* 263–269 (1957).

Mayer, D.J.; Wolfe, T.L.; Akil, H.; Carder, B.; Liebeskind, C.J.: Analgesia from electrical stimulation of the brain stem of the rat. Science *174:* 1351–1354 (1971).

Mazars, G.; Merienne, L.; Cioloca, C.: Control of dyskinesias due to sensory deafferentation by means of thalamic stimulation. Acta neurochir. *30:* suppl., pp. 239–244 (1980).

Mazars, G.; Merienne, L.; Cioloca, C.; Prendeville, M.: Intermittent thalamic stimulation in the management of intractable pain. Adv. Neurosurg. *3:* 243–245 (1975).

McCaul, I.R.: A method for the localization and production of discrete destructive lesions in brain. J. Neurol. Neurosurg. Psychiat. *22:* 109–112 (1959).

Mehler, W.H.; Feferman, M.E.; Nauta, W.J.H.: Ascending axon degeneration following anterolateral cordotomy. An experimental study in the monkey. Brain *83:* 718–750 (1960).

Melzack, R.; Wall, P.D.: Pain mechanisms: a new theory. Science *150:* 971–979 (1965).

Mempel, E.; Witkiewicz, B.; Stadnicki, R.; Luczywek, E.; Kicinski, L.; Pawlowski, G.; Nowak, J.: The effect of medial amygdalotomy and anterior hippocampotomy on behavior and seizures in epileptic patients. Acta neurochir. *30:* suppl., pp. 161–168 (1980).

Mettler, F.A.: Corticofugal fiber connections of the cortex of *Macaca mulatta.* The frontal region. J. comp. Neurol. *61:* 509–542 (1935).

Mettler, F.A.: Relation between pyramidal and extrapyramidal function. Res. Publs Ass. Res. nerv. ment. Dis. *21:* 150–227 (1942).

Mettler, F.A.: Fiber connections of the corpus striatum of the monkey and baboon. J. comp. Neurol. *82:* 169–204 (1945).

Mettler, F.A.: Anatomy and physiology of the extrapyramidal motor passage. Int. Congr. Sci. Neurol. Acta med. belg. *1:* 11–37 (1957).

Mettler, F.A.; Ades, H.W.; Lipman, E.; Culler, E.A.: The extrapyramidal system. Archs Neurol. Psychiat. *41:* 984–995 (1939).

Mettler, F.A.; Carpenter, M.B.: The modification of subthalamic hyperkinesia in primates. Trans. Am. neurol. Ass. *74:* 81–88 (1949).

Mettler, F.A.; Davidoff, L.M.; Grimes, R.: Static tremor with hemiplegia. Archs Neurol. Psychiat. *57:* 423–429 (1947).

Metzel, E.; Milios, E.; Pfeiffer, S.: Correlative investigations on the subjective horizontal and vertical before and after stereotaxic procedures, with special regard to the target point. Confinia neurol. *27:* 208–212 (1966).

Meyer, G.; McElhaney, M.; Martin, W.; McGraw, C.P.: Stereotactic cingulotomy with results of acute stimulation and serial psychological testing; in Laitinen, Livingston, Surgical approaches in psychiatry, pp. 39–58 (Medical and Technical Publishing, Lancaster 1973).

Meyers, R.: The modification of alternating tremors, rigidity and festination by surgery of the basal ganglia. Res. Publs Ass. Res. nerv. ment. Dis. *21:* 602–665 (1942).

Meyers, R.: Surgical experiments in the therapy of certain 'extrapyramidal diseases'. Acta psychiat. neurol. *67:* suppl., pp. 1–42 (1951).

Meyers, R.: Discussion of Mettler. Trans. Am. neurol. Ass. *82:* 32 (1957).

Meyers, R.: Historical background and personal experiences in the surgical relief of hyperkinesia and hypertonus; in Fields, Pathogenesis and treatment of parkinsonism, pp. 229–270 (Thomas, Springfield 1958).

Meyers, R.: Current neurosurgical researches and treatment referable to the hyperkinetic disorders. N.Y. St. J. Med. *62:* 2150–2166 (1962).

Meyers, R.: A contribution to the topology of the infracortical, suprasegmental, neural mechanism of emissive speech. Trans. Am. neurol. Ass. *91:* 55–60 (1966).

Meyers, R.; Fry, W.J.; Fry, F.J.; Dreyer, L.L.; Schultz, D.F.; Noyes, R.F.: Early experiences with ultrasonic irradiation of the pallidofugal and nigral complexes in hyperkinetic and hypertonic disorders. J. Neurosurg. *16:* 32–54 (1959).

Meyers, R.; Hayne, R.; Knott, J.: Electrical activity of the neostriatum, paleostriatum and neighboring structures in parkinsonism and hemiballism. J. Neurol. Neurosurg. Psychiat. *12:* 111–123 (1949).

Meyers, R.; Knott, J.R.; Hayne, R.A.; Sweeney, D.B.: The surgery of epilepsy. J. Neurosurg. *7:* 337 (1950).

Meyerson, B.A.: Biochemistry of the pain relieving effects of central nervous stimulation in man. Few facts and many hypotheses. Acta neurochir. *30:* suppl., pp. 229–238 (1980).

Meyerson, B.A.; Hakansson, S.: Alleviation of atypical trigeminal pain by stimulation of the Gasserian ganglion via an implanted electrode. Acta neurochir. *30:* suppl., pp. 303–310 (1980).

Minkowski, M.: Etude sur les connexions anatomiques des circonvolutions rolandiques, pariétales et frontales. Schweizer Arch. Neurol. Psychiat. *12:* 71–104; 227–268; *14:* 255–278; *15:* 97–132 (1923/24).

Miyazaki, Y.; Ervin, F.R.; Siegfried, J.; Richardson, E.P.; Mark, V.H.: Localized cooling in the central nervous system. II. Histopathological results. Archs Neurol., Chicago *9:* 392–399 (1963).

Modesti, L.; Blumetti, A.: Long-term effects of stereotaxic thalamotomy on parameters of cognitive functioning. Acta neurochir. *30:* suppl., pp. 401–404 (1980).

Monnier, M.: Appareil stéréotaxique et technique de repérage pour la coagulation du relais thalamique. Schweiz. med. Wschr. *82:* 206–216 (1952).

Montanelli, R.P.; Hassler, R.: Stimulation effects of the globus pallidus and nucleus entopeduncularis of the cat. Proc. 22nd Int. Physiol. Congr. Excerpta Medica Congr. Ser. No. 45, p. 1091 (1962).

Moore, R.Y.; Bratnagar, R.; Heller, A.: Anatomical and chemical studies of a nigrostriatal projection in the cat. Brain Res. *30:* 119–135 (1971).

Moran, C.J.; Naidich, T.P.; Gado, M.H.; Barier, J.Y.: CT-guided aspiration procedures in the central nervous system. J. Comput. assist. Tomogr. *3:* 571 (1979).

Moricca, G.: Chemical hypophysectomy for cancer pain. Adv. Neurol. *4:* 707–714 (1974).

Morison, R.S.; Dempsey, E.W.: A study of thalamocortical relations. Am. J. Physiol. *135:* 281–292 (1942).

Morison, R.S.; Dempsey, E.W.: Mechanism of thalamocortical augmentation and repetition. Am. J. Physiol. *138:* 297–308 (1943).

Moruzzi, G.: Effects at different frequencies of cerebellar stimulation upon postural tonus and myotatic reflexes. Electroenceph. Clin. Neurophysiol. *21:* 463–469 (1950).

Moruzzi, G.; Magoun, H.W.: Brain stem reticular formation and activation of the EEG. Electroenceph. clin. Neurophysiol. *1:* 455–473 (1949).

Moser, R.P.; Yap, J.C.; Fraley, E.E.: Stereotactic hypophysectomy for intractable pain secondary to metastatic prostate carcinoma. Appl. Neurophysiol. *43:* 145–149 (1980).

Mountcastle, V.B.; Henneman, E.: The representation of tactile sensibility in the thalamus of the monkey. J. comp. Neurol. *97:* 409–440 (1952).

Mountcastle, V.B.; Powell, T.P.S.: Central nervous mechanisms subserving position sense and kinesthesis. Bull. Johns Hopkins Hosp. *105:* 173–200 (1959).

Mullan, S.: Stereotactic thrombosis of intracranial aneurysms. Confinia neurol. *31:* 94 (1969).

Mullan, S.; Harper, P.V.; Hekmatpanah, J.; Torres, H.; Dobbin, G.: Percutaneous interruption of spinal pain tracts by means of a strontium-90 needle. J. Neurosurg. *20:* 931–939 (1963).

*Mullan, S.; Moseley, R.; Harper, P.V.: The creation of deep cerebral lesions by small beta ray sources implanted under guidance of fluoroscopic image intensifiers (as used in the treatment of Parkinson's disease). Am. J. Roentg. *82:* 613 (1959).

Mullan, S.; Vailati, G.; Karasick, J.; Mailis, M.: Thalamic lesions for the control of epilepsy. Archs Neurol., Chicago *16:* 277–285 (1967).

Müller, C.; Yasargil, M.G.: Zur Psychiatrie der stereotaktischen Hirnoperationen bei extrapyramidalen Erkrankungen. Schweizer Arch. Neurol. Psychiat. *84:* 136–154 (1959).

*Munari, C.; Talairach, J.; Bonis, A.; Szikla, G.; Bancaud, J.: Differential diagnosis between temporal and 'perisylvian' epilepsy in a surgical perspective. Acta neurochir. *30:* suppl., pp. 97–102 (1980).

Mundinger, F.: Stereotaxic intervention in the zona incerta area for treatment of extrapyramidal motor disturbances. Confinia neurol. *26:* 222–230 (1965).

Mundinger, F.: Stereotactic Curie therapy of pituitary adenomas. A long-term follow-up study. Acta neurochir. *21:* suppl., pp. 169–176 (1974).

Mundinger, F.: Die operative Behandlung des Intentionstremors und der Aktionsmyoclonie bei der multiplen Sklerose; in Bronisch, Multiple Sklerose, pp. 64–73 (Enke, Stuttgart 1975).

Mundinger, F.: Neue stereotaktisch-funktionelle Behandlungsmethode des Torticollis spasmodicus mit Hirnstimulatoren. Medsche. Klin. *72:* 1982–1986 (1977a).

Mundinger, F.: Die Behandlung chronischer Schmerzen mit Hirnstimulatoren. Dt. med. Wschr. *102:* 1724–1729 (1977b).

Mundinger, F.: Die stereotaktische Behandlung des Schmerzes durch intracerebrale Aus-schaltung und Stimulation; in Gottschaldt, Grass, Brock, Aktuelle Probleme der Neu-ropsychiatrie, pp. 88–103 (Springer, Berlin 1978).

Mundinger, F.; Becker, P.: Late results of central stereotactic intervention for pain. Acta neurochir. *24:* suppl., p. 229 (1977).

Mundinger, F.; Becker, P.; Groebner, E.; Bachschmid, G.: Late results of stereotactic sur-gery of epilepsy predominantly temporal lobe type. Acta neurochir. *23:* suppl., pp. 177–182 (1976).

Mundinger, F.; Birg, W.; Klar, M.: Computer assisted stereotactic brain operations. Appl. Neurophysiol. *41:* 169–182 (1978).

Mundinger, F.; Birg, W.; Ostertag, C.B.: Treatment of small cerebral gliomas with CT-aided stereotaxic curietherapy. Neuroradiology *16:* 564–567 (1978).

Mundinger, F.; Busam, B.: Stereotactic interstitial iridium-192 permanent irradiation of pi-tuitary adenomas. Abstr. Inserm Symp. Stereotactic Irradiations, Paris 1979, p. V 21.

Mundinger, F.; Busam, B.; Birg, W.; Schneider, J.: Life expectancy of inoperable gliomas after protracted long-term irradiation. (Interstitial iridium-192 permanent implanta-tion.) Abstr. Symp. Stereotactic Irradiations, Paris 1979, p. V 31.

*Mundinger, F.; Disselhoff, J.: Indications for stereotactic operations in torsion dystonia and choreoathetosis on the basis of long-term comparative studies; in Bushe, Spoerri, Shaw, Progress in paediatric neurosurgery, pp. 238–240 (Hippokrates, Stuttgart 1974).

Mundinger, F.; Hoefer, T.: Protracted long-term irradiation of inoperable midbrain tumors by stereotactic Curie-therapy using iridium-192. Acta neurochir. *21:* suppl., pp. 93–100 (1974).

Mundinger, F.; Ostertag, C.: Multilocular lesions in the therapy of cerebral palsy. Acta neurochir. *24:* suppl., pp. 11–14 (1977).

Mundinger, F.; Ostertag, C.; Birg, W.; Weigel, K.: Stereotactic treatment of brain lesions. Biopsy, interstitial radiotherapy (iridium-192 and iodine-125) and drainage proce-dures. Appl. Neurophysiol. *43:* 198–204 (1980).

Mundinger, F.; Reinke, M.A.; Hoefer, T.; Birg, W.: Determination of intracerebral struc-tures using osseous reference points for computer-aided stereotactic operations. Appl. Neurophysiol. *38:* 3–22 (1975).

Mundinger, F.; Riechert, T.: Ergebnisse der stereotaktischen Hirnoperationen bei extrapy-ramidalen Bewegungsstörungen auf Grund postoperativer und Langzeituntersu-chungen. Dt. Z. NervHeilk. *182:* 542–576 (1961).

Mundinger, F.; Riechert, T.: Stereotaxic irradiation procedure of brain tumors and pitu-itary adenomas by means of radioisotopes and its results. Confinia neurol. *22:* 190–203 (1962).

Mundinger, F.; Riechert, T.: Hypophysentumoren-Hypophysenektomie (Thieme, Stutt-gart 1967).

Mundinger, F.; Riechert, T.; Disselhoff, J.: Long-term results of stereotactic treatment of spasmodic torticollis. Confinia neurol. *34:* 41–46 (1972).

Mundinger, F.; Riechert, T.; Gabriel, E.: Untersuchungen zu den physikalischen und tech-nischen Voraussetzungen einer dosierten Hochfrequenz-Koagulation bei stereotak-tischen Hirnoperationen. Zentbl. Chir. *85:* 1051–1063 (1960).

Mundinger, F.; Salomao, J.F.: Deep brain stimulation in mesencephalic lemniscus me-dialis for chronic pain. Acta neurochir. *30:* suppl., pp. 245–258 (1980).

Mundinger, F.; Schildge, J.: Results of stereotaxic iridium-192 brachy-Curie therapy in cerebral tumors. Meeting of the European Society for Stereotactic and Functional Neurosurgery, Paris 1979. Abstr., p. V31.

Munk, H.: Verhalten der niederen Teile des Cerebrospinalsystems nach Ausschaltung oberer Teile. Sber. preuss. Akad. Wiss., pp. 1106–1133 (1909).

*Muratoff, W.: Sekundäre Degeneration nach Zerstörung der motorischen Sphäre des Gehirns in Verbindung mit der Frage von der Lokalisation der Gehirnfunktionen. Arch. Anat. Physiol. *1893:* 97–116.

Nádvornik, P.; Pogády, J.; Šramka, M.: The results of stereotactic treatment of the aggressive syndrome; in Laitinen, Livingston, Surgical approaches in psychiatry, pp. 125–127 (Medical and Technical Publishing, Lancaster 1973).

Nádvornik, P.; Šramka, M.; Gajdosova, D.; Kokavec, M.: Longitudinal hippocampectomy. Confinia neurol. *37:* 404–408 (1975).

Nádvornik, P.; Šramka, M.; Lisý, L.; Svicka, I.: Experiences with dentatectomy. Confinia neurol. *34:* 320–324 (1972).

Nakajima, H.; Ohye, C.: Electrophysiologically-guided stereotactic biopsy for symptomatic epileptic patients with CT-scan abnormality. Folia psychiat. neurol. jap. *34:* 377–378 (1980).

*Narabayashi, H.: Stereotaxic instrument for operation on the human basal ganglia. Psychiatria Neurol. jap. *54:* 669–671 (1952).

Narabayashi, H.: Neurophysiological ideas on pallidotomy and ventrolateral thalamotomy in hyperkinesia. Confinia neurol. *22:* 291–303 (1962).

Narabayashi, H.: Thalamic influences on the gamma motor system. Archs Neurol., Chicago *9:* 348–357 (1963).

Narabayashi, H.: Stereotaxic amygdalotomy; in Eleftheriou, The neurobiology of the amygdala, pp. 459–483 (Plenum Press, New York 1972).

Narabayashi, H.: Lessons from amygdaloid surgery in long-term observation. Acta neurochir. *23:* suppl., pp. 241–245 (1976).

Narabayashi, H.: Experiences of stereotaxic surgery on cerebral palsy patients. Acta neurochir. *24:* suppl., pp. 3–10 (1977).

Narabayashi, H.: Role of cerebellum in involuntary movements. Meeting of the European Society for Stereotactic and Functional Neurosurgery, Paris 1979. Abstr., p. J7.

Narabayashi, H.: Experiences of medial amygdalotomies in epileptics. Acta neurochir. *55:* suppl. 30, pp. 15–81 (1980).

Narabayashi, H.: Clinical analysis of akinesia. J. neural Transm. *16:* suppl., pp. 129–136 (1980).

Narabayashi, H.; Goto, A.; Miyazaki, S.; Kosaka, K.: Importance of the cerebellar hemisphere in production of tremulous movement or choreo-dystonic movements in monkeys. Acta neurochir. *21:* suppl., pp. 35–38 (1974).

Narabayashi, H.; Kondo, T.; Hayashi, A.; Suzuki, T.; Nagatsu, T.: L-Threo-3,4-dihydroxyphenylserine treatment for akinesia and freezing of parkinsonism. Proc. Japan. Acad. *57B:* 351–354 (1981).

Narabayashi, H.; Mizutani, T.: Epileptic seizures and the stereotaxic amygdalotomy. Confinia neurol. *32:* 289–297 (1970).

Narabayashi, H.; Nagao, T.; Saito, Y.; Yoshida, M.; Nagahata, M.: Stereotaxic amygdalotomy for behavior disorders. Archs Neurol., Chicago *9:* 1–16 (1963).

Narabayashi, H.; Ohye, C.: Importance of microstereoencephalotomy for tremor alleviation. Appl. Neurophysiol. *43:* 222–227 (1980).

Narabayashi, H.; Shimazu, H.; Fujita, Y.; Shikiba, S.; Nagao, T.; Nagahata, M.: Procaine-oil-wax pallidotomy for double athetosis and spastic states in infantile cerebral palsy. Neurology *10:* 61–69 (1960).

*Narabayashi, H.; Uno, M.: Long range results of stereotaxic amygdalotomy for behavior disorders. Confinia neurol. *27:* 168–171 (1966).

Nashold, B.S., Jr.: Ocular signs of brain stimulation in the human. Confinia neurol. *29:* 169–174 (1967).

Nashold, B.S., Jr.: Stereotactic neurosurgery: the present and future. Am. Surg. *36:* 85–93 (1970a).

Nashold, B.S., Jr.: Phosphenes resulting from stimulation of the midbrain in man. Archs Ophthal. *84:* 433–435 (1970b).

Nashold, B.S., Jr.; Friedman, H.: Dorsal column stimulation for control of pain. J. Neurosurg. *36:* 590–597 (1972).

Nashold, B.S., Jr.; Friedman, H.; Glenn, J.F.; Grimes, J.H.; Barry, W.F.; Avery, R.: Electromicturition in paraplegia. Archs Surg., Chicago *104:* 195–202 (1972).

Nashold, B.S., Jr.; Hanbery, J.; Olszewski, J.: Observations on the diffuse thalamic projections. Electroenceph. clin. Neurophysiol. *7:* 609–620 (1955).

Nashold, B.S., Jr.; Ostdahl, R.H.: Pain relief after dorsal root entry zone lesions. Acta neurochir. *30:* suppl., pp. 383–390 (1980).

Nashold, B.S., Jr.; Slaughter, D.G.: Effects of stimulating or destroying the deep cerebellar regions in man. J. Neurosurg. *31:* 172–186 (1969).

Nashold, B.S., Jr.; Slaughter, D.G.; Harrison, J.: A stereotaxic approach and evaluation of the cerebellar nuclei in man. Confinia neurol. *31:* 56 (1969).

Nashold, B.S., Jr.; Wilson, W.P.: Central pain. Observations in man with chronic implanted electrodes in the midbrain tegmentum. Confinia neurol. *27:* 30–44 (1966).

Nashold, B.S., Jr.; Wilson, W.P.; Fulghum, J.: Cerebellar stimulation and brain activity. Abstr. Symp. Stereotactic Treatment of Epilepsy, Bratislava, 1975, pp. 78–90.

Nashold, B.S., Jr.; Wilson, W.P.; Slaughter, D.C.: Sensations evoked by stimulation of the midbrain of man. J. Neurosurg. *30:* 14–24 (1966).

Nauta, W.H.: Hippocampal projections and related neural pathways to the midbrain in the cat. Brain *81:* 319 (1958).

Nauta, W.H.: Some neuronal pathways related to the limbic system; in Ramsey, O'Doherty, Electrical studies of the unanesthetized brain, pp. 1–16 (Hoeber, New York 1960).

Nauta, W.J.H.; Kuypers, H.G.J.M.: Some ascending pathways in the brain stem reticular formation; in Jasper, Reticular formation of the brain. Henry Ford Hospital Int. Symp., pp. 3–30 (Little, Brown, Boston 1958).

Nauta, W.J.H.; Mehler, W.R.: Some efferent connections of the lentiform nucleus in the monkey and cat. Anat. Rec. *139:* 260 (1961).

Newcombe, R.: The lesion in stereotactic subcaudate tractotomy. Br. J. Psychiat. *126:* 478–481 (1975).

Newman, R.R.; Jacobs, L.: Metoprolol in essential tremor. Archs Neurol., Chicago *37:* 596–597 (1980).

Nicoll, R.A.; Siggins, G.R.; Ling, N.; Bloom, F.E.; Guillemin, R.: Neuronal actions of endorphins and enkephalins among brain regions: a comparative microiontophoretic study. Proc. natn. Acad. Sci. USA *74:* 2584–2588 (1977).

Niemeyer, P.: Tratamento cirúrgica das discinesias. VIth Congr. Latinoam. Neurocirurgia, Montevideo 1955, pp. 424–456.

Nittner, K.: The combined thalamo-subthalamotomy. Confinia neurol. *32:* 93–99 (1970).

Nittner, K.; Petrovici, I.N.: Contributions to the pathogenesis of Parinaud's syndrome. Vertical gaze paralysis following bilateral stereotaxic lesions in the interstitial nucleus region. Acta neurochir. *21:* suppl., pp. 57–63 (1974).

Nordlie, R.; Denstad, I.; Sem-Jacobsen, C.W.; Herlofsen, H.; Hartviksen, K.: Om Parkinsons sykdom ok den neuro-kirurgiske dybdeelektrografiske behandling. Nord. Med. *68:* 1467–1471 (1962).

Norén, G.; Collins, V.P.: Stereotactic biopsies in acoustic tumors. Appl. Neurophysiol. *43:* 189–197 (1980).

Norén, G.; Leksell, L.: Stereotactic radiosurgery in acoustic neurinomas. Abstr. Symp. Stereotactic Irradiations, Paris 1979, p. V 25.

Noyes, A.P.: Modern clinical psychiatry; 4th ed. (Saunders, Philadelphia 1954).

Obrador, S.: A simplified neurosurgical technique for approaching and damaging the region of the globus pallidus in Parkinson's disease. J. Neurol. Neurosurg. Psychiat. *20:* 47–49 (1957).

Obrador, S.: Some physiopathological aspects related to subcortical therapeutical lesions. Confinia neurol. *22:* 283–290 (1962).

Obrador, S.; Dierssen, G.: Cirurgía de la región palidal. Revta clin. esp. Ano XVII *61:* 229–237 (1956).

Obrador, S.; Dierssen, G.: Sensory responses to subcortical stimulation and management of pain disorders by stereotaxic methods. Confinia neurol. *27:* 45–51 (1966).

Obrador, S.; Dierssen, G.: Mental changes induced by subcortical stimulation and therapeutic lesions. Confinia neurol. *29:* 168 (1967).

Ohmoto, T.; Mimura, Y.; Baba, Y.; Miyamoto, T.; Matsumoto, Y.; Nishimoto, A.; Matsumoto, K.: Thalamic control of spontaneous alpha rhythm and evoked responses. Appl. Neurophysiol. *41:* 188–192 (1978).

Ohye, C.; Nakajima, H.; Kawashima, Y.; Miyazaki, M.: Stereotactic CT-scan and its correlation with the neural activity of the deep structures. Appl. Neurophysiol. *43:* 183–188 (1980).

Ohye, C.; Nakamura, R.; Fukamachi, A.; Narabayashi, H.: Recording and stimulation of the ventralis intermedius nucleus of the human thalamus. Confinia neurol. *37:* 258 (1975).

Olianas, M.C.; De Montis, G.M.; Mulas, G.; Tagliamonte, A.: The striatal dopaminergic function is mediated by inhibition of a nigral, non-dopaminergic neuronal system via a strio-nigral gabaergic pathway. Eur. J. Pharmacol. *49:* 233–241 (1978).

Onofrio, B.M.: Radiofrequency percutaneous Gasserian ganglion lesion. J. Neurosurg. *42:* 132–139 (1975).

Organ, L.W.: Electrophysiological principles of radiofrequency lesion making. Appl. Neurophysiol. *39:* 69–76 (1976/77).

Orthner, H.: Die Beeinflussung der postenzephalitischen Schauanfälle durch die Pallidotomie. Confinia neurol. *26:* 456–457 (1965).

Orthner, H.; Roeder, F.D.: Das Parkinson Syndrom (Fischer, Stuttgart 1959).

Ostertag, C.; Kiessling, M.; Mennel, H.D.; Mundinger, F.; Weigel, K.: Stereotactic biopsy and smear preparation diagnosis of brain tumours in infants and children. Z. Kinderchir. *34:* 205–206 (1981).

Ostertag, C.; Mennel, H.D.; Kiessling, M.: Stereotactic biopsy of brain tumors. Surg. Neurol. *14:* 275–283 (1980).

Ostertag, C.; Weigel, K.; Birg, W.; Mundinger, F.: CT changes after long-term interstitial iridium-192 irradiation of cerebral gliomas. Abstr. Symp. Stereotactic Irradiations, Paris 1979, p. V 17.

Pagni, C.A.; Maspes, T.; Cassinari, V.: Etude stéréoélectroencéphalographique du lobe temporal. Revue neurol. *108:* 98–106 (1963).

Papez, J.W.: A proposed mechanism of emotion. Archs Neurol. Psychiat. *38:* 725–734 (1937).

Papez, J.W.: A summary of fiber connections of the basal ganglia. Res. Publs Ass. Res. nerv. ment. Dis. *21:* 21–68 (1942).

Peacock, S.M.: Studies on subcortical motor activity. I. Motor activity and inhibition from identical anatomical points. J. Neurophysiol. *17:* 144–154 (1954).

Peluso, F.; Gybels, J.: Computer calculation of two-target trajectory with center of arc-target stereotaxic equipment. Acta neurochir. *21:* 173–180 (1969).

Penfield, W.; Jasper, H.: Epilepsy and the functional anatomy of the brain (Little, Brown, Boston 1954).

Penfield, W.; Milner, B.: Memory deficit produced by bilateral lesions in the hippocampal zone. Archs Neurol. Psychiat. *79:* 475–497 (1958).

Penfield, W.; Perot, P.: The brain's record of auditory and visual experience. Brain *86:* 595–696 (1963).

Penfield, W.; Rasmussen, T.: The cerebral cortex of man (Macmillan, New York 1950).

Penn, R.D.; Whisler, W.W.; Smith, C.A.; Yasnoff, W.A.: Stereotactic surgery with image processing of computerized tomographic scans. Neurosurgery *3:* 157–163 (1978).

Perloff, W.H.; Levy, L.M.; Despopoulos, A.: The eosinophil response to stress of patients with surgically produced thalamic and hypothalamic lesions. J. clin. Endocr. Metab. *12:* 36–41 (1952).

Perry, J.H.; Rosenbaum, A.E.; Lunsford, L.D.; Swink, C.A.; Zorub, D.S.: Computed tomography-guided stereotactic surgery: conception and development of a new stereotactic methodology. Neurosurgery *7:* 376–381 (1980).

Pertuiset, B.; Hirsch, J.; Sachs, M.; Landau, F.J.: Selective stereotactic interventions in grand mal epilepsy. Excerpta Med. Int. Congr. Ser. *193:* p. 72 (1969).

Peters, G.: Spezielle Pathologie der Krankheiten des zentralen und peripheren Nervensystems (Thieme, Stuttgart 1951).

Piskun, W.S.; Stevens, E.A.; MaMorgese, J.R.; Paullus, W.S.; Meyers, P.W.: A simplified method of CT assisted localization and biopsy of intracranial lesions. Surg. Neurol. *11:* 413–417 (1979).

Poblete, M.; Mancini, R.; Aranda, L.: Stereotaxic posterior capsulotomy in hemiballismus. Meeting of the World Society for Stereotactic and Functional Neurosurgery, São Paulo 1977, p. 63.

*Poblete, M.; Palestini, M.; Figueroa, E.; Gallardo, R.; Rojas, J.; Covarrubias, M.I.; Doyharcabal, Y.: Stereotaxic thalamotomy (lamella medialis) in aggressive psychiatric patients. Confinia neurol. *32:* 326–331 (1970).

Poblete, M.; Zamboni, R.: Stereotactic pituitary implantation of radioisotopes by transfrontal route. Acta neurochir., *21:* suppl., pp. 159–163 (1974).

Poirier, L.J.: Production expérimentale du tremblement postural. Revue can. Biol. *20:* 137–142 (1964).

Poirier, L.J.; Sourkes, T.L.: Influence of the substantia nigra on the catecholamine content of striatum. Brain *88:* 181–192 (1965).

Pollock, L.J.; Davis, L.: Muscle tone in parkinsonian states. Archs Neurol. Psychiat., Chicago *23:* 303–317 (1930).

Pool, J.L.; Ransohoff, J.: Autonomic effects on stimulating rostral portion of cingulate gyri in man. J. Neurophysiol. *12:* 385–392 (1949).

Pötzl, O.: Optisch-agnostische Störungen (Deuticke, Vienna 1928).

Powell, T.P.S.; Cowan, M.: A study of thalamocortical relations in the monkey. Brain *79:* 364–390 (1956).

Pribram, K.H.; Kruger, L.: Functions of the 'olfactory' brain. Ann. N.Y. Acad. Sci. *58:* 109–138 (1954).

*Price, P.; Baxter, R.C.H.; Parkes, J.D.; Marsden, C.D.: Opiate antagonists and Parkinson's disease. Archs Neurol. *36:* 661 (1979).

*Puech, P.; Guilly, P.; Lairy-Bounes, G.C.: Introduction à la psychochirurgie (Masson, Paris 1950).

Rähn, T.; Hall, K.; Thorén, M.; Backlund, E.O.: Stereotactic radiosurgery in treatment of morbus Cushing. Abstr. Inserm Symp. on Stereotactic Irradiation, Paris 1979, p. V 23.

Ramamurthi, B.; Davidson, A.: Central median lesions. Confinia neurol. *37:* 63–72 (1975).

Ramamurthi, B.; Kalayanaraman, S.: Stereotaxic thalamotomy for pain relief. Excerpta med. *93:* 102–103 (1965).

Ramamurthi, B.; Mascreen, M.; Valmikinathan, K.: Role of the amygdala and hypothalamus in the control of gastric secretion in human beings. Acta. neurochir. *24:* suppl., pp. 187–190 (1977).

Ramani, S.V.; Yap, J.C.; Gummit, R.J.: Stereotactic fields of Forel interruption for intractable epilepsy. Appl. Neurophysiol. *43:* 104–108 (1980).

Rand, R.W.: Substantia nigralysis. Bull. Los Angeles. neurol. Soc. *24:* 214 (1959).

Rand, R.W.: A stereotaxic instrument for pallidothalamectomy. J. Neurosurg. *18:* 258–260 (1961).

Rand, R.W.; Crandall, P.H.; Adey, W.P.; Walter, R.D.; Markham, C.H.: Electrophysiologic investigations in Parkinson's disease and other dyskinesias in man. Neurology *12:* 754–770 (1962a).

Rand, R.W.; Dashe, A.M.; Paglia, D.E.; Conway, L.W.; Solomon, D.H.: Stereotactic cryohypophysectomy. J. Am. med. Ass. *189:* 255–259 (1964).

Rand, R.W.; Dashe, A.M.; Solomon, D.H.; Westover, J.L.; Crandall, P.H.; Brown, J.; Tranquada, R.: Stereotaxic yttrium-90 hypophysectomy for metastatic mammary carcinoma. Ann. Surg. *156:* 989–993 (1962b).

Ranson, S.W.; Ranson, M.: Pallidofugal fibers in the monkey. Archs Neurol. Psychiat. *42:* 1059–1067 (1939).

*Rasmussen, T.: Surgical aspects of temporal lobe epilepsy. Meeting of the European Society for Stereotactic and Functional Neurosurgery, Paris 1979. Abstr., p. J2.

Ray, C.D.: Control of pain by electrical stimulation. Adv. Neurosurg. *3:* 216–224 (1975).

Ray, C.D.; Burton, C.V.: Deep brain stimulation for severe chronic pain. Meeting of the European Society for Stereotactic and Functional Neurosurgery, Paris 1979, p. S16.

Rees, W.L.: Schizophrenia: current views of its psycho-biology and arcanum. Trans. Stud. Coll. Physns Philad. Ser. V *3:* 125–147 (1981).

Rémond, A.: A stereotaxic instrument for man. Demonstration Am. EEG Ass., Atlantic City 1952.

Rémond, A.; Houdart, R.; Lecasble, R.; Dondey, M.; Aubert, P.: Recherche sur l'approche stéréotaxique des structures pallidales. Revue neurol. *99:* 355–384 (1958).

Rexed, B.; Mair, W.; Sourander, P.; Larsson, B.; Leksell, L.: Effect of high energy protons on the brain of the rabbit. Acta radiol. *53:* 289 (1960).

Reynolds, D.V.: Surgery in the rat during electrical analgesia induced by focal brain stimulation. Science *164:* 444–445 (1969).

Reynolds, A.R.; Hardy, T.L.: Cerebellar stimulation in four patients with cerebral palsy. Appl. Neurophysiol. *43:* 114–117 (1980).

Rhoton, A.L.; Manischico, G.E.: Percutaneous stereotactic radiofrequency lesions for trigeminal neuralgia. J. Fla med. Ass. *64:* 488–493 (1977).

Richardson, D.E.: Thalamotomy for intractable pain. Confinia neurol. *29:* 139–145 (1967).

*Richardson, D.E.: Thalamotomy for control of chronic pain. Acta neurochir. *21:* suppl., pp. 77–88 (1974).

Richardson, D.E.; Akil, H.: Pain relief by electrical stimulation of the brain in human patients. Excerpta med. *293* (1973).

Richardson, D.E.; Zorub, D.S.: Sensory function of the pulvinar. Confinia neurol. *32:* 165–173 (1970).

Richet, C.: Fièvre traumatique. C.r. hebd. Séanc. Acad. Sci., Paris *99:* 279 (1884).

Richter, R.: Degeneration of the basal ganglia in monkeys from chronic carbon disulfide poisoning. J. Neuropath. exp. Neurol. *4:* 324 (1945).

Riechert, T.: Die psychochirurgischen Eingriffe mit besonderer Berücksichtigung der gezielten Hirnoperationen. Arch. klin. Chir. *276:* 101–108 (1953a).

Riechert, T.: Neurochirurgische Therapie; in Handbuch der inneren Medizin; 4th ed., vol. 5, part I, pp. 1472–1543 (Springer, Berlin 1953b).

Riechert, T.: Die Entfernung von Hirnstecksplittern mit Hilfe des stereotaktischen Operationsverfahrens. Zentbl. Neurochir. *15:* 159–164 (1955).

Riechert, T.: Die stereotaktischen Hirnoperationen in ihrer Anwendung bei den Hyperkinesen (mit Ausnahme des Parkinsonismus), bei Schmerzzuständen und einigen weiteren Indikationen (Einführen von radioaktiven Isotopen usw.). 1er Congr. de Neurochirurgie. Acta med. belg., pp. 121–160 (1957a).

Riechert, T.: Die chirurgische Behandlung des Parkinsonismus. Arch. klin. Chir. *287:* 660–666 (1957b).

Riechert, T.: Moderne Chirurgie des Zentralnervensystems (inductive heating). Therapiewoche *9:* 430–435 (1959).

Riechert, T.: Die chirurgische Behandlung der zentralen Schmerzzustände. Acta neurochir. *8:* 136–152 (1960).

Riechert, T.: Eine neue Methode zur Behandlung bisher inoperabler arteriovenöser

Angiome. Die Operation auf stereotaktischem Wege. Czechoslovakian Med. Congr., Prague 1962a.

Riechert, T.: Long-term follow-up of results of stereotaxic treatment of extrapyramidal disorders. Confinia neurol. *22:* 356–363 (1962b).

Riechert, T.: Relief of certain types of intractable pain; in Knighton, Dumke, Pain, pp. 519–529 (Little, Brown, Boston 1966).

Riechert, T.: Development of human stereotactic surgery. Confinia neurol. *37:* 399–409 (1975).

Riechert, T.: Stereotactic brain operations (Huber, Bern 1980).

Riechert, T.; Gabriel, E.; Asai, A.: Die Ausschaltung biologischen Gewebes mittels induktiver Erwärmung. Acta neurochir. *16:* 299–300 (1967).

Riechert, T.; Hassler, R.; Mundinger, F.; Bronisch, F.; Schmidt, K.: Pathologic-anatomic findings and cerebral localization in stereotactic treatment of extrapyramidal motor disturbances in multiple sclerosis. Confinia neurol. *37:* 24–40 (1975).

Riechert, T.; Kapp, H.; Krainick, J.U.; Schmidt, C.L.; Thoden, U.: Operative relief of chronic pain by electrostimulation of the dorsal column. Germ. med. Mon. *3:* 144–145 (1973a).

Riechert, T.; Krainick, J.U.; Thoden, U.: Experience with dorsal column stimulation, especially in phantom and stump pain. Seminar on Electrical Stimulation of the Human Nervous System for Control of Pain, Minneapolis 1973b.

Riechert, T.; Mundinger, F.: Beschreibung und Anwendung eines Zielgerätes für stereotaktische Hirnoperationen (II. Modell). Acta neurochir. *3:* suppl., pp. 308–337 (1955).

Riechert, T.; Wolff, M.: Die Entwicklung und klinische Bedeutung der gezielten Hirnoperationen. Medsche Klin. *46:* 609–611 (1951).

Riklan, M.; Levita, E.: Subcortical correlates of human behavior (Williams & Wilkins, Baltimore 1969).

Rinaldi, F.; Himwich, H.E.: The site of action of antiparkinson drugs. Confinia neurol. *15:* 209–224 (1955).

Roberts, T.S.; Brown, R.: Technical and clinical aspects of CT-directed stereotaxis. Appl. Neurophysiol. *43:* 170–171 (1980).

Robinson, B.W.; Tompkins, E.: Impedance method for localizing brain structures. Archs Neurol., Chicago *10:* 563–574 (1964).

Roeder, F.D.: Stereotaxic lesions of the tuber cinereum in sexual deviation. Confinia neurol. *27:* 162–163 (1966).

Roeder, F.D.: Stereotactische Therapie der Suchten; in Nass, Vorbeugung und Behandlung bei Kriminellen und Süchtigen, pp. 3–35 (Gesellschaft für vorbeugende Verbrechensbekämpfung, Kassel 1974).

Roeder, F.; Müller, D.: Zur stereotaktischen Heilung der paedophilen Homosexualität. Dt. med. Wschr. *94:* 409 (1969).

Roeder, F.; Müller, D.; Orthner, H.: Further results of stereotaxis in human hypothalamus in sexual deviation and other behavioral disorders (addictions). Abstr. 3rd Wld Congr. Psychosurgery, Cambridge 1972a, p. 36.

Roeder, F.; Orthner, H.: Pallidotomy in hemiballism, paralysis agitans, etc. 1st Int. Congr. Neurol. Surg., Brussels. Excerpta med. *1957:* 75–76.

Roeder, F.; Orthner, H.: Über zentrale Schmerzoperationen, insbesondere mediale Mesencephalotomie bei thalamischer Hyperpathie und bei Anaesthesia dolorosa. Confinia neurol. *21:* 51–97 (1961).

Roeder, F.; Orthner, H.; Müller, D.: The stereotaxic treatment of pedophilic homosexuality and other sexual deviations. 2nd Int. Conf. Psychosurgery, Copenhagen 1971, pp. 87–111.

Roeder, F.D.; Orthner, H.; Müller, D.: Treatment of sexual perversion by stereotactic lesion of the ventromedial hypothalamic nucleus (Cajal); in Hitchcock, Vaernet, Int. Conf. Psychosurgery (Thomas, Springfield 1972b).

Rosegay, H.: An experimental investigation of the connnections between the corpus striatum and substantia nigra in the cat. J. comp. Neurol. 80: 293–321 (1944).

Rosenbaum, A.; Lunsford, D.L.; Perry, J.: Computerized tomography guided stereotaxis: a new approach. Appl. Neurophysiol. 43: 172–173 (1980).

Rosomoff, H.L.; Brown, C.J.; Sheptak, P.: Percutaneous radio-frequency cervical cordotomy. J. Neurosurg. 23: 639–645 (1965).

Ross, J.E.: The cortical connections of the reticular complex of the thalamus; in Patterns of organization of the central nervous system. Res. Publs Ass. Res. nerv. ment. Dis. 30: 454–479 (1952).

Rosvold, H.E.; Delgado, J.M.R.: Effect on delayed-alternation test of performance of stimulating or destroying electrically structures within frontal lobes of monkey's brain. J. comp. physiol. Psychol. 49: 365–372 (1956).

Rubin, R.T.; Mandell, A.J.; Crandell, P.H.: Corticosteroid responses to limbic stimulation in man: localization of stimulus sites. Science 153: 767–768 (1966).

Rümler, B.; Schaltenbrand, G.; Spuler, H.; Wahren, W.: Somatotopic array of the ventrooral nucleus of the thalamus based on electrical stimulation during stereotactic procedures. Confinia neurol. 34: 197–199 (1972).

Rushworth, R.G.: Stereotactic guided biopsy in the computerized tomographic scanner. Surg. Neurol. 14: 451–454 (1980).

Rylander, G.: The renaissance of psychosurgery; in Laitinen, Livingston, Surgical approaches in psychiatry, pp. 3–12 (Medical and Technical Publishing, Lancaster 1973).

Saito, Y.; Ohye, C.: Automatically controlled recording and processing of thalamic unit discharges in human stereotaxic operation. Confinia neurol. 36: 314–325 (1974).

Salcman, M.; Correll, J.; Defendini, R.; Gilman, S.: Morphological abnormalities in cerebellar biopsies of epileptic patients. Trans. Am. neurol. Ass. 1976: 26–29.

Samanin, R.; Valzelli, L.: Increase of morphine-induced analgesia by stimulation of the nucl. raphe dorsalis. Eur. J. Pharmacol. 16: 298–302 (1971).

Sano, K.: Sedative neurosurgery with special reference to posteromedial hypothalamotomy. Neurol. med. chir. 4: 112–142 (1962).

Sano, K.; Mayanagi, Y.; Sekino, H.; Ogashiwa, M.; Ishijima, B.: Results of stimulation and destruction of the posterior hypothalamus in man. J. Neurosurg. 33: 689–707 (1970a).

Sano, K.; Sekino, H.; Hashimoto, I.; Amano, K.; Sugiyama, H.: Postero-medial hypothalamotomy in the treatment of intractable pain. Confinia neurol. 37: 285–290 (1975).

Sano, K.; Yoshioka, M.; Mayanagi, Y.; Sekino, H.; Yoshimasu, N.; Tsukamoto, Y.: Stimulation and destruction of and around the interstitial nucleus of Cajal in man. Confinia neurol. 32: 118–125 (1970b).

Sano, K.; Yoshioka, M.; Ogashiwa, M.; Ishijima, B.; Ohye, C.: Thalamolaminotomy. A new operation for relief of intractable pain. Confinia neurol. 27: 63–66 (1966a).

Sano, K.; Yoshioka, M.; Ogashiwa, M.; Ishijima, B.; Ohye, C.: Posteromedial hypothalamotomy in the treatment of aggressive behavior. Confinia neurol. *27:* 164–167 (1966b).

Sano, K.; Yoshioka, M.; Ogashiwa, M.; Ishijima, B.; Ohye, C.; Sekino, H.; Mayanagi, Y.: Central mechanisms of neck movements in the human brain stem. Confinia neurol. *29:* 107–111 (1967a).

Sano, K.; Yoshioka, M.; Ogashiwa, M.; Ishijima, B.; Ohye, C.; Sekino, H.; Mayanagi, Y.: Autonomic, somatomotor and electroencephalographic responses upon stimulation of the hypothalamus and the rostral brain stem in man. Confinia neurol. *29:* 257–261 (1967b).

Scarabin, J.M.; Pecker, J.; Bucher, J.M.; Vallee, B.; Guegan, Y.; Faivre, J.; Simon, J.: Stereotaxic exploration in 200 supratentorial brain tumors. Its value in addition to computerized tomography. Neuroradiology *16:* 591–593 (1978).

Schaltenbrand, G.: The effect of stereotactic electric stimulation of the depth of the brain. Brain *88:* 835–840 (1965).

Schaltenbrand, G.; Bailey, P.: Introduction to stereotaxis with an atlas of the human brain (Thieme, Stuttgart 1959).

Schaltenbrand, G.; Spuler, H.; Nadjmi, M.; Hoff, H.C.; Wahren, W.: Die stereotaktische Behandlung der Epilepsien. Confinia neurol. *27:* 111–113 (1966).

Schaltenbrand, G.; Spuler, H.; Wahren, W.: Electroanatomy of the corpus callosum radiation according to the facts of stereotactic stimulation in man. Z. Neurol. *198:* 70–92 (1970).

Schaltenbrand, G.; Walker, A.E.: Stereotaxy of the human brain (Thieme, Stuttgart 1982).

Schaub, C.; Askienazi, S.; Szikla, G.: Endocavitary beta irradiation of glioma cysts with colloidal 186-rhenium. Abstr. Symp. Stereotactic Irradiations, Paris 1979a, p. V 30.

Schaub, C.; Betti, O.; Szikla, G.; Talairach, J.: Selective blockade of growth hormone secretion by interstitial gamma irradiation of the pituitary in acromegaly and diabetic retinopathy. Abstr. Symp. Stereotactic Irradiations, Paris 1979b, p. V 24.

Schilder, P.; Stengel, E.: Asymbolia for pain. Archs Neurol. Psychiat. *25:* 598–600 (1932).

Schlegel, W.; Scharfenberg, H.; Sturm, V.; Penzholz, H.; Lorenz, W.J.: Direct visualization of tumours in stereotactic and angiographic films by computer calculation of longitudinal CT-sections: a new method for stereotactic localization of tumour outlines. Acta neurochir. *58:* 27–35 (1981).

Schmidt, K.: Kreislauf und Atmung beim Parkinsonsyndrom und deren Beeinflussung durch umschriebene und akute Ausschaltung im Stammganglienbereich. Fortschr. Med. *84:* 805–808 (1966).

Schvarcz, J.R.: Stereotactic extralemniscal myelotomy. J. Neurol. Neurosurg. Psychiat. *39:* 53–57 (1976).

Schvarcz, J.R.: Functional exploration of the spinomedullary junction. Acta neurochir. *24:* suppl., pp. 179–195 (1977a).

Schvarcz, J.R.: Spinal cord stereotactic techniques re trigeminal nucleotomy and extralemniscal myelotomy. Appl. Neurophysiol. *41:* 99–112 (1978).

Schvarcz, J.R.: Paraqueductal mesencephalotomy for facial central pain. Acta neurochir. *24:* suppl., p. 227 (1977b).

Schvarcz, J.R.: Chronic stimulation of the periaqueductal and periventricular region for deafferentation pain. Meeting of the European Society for Stereotactic and Functional Neurosurgery, Paris 1979. Abstr., p. S17.

Schvarcz, J.R.; Sica, R.E.; Morita, E.: Chronic self-stimulation of the dentate nucleus for treatment of spasticity. Acta neurochir. *30:* suppl., pp. 351–362 (1980).

Schwartz, J.C.; Pollard, H.; Llorens, C.; Malfroy, B.; Gros, C.; Pradelles, P.; Dray, F.: Endorphins and endorphin receptors in striatum. Relationship with dopaminergic neurons; in Costa, Trabucchi, The endorphins, pp. 245–264 (Raven Press, New York 1978).

Scoville, W.B.: Selective cortical undercutting as a means of modifying and studying frontal lobe function in man. J. Neurosurg. *6:* 65–73 (1949).

Scoville, W.B.: Surgical locations for psychiatric surgery with special reference to orbital and cingulate operations; in Laitinen, Livingston, Surgical approaches in psychiatry, pp. 29–36 (Medical and Technical Publishing, Lancaster 1973).

Segundo, J.P.; Machne, X.: Unitary responses to afferent volleys in lenticular nucleus and claustrum. J. Neurophysiol. *19:* 325–339 (1956).

Selby, G.: Stereotactic surgery for the relief of Parkinson's disease. J. neurol. Sci. *5:* 315–342, 343–375 (1967).

Sem-Jacobsen, C.W.: Depth electrographic stimulation of the human brain and behavior; from fourteen years of studies and treatment of Parkinson's disease and mental disorders with implanted electrodes (Thomas, Springfield 1968).

Sem-Jacobsen, C.W.; Torkildsen, A.: Depth recording and electrical stimulation in the human brain; in Ramey, O'Doherty, Electrical studies on the unanesthetized brain, pp. 275–287 (Hoeber, New York 1960).

Shay, H.: Quoted by Spiegel and Wycis (1962).

Shealy, C.N.: Transcutaneous electro-analgesia. Surg. Forum *23:* 419–421 (1970).

Shealy, C.N.: Transcutaneous electrical stimulation for control of pain. Clin. Neurosurg. *21:* 269–277 (1974).

Shealy, C.N.; Mortimer, J.T.; Hagfors, N.R.: Dorsal column electroanalgesia. J. Neurosurg. *32:* 560–564 (1970).

Shealy, C.N.; Mortimer, J.T.; Reswick, J.B.: Electrical inhibition of pain by stimulation of the dorsal columns. Anaesth. Analg. *46:* 489–491 (1967).

Shelden, C.H.; Jacques, S.; McCann, G.: The Shelden CT-based microneurosurgical stereotactic system: its application to CNS pathology. Appl. Neurophysiol. *45:* 341–346 (1982).

Shelden, C.H.; McCann, G.; Jacques, S.; Lutes, H.R.; Frazier, R.E.; Katz, R.; Kuki, R.: Development of a computerized microstereotaxic method for localization and removal of minute CNS lesions under direct 3-D vision. Technical report. J. Neurosurg. *52:* 21–27 (1980).

Sheldon, C.H.; Pudenz, R.H.; Doyle, J.: Electrical control of facial pain. Am. J. Surg. *114:* 209–212 (1967).

Sherrington, C.S.: Decerebrate rigidity and reflex coordination of movements. J. Physiol., Lond. *22:* 319–332 (1898).

Showers, M.J.C.: Correlation of medial thalamic nuclear activity with cortical and subcortical neuronal arcs. J. comp. Neurol. *109:* 261–315 (1958).

Siegfried, J.: Thalamic surgery in the treatment of pain; in Fusek, Kunc, Present limits of neurosurgery, pp. 521–524 (Avicenum, Prague 1972).

Siegfried, J.: The place of L-dopa in the treatment of Parkinson's disease. Prog. neurol. Surg., vol. 5, pp. 387–405 (Karger, Basel 1973).

Siegfried, J.; Ben-Shmuel, A.: Long-term assessment of stereotactic amygdalotomy for aggressive behavior; in Laitinen, Livingston, Surgical approaches in psychiatry, pp. 138–141 (Medical and Technical Publishing, Lancaster 1973).

Siegfried, J.; Esslen, E.; Gretener, V.; Ketz, E.; Perret, E.: Functional anatomy of the dentate nucleus in the light of stereotaxic operations. Confinia neurol. *32:* 1–10 (1970).

Siegfried, J.; Fisch, U.: Influence du thalamus sur les centres vestibulaires et auditifs. Revue Oto-Neuro-Ophtal. *39:* 301–304 (1967).

Siegfried, J.; Krainick, J.U.; Hass, H.; Adorjani, C.; Meyer, M.; Thoden, U.: Electrical spinal cord stimulation for spastic movement disorders. Appl. Neurophysiol. *41:* 134–141 (1978).

Siegfried, J.; Lazorthes, K.; Sedan, R.: Indications and ethical considerations of deep brain stimulation. Acta neurochir. *30:* suppl., pp. 269–274 (1980).

Siegfried, J.; Verdie, J.C.: Long-term assessment of stereotaxic dentatotomy for spasticity and other disorders. Acta neurochir. *24:* suppl., pp. 41–48 (1977).

Siegfried, J.; Wiesendanger, M.: Respiratory alterations produced by thalamic stimulation during stereotaxic operations. Confinia neurol. *29:* 220–223 (1967).

Sjoqvist, O.: Eine neue Operationsmethode bei der Trigeminusneuralgie: Durchschneidung des Tractus spinalis trigemini. Zentbl. Neurochir. *2:* 274–281 (1938).

Slaughter, D.G.; Nashold, B.S., Jr.: Intracranial measurements for stereotactic surgery. Confinia neurol. *32:* 250–254 (1970).

Smith, M.C.: Certain fibre groups of the human internal capsule; in Gillingham, Donaldson, 3rd Symp. Parkinson's Disease, pp. 87–94 (Livingstone, Edinburgh 1969).

Snider, R.S.; Cooke, P.M.: Cerebellar activity in relation to the electrocorticogram before, during and after seizure states. Electroenceph. clin. Neurophysiol. *5:* suppl. 3, p. 78 (1953).

Spatz, H.: Physiologie und Pathologie der Stammganglien; in Bethe, Bergmann, Handbuch der normalen und pathologischen Physiologie, Bd. 10, pp. 318–417 (Springer, Berlin 1927).

Spiegel, E.A.: Die Kerne im Vorderhirn der Säuger. Arb. neurol. Inst. Wien Univ. *22:* 418–497 (1919).

Spiegel, E.A.: Der Tonus der Skelettmuskulatur (Springer, Berlin 1927).

Spiegel, E.A.: Comparative study of the thalamic, cerebral and cerebellar potentials. Am. J. Physiol. *118:* 569–579 (1937).

Spiegel, E.A.: Physiology of the striopallidum in relation to extrapyramidal function and disorders; in Biochemical and neurophysiological correlations of centrally acting drugs. Proc. 2nd Int. Pharmacol. Meet., Prague 1963, pp. 3–34 (Pergamon Press, Oxford 1964).

Spiegel, E.A.: Methodological problems in stereoencephalotomy. Confinia neurol. *26:* 125–132 (1965a).

Spiegel, E.A.: Die Bedeutung des Forelschen Feldes für die Neurochirurgie und Neurophysiologie. Acta neurochir. *13:* 292–304 (1965b).

Spiegel, E.A.: Discussion of Hassler; in Purpura, Yahr, The thalamus, p. 437 (Columbia University Press, New York 1966).

*Spiegel, E.A.: Indications for stereoencephalotomies. Confinia neurol. *31:* 5–10 (1969).

Spiegel, E.A.: Relief of pain and spasticity by posterior column stimulation. Archs Neurol., Chicago *39:* 184–185 (1982).

*Spiegel, E.A.; Baird, H.W.: Athetotic syndromes; in Vinken, Bruyn, Handbook of clinical neurology, vol. 6; Diseases of the basal ganglia, pp. 440–475 (North-Holland, Amsterdam 1968).

Spiegel, E.A.; Kletzkin, M.; Szekely, E.G.: Pain reactions on stimulation of the quadrigeminal region. Fed. Proc. *12:* No. 1 (1953).

Spiegel, E.A.; Kletzkin, M.; Szekely, E.G.: Pain reactions upon stimulation of the tectum mesencephali. J. Neuropath. exp. Neurol. *13:* 212–220 (1954a).

Spiegel, E.A.; Kletzkin, M.; Szekely, E.G.; Wycis, H.T.: Role of hypothalamic mechanisms in thalamic pain. Neurology, Minneap. *4:* 739–751 (1954b).

Spiegel, E.A.; Miller, H.R.; Oppenheimer, M.J.: Forebrain and rage reactions. J. Neurophysiol. *3:* 538–548 (1940).

Spiegel, E.A.; Reynolds, R.: Wirkung von Stichverletzungen des Corpus striatum und seiner Nachbarschaft auf die Diurese. Z. ges. exp. Med. *70:* 504–512 (1930).

Spiegel, E.A.; Szekely, E.G.: Prolonged stimulation of the head of the caudate nucleus. Archs Neurol. *4:* 55–65 (1961).

Spiegel, E.A.; Szekely, E.G.: Strio-pallidal relationships. Am. J. med. Sci. *243:* 534 (1962).

Spiegel, E.A.; Szekely, E.G.; Baker, W.W.: Electrographic study of thalamic impulses to the striatum and pallidum. Electroenceph. clin. Neurophysiol. *9:* 291–299 (1957a).

Spiegel, E.A.; Szekely, E.G.; Gildenberg, P.L.: Vestibular responses in midbrain, thalamus, and basal ganglia. Archs Neurol., Chicago *12:* 258–269 (1965a).

Spiegel, E.A.; Szekely, E.G.; Kirby, A.R.: Influence of the corpus striatum upon electrical potentials of the liver. Expl Neurol. *7:* 246–257 (1963a).

Spiegel, E.A.; Szekely, E.G.; Zanes, C.: The striatoamygdaloid system. Expl Neurol. *11:* 182–189 (1965b).

Spiegel, E.A.; Szekely, E.G.; Zivanovic, D.: The effect of intracaudate injection of *L*-dopa upon bradykinesia; in Progress in neurogenetics. Proc. 2nd Int. Congr. Neurogenetics and Neuro-Ophthalmology, Montreal 1967, vol. 1. Excerpta Med. Int. Congr. Ser., No. 175, pp. 324–330 (1967).

Spiegel, E.A.; Takano, K.: Zur Analyse der vom Streifenhügel erhaltenen Reizwirkungen. Z. ges. Neurol. Psychiat. *118:* 429–432 (1929).

Spiegel, E.A.; Wycis, H.T.: Mesencephalotomy for relief of pain; in Anniversary volume for O. Poetzl, p. 438 (Vienna, 1948).

Spiegel, E.A.; Wycis, H.T.: Thalamic recordings in man with special reference to seizure discharges. Electroenceph. clin. Neurophysiol. *2:* 23–27 (1950a).

Spiegel, E.A.; Wycis, H.T.: Pallido-thalamotomy in chorea. Philadelphia Neurol. Soc. 1949. Archs Neurol. Psychiat., Chicago *64:* 495–496 (1950b).

*Spiegel, E.A.; Wycis, H.T.: Effect of thalamic and pallidal lesions upon involuntary movements in choreoathetosis. Trans. Am. neurol. Ass. *75:* 234–236 (1950c).

Spiegel, E.A.; Wycis, H.T.: The central mechanism of emotion. Am. J. Psychiat. *108:* 426–431 (1951).

Spiegel, E.A.; Wycis, H.T.: Mesencephalotomy in treatment of 'intractable' facial pain. Archs Neurol. Psychiat., Chicago *69:* 1–13 (1953).

Spiegel, E.A.; Wycis, H.T.: Ansotomy in paralysis agitans. Transact. Am. neurol. Ass. *78:* 178–180 (1953a).

Spiegel, E.A.; Wycis, H.T.: Ansotomy in paralysis agitans. Archs Neurol. Psychiat., Chicago *71:* 598–614 (1954).

Spiegel, E.A.; Wycis, H.T.: Pallido-ansotomy. Anatomic-physiologic foundation and histopathologic control; in Fields, Pathogenesis and treatment of parkinsonism, pp. 86–105 (Thomas, Springfield 1958).

Spiegel, E.A.; Wycis, H.T.: Stimulation of the brainstem and basal ganglia in man; in Sheer, Electrical stimulation of the brain, pp. 487–497 (University of Texas Press, Austin 1961).

Spiegel, E.A.; Wycis, H.T.: Stereoencephalotomy; parts I/II (Grune & Stratton, New York 1952/1962).

Spiegel, E.A.; Wycis, H.T.: Present status of stereoencephalotomies for pain relief. Confinia neurol. *27:* 7–17 (1966).

Spiegel, E.A.; Wycis, H.T.: Stereotaxic neurosurgical techniques; in Engineering in the practice of medicine, pp. 466–474 (Williams & Wilkins, Baltimore 1967).

Spiegel, E.A.; Wycis, H.T.: Multiplicity of subcortical localization of various functions. J. nerv. ment. Dis. *147:* 45–48 (1968).

Spiegel, E.A.; Wycis, H.T.; Baird, H.W.: Pallidotomy and pallidoamygdalotomy in certain types of convulsive disorders. Archs Neurol. Psychiat., Chicago *80:* 714–728 (1958a).

Spiegel, E.A.; Wycis, H.T.; Baird, H.W., III: Long range effects of electropallido-ansotomy in extrapyramidal and convulsive disorders. Neurology *8:* 734–740 (1958b).

*Spiegel, E.A.; Wycis, H.T.; Baird, H.W.; Rovner, D.; Thur, C.: Pallidum and muscle tone. Neurology, Minneap. *6:* 350–356 (1956a).

Spiegel, E.A.; Wycis, H.T.; Baird, H.W.; Szekely, E.G.: Functional state of the basal ganglia in extrapyramidal and convulsive disorders. Archs Neurol. Psychiat. *75:* 167–174 (1956b).

Spiegel, E.A.; Wycis, H.T.; Freed, H.; Orchinik, O.: The central mechanism of emotions. Am. J. Psychiat. *108:* 426–431 (1951a).

Spiegel, E.A.; Wycis, H.T.; Freed, H.; Orchinik, C.W.: A follow-up study of patients treated by thalamotomy and by combined frontal and thalamic lesions. J. nerv. ment. Dis. *124:* 399–404 (1956c).

Spiegel, E.A.; Wycis, H.T.; Goode, R.: Studies in stereoencephalotomy. V. A universal stereoencephalotome (model V) for use in man and experimental animals. J. Neurosurg. *13:* 305–309 (1956d).

Spiegel, E.A.; Wycis, H.T.; Henny, G.C.; Stauffer, H.M.; Goode, R.: Radiographic observations of the electrode position during stereoencephalotomy. Br. J. Radiol. *30:* 278–280 (1957b).

Spiegel, E.A.; Wycis, H.T.; Kletzkin, M.; Thur, C.: A new procedure for exploration and elimination of subcortical structures. Electroenceph. clin. Neurophysiol. *5:* 309–311 (1953a).

Spiegel, E.A.; Wycis, H.T.; Marks, M.; Lee, A.J.: Stereotaxic apparatus for operations on the human brain. Science *106:* 349–350 (1947).

Spiegel, E.A.; Wycis, H.T.; Orchinik, C.: Thalamotomy and hypothalamotomy for the treatment of psychoses; in Psychiatric treatment. Proc. Ass. Res. nerv. ment. Dis. *31:* 379–391 (1953b).

Spiegel, E.A.; Wycis, H.T.; Orchinik, C.; Freed, H.: Thalamic chronotaraxis. Am. J. Psychiat. *113:* 97–105 (1956e).

Spiegel, E.A.; Wycis, H.T.; Reyes, V.: Diencephalic mechanisms in petit mal epilepsy. Electroenceph. clin. Neurophysiol. *3:* 473–475 (1951b).

Spiegel, E.A.; Wycis, H.T.; Szekely, E.G.; Adams, J.; Flanagan, M.; Baird, H.W.: Campotomy in various extrapyramidal disorders. J. Neurosurg. *20:* 871–881 (1963b).

Spiegel, E.A.; Wycis, H.T.; Szekely, E.G.; Baird, H.W.: Physiopathologic observations on the basal ganglia; in Ramey, O'Doherty, Electric studies on the unanesthetized brain, pp. 192–202 (Hoeber, New York 1960a).

Spiegel, E.A.; Wycis, H.T.; Szekely, E.G.; Constantinovici, A.; Egyed, J.J.; Gildenberg, P.; Lehman, R.; Werthan, M.: Role of the caudate nucleus in parkinsonian bradykinesia. Confinia neurol. *26:* 336–341 (1965c).

Spiegel, E.A.; Wycis, H.T.; Szekely, E.G.; Gildenberg, P.L.: Medial and basal thalamotomy in so-called intractable pain; in Knighton, Dumke, Pain, pp. 503–517 (Little, Brown, Boston 1966).

Spiegel, E.A.; Wycis, H.T.; Szekely, E.G.; Gildenberg, P.; Zanes, C.: Combined dorsomedial, intralaminar and basal thalamotomy for relief of so-called intractable pain. J. int. Coll. Surg. *42:* 160–168 (1964a).

Spiegel, E.A.; Wycis, H.T.; Szekely, E.G.; Rusy, B.; Baird, H.W.: Study of the mesencephalic tegmentum in paralysis agitans and parkinsonism. Archs Neurol., Chicago *2:* 46–54 (1960b).

Spiegel, E.A.; Wycis, H.T.; Szekely, E.G.; Soloff, L.; Adams, J.; Gildenberg, P.; Zanes, C.: Stimulation of Forel's field during stereotaxic operations in the human brain. Electroenceph. clin. Neurophysiol. *16:* 537–548 (1964b).

Spiegel, E.A.; Wycis, H.T.; Thur, C.: The stereoencephalotome. (Model III of our stereotaxic apparatus for operations on the human brain.) J. Neurosurg. *8:* 452–453 (1951c).

Spiegel-Adolf, M.; Wycis, H.T.: Enzymatic action of fluids from cystic brain tumors. J. Neuropath. exp. Neurol. *12:* 601–607 (1954).

Spiegel-Adolf, M.; Wycis, H.T.: Enzymatic action of fluids from cystic brain tumors. J. Neuropath. exp. Neurol. *16:* 404–409 (1957).

*Sprague, J.M.; Chambers, W.W.: Control of posture by reticular formation and cerebellum in the intact, anesthetized and unanesthetized and in the decerebrated cat. Am. J. Physiol. *176:* 52–64 (1954).

Spuler, H.; Szekely, E.G.; Spiegel, E.A.: Stimulation of the ventrolateral region of the thalamus. Archs Neurol., Chicago *6:* 208–219 (1962).

Šramka, M.; Fritz, G.; Galanda, M.; Nádvornik, P.: Some observations in treatment stimulation of epilepsy. Acta neurochir. *23:* suppl., pp. 257–262 (1976).

Šramka, M.; Fritz, G.; Nádvornik, P.: Results of therapeutic stimulation for epilepsy. Acta neurochir. *30:* suppl., pp. 183–188 (1980).

Starzl, T.E.; Magoun, H.W.: Organization of the diffuse thalamic projection system. J. Neurophysiol. *14:* 133–146 (1951).

Starzl, T.E.; Taylor, C.W.; Magoun, H.W.: Ascending conduction in reticular activating system, with special reference to the diencephalon. J. Neurophysiol. *14:* 461–477 (1951).

Starzl, T.E.; Whitlock, D.G.: Diffuse thalamic projection system in monkey. J. Neurophysiol. *15:* 449–468 (1952).

Stavraky, G.W.: Supersensitivity following lesions of the nervous system (University of Toronto Press, Toronto 1961).

Steck, H.: Zur pathologischen Anatomie der echten posthemiplegischen Athetose. Schweizer Arch. Neurol. Psychiat. *8:* 75 (1921).

Stein, L.; Belluzzi, J.D.: Brain endorphins and the sense of well being. A psychobiological hypothesis; in Costa, Trabucchi, The endorphins, pp. 299–311 (Raven Press, New York 1978).

Steiner, L.; Backlund, E.O.; Greitz, T.; Leksell, L.; Norén, G.; Röhn, T.: Radiosurgery in the treatment of inoperable arteriovenous malformations of the brain. Abstr. Symp. Stereotactic Irradiations, Paris 1979, p. V 27.

Steiner, L.; Leksell, L.; Forster, D.M.C.; Greitz, T.; Backlund, E.O.: Stereotactic radiosurgery in intracranial arteriovenous malformation. Acta neurochir. *21:* suppl., pp. 195–209 (1974).

Stern, J.; Ward, A., Jr.: Inhibition of muscle spindle discharges by ventrolateral thalamic stimulation. Archs Neurol. *3:* 193–204 (1960).

Stevens, J.R.; Kim, C.; MacLean, P.D.: Stimulation of caudate nucleus. Archs Neurol. *4:* 47–54 (1961).

Stevens, J.R.; Mark, V.H.; Ervin, F.; Pacheco, P.; Suematsu, K.: Deep temporal stimulation in man. Long latency, long lasting psychological changes. Archs Neurol., Chicago *21:* 157–169 (1969).

Stowsand, D.; Markakis, E.; Laubner, P.: Zur Elektrokoagulation des Ganglion Gasseri bei der idiopathischen Trigeminus Neuralgie. Nervenarzt *44:* 44 (1973).

Strassburger, R.H.; French, L.A.: Experimental production of tremor. Lancet *i:* 86–89 (1961).

Struppler, A.: Contributions of electromyography to stereotaxy; in Schaltenbrand, Walker, Stereotaxy of the human brain, pp. 436–448 (Thieme, Stuttgart 1982).

Struppler, A.; Struppler, E.: Veränderungen der Motoneuronaktivität auf elektrischen Reiz eines Thalamuskerns (V.o.a.) während stereotaktischer Thalamusoperationen. Z. ges. Neurol. *203:* 483–499 (1962).

Sugita, K.; Doi, T.: The effect of electrical stimulation on the motor and sensory system during stereotaxic operations. Confinia neurol. *29:* 224–229 (1967).

Sweet, W.H.: Pain; in Field, Magoun, Hall, Handbook of physiology, Section I: Neurophysiology, vol. 1, pp. 459–506 (American Physiological Society, Washington 1959).

Sweet, W.H.: Central mechanisms of chronic pain. Res. Publs Ass. Res. nerv. ment. Dis. *58:* 287–303 (1980).

Sweet, W.H.; Mark, V.H.; Hamlin, H.: Radiofrequency lesions in the CNS of man and cat. J. Neurosurg. *17:* 213–225 (1960).

Sweet, W.H.; Wepsic, J.G.: Treatment of chronic pain by stimulation of fibers of primary afferent neuron. Trans. Am. neurol. Ass. *93:* 103–107 (1968).

Sweet, W.H.; Wepsic, J.G.: Controlled thermocoagulation of trigeminal ganglion and rootlets for differential destruction of pain fibers. J. Neurosurg. *39:* 143–156 (1974).

Szekely, E.G.: Cortical recruiting on thalamic stimulation after elimination of the pallidum. Confinia neurol. *17:* 243–249 (1957).

Szikla, G.; Bouvier, G.; Hori, T.; Petrov, V.: Three-dimensional angiography for stereotactic localization of normal and pathological cortical structures. Meeting of the European Society for Stereotactic and Functional Neurosurgery, Paris 1979a, Abstr. p. J. 27.

Szikla, G.; Schlienger, M.; et al.: Combined interstitial and external irradiation of gliomas:

a progress report. Abstr. Inserm Symp. Stereotactic Irradiations, Paris 1979b, p. V 33.

Takebayashi, H.; Komai, N.: Stereotaxic operation as treatment of ataxia and cerebral spastic palsy. Confinia neurol. *27:* 225–229 (1966).

Talairach, J.: Destruction du noyau ventral antérieur thalamique dans le traitement des maladies mentales. Revue neurol. *87:* 352–357 (1952).

Talairach, J.: Three-dimensional investigation of the brain. Utilization of stereotactic data in open surgery. Meeting of the European Society for Stereotactic and Functional Neurosurgery, Paris 1979, abstr., p. J 4.

Talairach, J.; Aboulker, J.; Tournoux, P.; David, M.: Technique stéréotaxique de la chirurgie hypophysaire par voie nasale. Neuro-Chirurgie *2:* 3–23 (1956).

Talairach, J.; Bancaud, J.: Stereotactic approach to epilepsy. Prog. neurol. Surg., vol. 5, pp. 297–354 (Karger, Basel 1973).

Talairach, J.; Bonis, A.; Szikla, G.; Schaub, G.; Bancaud, J.; Covellod Bordas-Ferrer, M.: Stereotaxic implantation of radioactive isotopes in functional pituitary surgery; in Yen Wang, Paoletti, Radionucleide application in neurology and neurosurgery, pp. 267–299 (Thomas, Springfield 1970).

Talairach, J.; David, M.; Tournoux, P.: L'exploration chirurgicale stéréotaxique du lobe temporal dans l'épilepsie temporale (Masson, Paris 1958).

Talairach, J.; David, M.; Tournoux, P.; Corredor, H.; Kvasina, T.: Atlas d'anatomie stéréotaxique (Masson, Paris 1957).

Talairach, J.; Hécaen, H.; David, M.; Monnier, M.; Ajuriaguerra, J.: Recherches sur la coagulation thérapeutique des structures souscorticales chez l'homme. Revue neurol. *81:* 4–24 (1949).

Talairach, J.; Paillas, J.E.; David, M.: Dyskinésie du type hémiballique traitée par cortectomie frontale, limitée, puis par coagulation de l'anse lenticulaire et de la portion interne du globus pallidus. Revue neurol. *83:* 440–451 (1950).

Talairach, J.; Ruggiero, G.; Aboulker, J.; David, M.: A method of treatment of inoperable brain tumours by stereotaxic implantation of radioactive gold. Br. J. Radiol. *28:* 62–74 (1955).

Talairach, J.; Szikla, G.; Bonis, A.; Tournoux, P.; Bancaud, J.; Mempel, E.: Destruction stéréotaxique de l'hypophyse non-tumorale par les isotopes radioactifs. Presse méd. *70:* 1399–1402, 1449–1451 (1962).

Talairach, J.; Tournoux, P.: Appareil de stéréotaxie hypophysaire pour voie d'abord nasale. Neuro-Chirurgie *1:* 127–131 (1955).

Talairach, J.; Tournoux, P.; Bancaud, J.: Chirurgie pariétale de la douleur. Acta neurochir. *8:* 153–250 (1960).

Tasker, R.R.; Emmers, R.: A double somatotopic representation in the human thalamus. Its application in localization during thalamotomy for Parkinson's disease; in Gillingham, Donaldson, 3rd Symp. on Parkinson's Disease, pp. 94–99 (Livingstone, Edinburgh 1969).

Tasker, R.R.; Hawrylyshyn, P.; Organ, L.W.: Computerized graphic display of physiological data collected during human stereotactic surgery. Appl. Neurophysiol. *41:* 183–187 (1978).

Tasker, R.R.; Hawrylyshyn, P.; Rowe, I.H.; Organ, L.W.: Computerized graphic display of results of subcortical stimulation during stereotactic surgery. Acta. neurochir. *24:* suppl., pp. 85–98 (1977).

Tasker, R.R.; Organ, L.W.; Hawrylyshyn, P.: Visual phenomena evoked by electrical stimulation of the human brain stem. Appl. Neurophysiol. *43:* 89–95 (1980).

Terenius, L.: Significance of endorphins in endogenous antinociception; in Costa, Trabucchi, The endorphins, pp. 321–332 (Raven Press, New York 1978).

Teuber, H.L.; Corkin, S.; Twitchell, T.E.: A study of cingulotomy in man. Appendix to Psychosurgery. Reports prepared for the National Commission for the Protection of Human Subjects of Biomedical and Behavioral Research. US Dept. Hlth Educ. Welf. No. (OS) 77–0002. *3:* 1–115 (1977).

Tew, J.M., Jr.: Percutaneous stereotactic trigeminal rhizotomy. Appl. Neurophysiol *41:* 146–157 (1978).

Teychenne, P.F.: Bromocriptine: low dose therapy in Parkinson's disease; in Symp. Am. Acad. of Neurology, 1981.

Thompson, R.L.: Effects of lesions in the caudate nuclei and dorsofrontal cortex on conditioned avoidance behavior in cats. J. comp. physiol. Psychol. *52:* 650–659 (1959).

Tobias, C.A.; Roberts, J.E.; Lawrence, J.H.; Lew-Beer, B.V.A.; Anger, H.O.; Born, J.L.; McCombs, R.; Huggins, C.: Peaceful uses of atomic energy. Proc. Int. Conf., Geneva *10:* 95 (1955).

Todd, E.M.: Todd-Wells manual of stereotaxic procedures (Codman & Shurtleff, Randolph 1967).

Todd, E.M.; Crue, B.I.; Carregal, E.J.A.: Posterior percutaneous tractotomy and cordotomy. Confinia neurol. *31:* 106–115 (1969).

Tokay, L.: Wirkung von Stichverletzungen des Corpus striatum auf die Molenausscheidung mit dem Harn. Z. ges. Neurol. Psychiat. *136:* 47–61 (1931).

Tolosa, E.S.; Loewenson, R.B.: Essential tremor. Treatment with propranolol. Neurology *25:* 1041–1044 (1975).

Tóth, S.: The effect of removal of the nucleus dentatus on the parkinsonian syndrome. J. Neurol. Neurosurg. Psychiat. *24:* 143–147 (1961).

Tóth, S.; Vajda, J.: Multitarget technique in Parkinson surgery. Appl. Neurophysiol. *43:* 109–113 (1980).

Trendelenburg, W.: Untersuchungen über reizlose, vorübergehende Ausschaltung am ZNS. Pflügers Arch. ges. Physiol. *133:* 305–312 (1910).

Trétiakoff, C.: Contribution à l'étude de l'anatomie pathologique du locus niger de Soemmering avec quelques déductions relatives à la pathogénie des troubles du tonus musculaire de la maladie de Parkinson; thèse Paris (1919).

Turner, J.W.; Shaw, A.: A versatile stereotaxic system based on cylindrical coordinates and using absolute measurements. Acta neurochir. *21:* suppl., pp. 211–220 (1974).

Uchimura, Y.; Narabayashi, H.; Shiotsuki, M.: Two new instruments in neurosurgery: (1) stereoencephalotome, (2) polygraph. Psychiatria Neurol. jap. *52:* 86 (1950).

Uhl, G.R.; Goodman, R.R.; Kuhar, M.J.; Snyder, S.H.: Localization and identification of an amygdalofugal pathway; in Costa, Trabucchi, The endorphins, pp. 71–87 (Raven Press, New York 1978).

Umbach, W.: Elektrophysiologische und vegetative Phänomene bei stereotaktischen Hirnoperationen (Springer, Berlin 1966).

Umbach, W.; Riechert, T.: The stereotactic coagulation of the fornix as treatment of temporal lobe epilepsy. Proc. 1st Int. Congr. Neurol. Sci., vol. 3, pp. 565–578 (Pergamon Press, London 1959).

Umbach, W.; Riechert, T.: Elektrophysiologische und klinische Ergebnisse stereotaktischer Eingriffe im limbischen System bei temporaler Epilepsie. Nervenarzt *35:* 482–488 (1964).

Upton, A.R.M.; Cooper, I.S.; Rappaport, Z.H.: Correlation of clinical and physiological effects of cerebellar stimulation (Abstract). Meet. Eur. Soc. for Functional and Stereotactic Neurosurgery, Paris 1979, p. S12.

Usunoff, K.G.; Hassler, R.; Romansky, K.; Usunova, P.; Wagner, A.: The nigrostriatal projection in the cat. I. Silver impregnation study. J. neurol. Sci. *28:* 265–288 (1974).

Vaernet, K.: Chronic cerebellar stimulation in spastic choreo-athetosis. Acta neurochir. *24:* suppl., pp. 59–63 (1977).

Vaernet, K.; Madsen, A.: Stereotaxic amygdalectomy and basofrontal tractotomy in psychotics with aggressive behavior. J. Neurol. Neurosurg. Psychiat. *33:* 858 (1970).

Van Buren, J.M.: Speech disturbances and confusion produced by stimulation in the vicinity of the caudate head. Electroenceph. clin. Neurophysiol. *14:* 586 (1962).

Van Buren, J.M.: Confusion and disturbance of speech from stimulation in vicinity of the head of the caudate nucleus. J. Neurosurg. *20:* 148–157 (1963).

Van Buren, J.M.; Borke, R.C.: Variations and connections of the human thalamus. 2. Variations of the human diencephalon (Springer, New York 1972).

Van Buren, J.M.; Maccubin, D.A.: An outline atlas of the human basal ganglia with estimation of anatomical variation. J. Neurosurg. *19:* 811–839 (1962).

Van Manen, J.: Stereotaxic operations in cases of hereditary and intention tremor. Acta neurochir. *21:* suppl., pp. 49–50 (1974).

Van Manen, J.; Van Hoytema, G.J.: A Dutch stereotaxic apparatus. Psychiatria Neur. Neurochir. *65:* 81–91 (1962).

Velasco-Suarez, M.M.; Escobedo, F.R.: Vegetative symptoms in parkinsonism and their modification after thalamotomy. Confinia neurol. *29:* 123–126 (1967).

Velasco-Suarez, M.M.; Escobedo, F.R.: Stereotaxic intracerebral instillation of dopa. Confinia neurol. *32:* 149–157 (1970).

Vogt, C.: Quelques considérations générales à propos du syndrome du corps strié. J. Psychol. Neurol., Lpz. *18:* 479–488 (1911).

Vogt, C.; Vogt, O.: Zur Lehre der Erkrankungen des striären Systems. J. Psychol. Neurol., Lpz. *25:* suppl. 3, pp. 627–846 (1920).

Voneida, T.J.: An experimental study of the course and destination of fibers arising in the head of caudate nucleus in the cat and monkey. J. comp. Neurol. *115:* 75–87 (1960).

Voris, H.C.; Whisler, W.W.: Results of stereotaxic surgery for intractable pain. Confinia neurol. *37:* 86–96 (1975).

Wada, V.; Endo, K.: Dorsomedial thalamotomy. Folia psychiat. neurol. jap. *4:* 309–319; *5:* 61–66 (1951).

Wagner, A.: Veränderungen der Gamma-Activität durch Reizungen im Zwischen- und Mittelhirn bei der Katze; in Bargmann, Schade, Progress in brain research, vol. 5, pp. 67–73 (Elsevier, Amsterdam 1964).

Walker, A.E.: An oscillographic study of the cerebro-cerebellar relationships. J. Neurophysiol. *1:* 16–23 (1938a).

Walker, A.E.: The primate thalamus (University of Chicago Press, Chicago 1938b).

Walker, A.E.: Physiological principles and results of neurosurgical interventions in extra-

pyramidal diseases. 1st Congr. Int. Sci. Neurol., Brussels. Acta med. belg., Bruxelles
1: 118–137 (1957).

Walker, A.E.: Summary of symposium; in Fields, Pathogenesis and treatment of parkinsonism, pp. 364–372 (Thomas, Springfield 1958a).

Walker, A.E.: Survey of surgery in and about the brain stem. Congr. Neurol. Surg., San
Francisco 1958b.

Walker, A.E.: Posttraumatic epilepsy – an inquiry into the evolution and dissolution of
convulsions following head injury. Clin. Neurosurg. *6:* 69–103 (1958c).

Walker, A.E.: Internal structure and afferent-efferent relations of the thalamus; in Purpura,
Yahr, The thalamus, pp. 1–12 (Columbia University Press, New York 1966).

Walker, A.E.; Burton, C.V.: Radiofrequency telethermocoagulation. J. Am. med. Ass. *197:*
108–112 (1966).

Walker, A.E.; Marshall, N.C.: Stimulation and depth recording in man; in Sheer, Electrical
stimulation of the brain, pp. 498–518 (Hogg Foundation, Austin 1961).

Walker, A.E.; Poggio, G.F.; Andy, O.J.: Structural spread of cortically induced epileptic
discharges, Neurology *6:* 616–626 (1956).

Wall, P.D.; Sweet, W.H.: Temporary abolition of pain in man. Science *155:* 108–109
(1967).

Walsh, P.R.; Larson, S.J.; Rytel, M.W.; Maiman, D.J.: Stereotactic aspiration of deep
cerebral abscesses after CT-directed labeling. Appl. Neurophysiol. *43:* 205–209
(1980).

Walsh, L.W.; Till, K.: A comparison of the results of treating parkinsonism by Leksell's
stereotactic machine and using Cooper's technique. J. Neurol. Neurosurg. Psychiat.
23: 84 (1960).

*Walter, R.P.; Rand, R.W.; Crandall, P.H.; Markam, C.H.; Adey, W.R.: Depth electrode
studies of thalamus and basal ganglia. Archs Neurol., Chicago *8:* 388–397 (1963).

Walter, W.G.: Intrinsic rhythms of the brain; in Handbook of physiology, section I, Neurophysiology, vol. 1, pp. 279–313 (American Physiological Society, Washington
1959).

Walter, W.G.; Crow, H.J.: Depth recordings from the human brain. Electroenceph. clin.
Neurophysiol. *16:* 68–72 (1964).

Wang, G.H.; Akert, R.K.: Behavior and reflexes of chronic striatal cats. Archs ital. Biol.
100: 48–85 (1962).

Wang, G.H.; Brown, W.W.: Suprasegmental inhibition of an autonomic reflex. J. Neurophysiol. *19:* 564–572 (1956).

Ward, A.A., Jr.: The anterior cingulate gyrus and personality; Res. Publs Ass. Res. nerv.
ment. Dis. *27:* 438–445 (1948).

Ward, A.A. Jr.; McCulloch, W.S.; Magoun, H.W.: Production of an alternating tremor at
rest in monkeys. J. Neurophysiol. *11:* 317–330 (1948).

Warwick, R.: Oculomotor organization; in Bender, The oculomotor system, pp. 173–202
(Hoeber, New York 1964).

Watson, S.J.; Akil, H., et al.: Some observations on the opiate peptides and schizophrenia,
Archs gen. Psychiat. *36:* 25–41 (1979).

Watson, W.S.; Naughton, J.N.: Surgical management of the dyskinesias. J. Neurol. Neurosurg. Psychiat. *23:* 348–349 (1960).

Weigel, K.; Mundinger, F.: Iodine-125 or iridium-192 permanent implantation in tumors
of the pineal region. Abstr. Symp. Stereotactic Irradiations, Paris 1979, p. V 29.

Weiner, J.: Drug holidays; in Symp. Am. Acad. of Neurology, 1981.

Weingarten, S.; Charlow, D.G.; Holmgren, E.: The relationship of hallucination to the depth structures of the temporal lobe. Acta neurochir. *24:* suppl., pp. 199–216 (1977).

Wertheimer, P.; Lapras, C.; Lévy, A.: Essais de chirurgie thalamique. Neuro-Chirurgie *6:* 8–112 (1960).

Wester, K.; Sortland, O.; Hauglie-Hanssen, E.: A simple and inexpensive method for CT-guided stereotaxy. Neuroradiology *20:* 255–256 (1981).

White, J.C.; Sweet, W.H.: Pain and the neurosurgeon (Thomas, Springfield 1969).

White, R.P.; Himwich, H.E.: Circus movements and excitation of striatal and mesodien-cephalic centers in rabbits. J. Neurophysiol. *20:* 81–90 (1957).

Whitty, C.M.M.; Duffield, J.E.; Tow, P.M.; Cairns, H.: Anterior cingulectomy in the treatment of mental disease. Lancet *i:* 475–481 (1952).

Williams, D.: The thalamus and epilepsy. Brain *88:* 539–556 (1965).

Williams, M.; Zangwill, M.A.: Disorders of temporal judgment associated with amnesic states. J. ment. Sci. *96:* 484–493 (1950).

Wilson, D.H.; Chang, A.E.: Bilateral anterior cingulectomy for the relief of intractable pain. Confinia neurol. *36:* 61–68 (1974).

Wilson, S.A.K.: An experimental research into the anatomy and physiology of the corpus striatum. Brain *36:* 427–492 (1914).

Winkler, G.F.; Young, R.R.: Efficiency of chronic propranolol therapy on action tremor of the familial, senile or essential variety. New Engl. J. Med. *290:* 984–988 (1974).

Wise, B.L.; Gleason, C.A.: CT-directed stereotactic surgery in the management of brain abscess. Ann. Neurol. *6:* 457 (1979).

Woolsey, C.N.: Discussion of Walker; in Purpura, Yahr, The thalamus, pp. 11–12 (Columbia University Press, New York 1966).

Woringer, E.; Chambon, P.; Brain, J.: A stereotaxic apparatus with optic aiming. J. Neurol. Neurosurg. Psychiat. *23:* 352–353 (1960).

Wycis, H.T.; Gildenberg, P.L.: Further observations on campotomy in various extrapyramidal disorders; in Barbeau, Doshay, Spiegel, Parkinson's disease, pp. 134–148 (Grune & Stratton, New York 1965).

Wycis, H.T.; Lee, A.J.; Spiegel, E.A.: Simultaneous records of thalamic and cortical potentials in schizophrenics and epileptics. Confinia neurol. *9:* 264–272 (1949).

Wycis, H.T.; Robbins, R.; Spiegel-Adolf, M.; Meszaros, J.; Spiegel, E.A.: Treatment of a cystic craniopharyngioma by injection of radioactive ^{32} P. Confinia neurol. *14:* 193–202 (1954).

Wycis, H.T.; Spiegel, E.A.: Ansotomy in paralysis agitans. Confinia neurol. *12:* 245–246 (1952).

Wycis, H.T.; Spiegel, E.A.: Parkinsonism with oculogyric crises. Stimulation and partial elimination of periaqueductal grey and mesencephalic tegmentum. Confinia neurol. *13:* 385–393 (1953).

Wycis, H.T.; Spiegel, E.A.: Long range results in the treatment of intractable pain by stereotaxic midbrain surgery. J. Neurosurg. *19:* 101–107 (1962).

Wycis, H.T.; Spiegel, E.A.: Campotomy in myoclonia. J. Neurosurg. *30:* 708–713 (1969).

Wycis, H.T.; Szekely, E.G.; Spiegel, E.A.: Tremor on stimulation of the midbrain tegmentum after degeneration of the brachium conjunctivum. J. Neuropath. exp. Neurol. *16:* 79–84 (1957).

Wyss, O.A.M.: Hochfrequenz Koagulationsgerät zur reizlosen Ausschaltung. Helv. physiol. pharmacol. Acta *3:* 437–443 (1945).

Yang, H.Y.T.; Hong, G.F.; Fratta, W.; Costa, E.: Rat brain enkephalins; in Costa, Trabucchi, The endorphins, pp. 149–159 (Raven Press, New York 1978).

*Yasargil, M.G.; Wyss, A.M.; Krayenbühl, H.: Beitrag zur Behandlung extrapyramidaler Erkrankungen mittels gezielter Hirnoperationen. Schweiz. med. Wschr. *6:* 143–150 (1959).

Yoshida, M.; Yanagisawa, N.; Shimazu, H.; Givre, A.; Narabayashi, H.: Physiological identification of the thalamic nucleus. Archs Neurol., Chicago *11:* 435–443 (1964).

Yoshii, N.; Kudo, T.; Shimizu, S.: Clinical and experimental studies of thalamic pulvinotomy. Confinia neurol. *37:* 97–98 (1975).

*Yoshii, N.; Mizokami, T.; Ushikubo, T.; Kuramitsu, T.; Fukuda, S.: Long-term follow-up study after pulvinotomy for intractable pain. Appl. Neurophysiol. *43:* 128–132 (1980).

Zervas, N.T.: Technique of radio-frequency hypophysectomy. Confinia neurol. *26:* 157–160 (1965).

Zervas, N.T.: Paramedial cerebellar nuclear lesions. Confinia neurol. *32:* 114–117 (1970).

Zervas, N.T.: Long-term review of dentatectomy in dystonia musculorum deformans and cerebral palsy. Acta neurochir. *24:* suppl., pp. 49–51 (1977).

Zervas, N.T.; Hamlin, H.: Stereotaxic thermal pituitary ablation. Acta neurochir. *21:* suppl., pp. 165–168 (1974).

Zervas, N.T.; Horner, F.A.; Pickren, K.S.: The treatment of dyskinesia by stereotaxic dentatectomy. Confinia neurol. *29:* 93–100 (1967).

Zimmermann, M.: Neurophysiological models for nociception, pain and pain therapy; in Advances in neurosurgery, vol. 3, pp. 199–209 (Springer, Berlin 1975).

Subject Index